Facts and Ideas from Anywhere
2011 to 2015

WILLIAM CLIFFORD ROBERTS, MD

BAYLOR HEART AND VASCULAR INSTITUTE
BAYLOR UNIVERSITY MEDICAL CENTER
DALLAS, TEXAS

BAYLOR SCOTT AND WHITE HEALTH • DALLAS, TEXAS

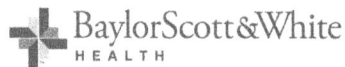

BaylorScott&White
H E A L T H

3500 Gaston Avenue
Dallas, Texas 75246
1-800-4BAYLOR
www.BaylorHealth.com

ISBN: 978-0-9845237-7-1
Printed in the United States of America on acid-free paper.

Introduction

The first volume of *Facts and Ideas from Anywhere* appeared in 2000, the second in 2005, the third in 2010, and now 2015 brings the fourth volume. Volume 1 (2000) included 25 column containing 560 subject items; volume 2 (2005) included 22 columns containing 431 subject items; volume 3 (2010) included 20 columns and 540 subject items; and the current volume includes 20 columns and 461 subject items. The columns have been both fun and intellectually rewarding to produce. I hope that they bring both pleasant and rewarding reading.

I am indebted to Cynthia D. Orticio, managing editor, *Baylor University Medical Center Proceedings*, for making the journal what it is and for making me "look good"; to my assistant, Rebecca Banks, for producing so pleasantly and so efficiently these many columns; and to Joel T. Allison, president and CEO, Baylor Scott & White Health, for his continued and unqualified support of the journal and of me.

BUMC Proceedings has about 7000 subscribers, most in northeast Texas. Its manuscripts are peer-reviewed, and each article in the *BUMC Proceedings* is published on acid-free paper.

BACKGROUND: INTRODUCTION TO THE FIRST VOLUME

In the early 1990s, when I was working at the National Institutes of Health in Bethesda, Maryland, I noticed on the library's shelf of "newly received journals" a small blue and white journal called *Baylor University Medical Proceedings*, Dallas. The first issue appeared in January 1988 and contained 48 pages with relatively large type, and each page was only 21.5 × 14 cm (8.5 × 5.5 inches) in size. The first issue contained a brief editorial entitled "Why a Baylor Scientific Journal?" by Dr. George J. Race, who was the journal's founder and first editor. He indicated that the journal was "intended to serve as a forum for scientific communication and education." Initially, the journal was distributed at no cost to approximately 1600 physicians and other interested individuals in the Baylor Health Care System. One year after its beginning, the journal's size was increased to 28.0 × 21.5 cm (11.0 × 8.5 inches); the page count and type size were not changed.

In March 1992, the American College of Cardiology met in Dallas, Texas, and during that time the editorial board of *The American Journal of Cardiology* met. (I have been editor in chief of *The American Journal of Cardiology* since 1982.) I told a friend at Baylor University Medical Center about the editorial board meeting, and she attended along with Dr. George J. Race, the editor of the *BUMC Proceedings*, and Ms. Rose Kraft, its managing editor. Thus, I met George Race and Rose Kraft for the first time.

In August 1992, I was invited to give medical grand rounds at Baylor University Medical Center in Dallas, and not long afterwards I was offered my present position of executive director of the Baylor Heart and Vascular Institute. Shortly after I came to Baylor permanently in March 1993, George Race indicated that he wanted to retire from the editorship of the *BUMC Proceedings* and that he would support my being his successor. Thus, in February 1994, I was appointed editor in chief of the *BUMC Proceedings*. The first issue I was responsible for was the April 1994 one. Before that issue appeared, we made a number of format changes, including decreasing the size of the type and increasing considerably the amount of information per page.

I also wanted to write an editorial or some type of article in each of the quarterly issues as a way of putting my "stamp" on the journal. The result was a column initially entitled "Ideas and facts from elsewhere." (It subsequently was changed to "Facts and ideas from anywhere.") That column has appeared in each of the subsequent issues. Each column discussed anywhere from 12 to 47 subjects. Most, of course, concerned health problems, but many concerned items with only an indirect effect on medicine. Many topics concerned injuries or diseases or death to people before they had an opportunity to go to a physician. For example, a number of articles have concerned guns and the resulting damage. One or more concerned the importance of helmets for cyclists. Physicians mainly respond to diseases and injuries in persons without playing much of a role in preventing them from occurring in the first place. Thus, many of the pieces hopefully underline the importance of physicians' getting involved in prevention of disease and injury so that patients won't end up in the accident rooms with diseases and injuries that should not have occurred in the first place.

—William Clifford Roberts, MD

Table of Contents

Chapter 1

January 2011

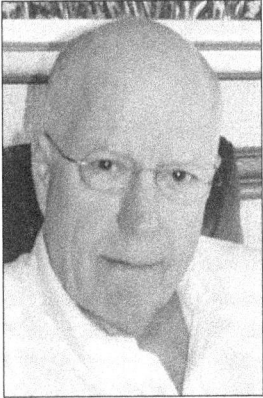

William C. Roberts, MD

IT'S THE CHOLESTEROL, STUPID!

During the 1992 presidential campaign in the USA, the Clinton campaign slogan was "*It's the economy, stupid*," and that phrase apparently was helpful in getting Mr. Clinton elected president. Several recent publications have been highly critical of some lipid-lowering trials using statin drugs and also have debased the cholesterol "hypothesis" on atherosclerosis (1–3).

What is the evidence that "elevated cholesterol" causes atherosclerosis? There are four supporting arguments in my view (4–7). 1) *Atherosclerotic plaques are easily produced experimentally in herbivores (e.g., rabbits, monkeys) simply by feeding these animals cholesterol (e.g., egg yokes) or saturated fats.* Indeed, atherosclerosis is probably the second easiest disease to produce experimentally. (The first is an endocrine deficiency—simply excise an endocrine gland.) 2) *Cholesterol is present in atherosclerotic plaques in experimentally produced atherosclerosis and in plaques in human beings.* 3) *Societies and individuals with high serum cholesterol levels (total and low-density lipoprotein [LDL] cholesterol) compared to populations and individuals with low levels have a high frequency of atherosclerotic events, a high frequency of dying from these events, and a large quantity (burden) of plaque in their arteries.* (The best study in my view supporting this thesis is the Seven Countries study [8–10].) 4) *Lowering total and LDL cholesterol levels decreases the frequency of atherosclerotic events, the chances of dying from these events, and the quantity of plaques in the arteries.* No one has produced atherosclerosis experimentally by increasing the arterial blood pressure or glucose levels or by blowing smoke in the faces of rabbits their entire lifetime or by stressing these animals. The only way to produce atherosclerosis experimentally is by feeding high-cholesterol and/or high-saturated-fat diets to herbivores. (Atherosclerosis is not a disease of carnivores, and it is not possible to produce atherosclerosis in carnivores [dogs, cats, tigers, lions, etc.] unless the thyroid gland is removed or made dysfunctional before a high-cholesterol or high-saturated-fat diet is administered [11]).

Why has the proven causal relation between abnormal serum LDL cholesterol and atherosclerosis been so difficult to accept by so many extremely intelligent physicians? One factor, in my view, is that this cholesterol-atherosclerosis causal relation has been diluted by the concept of multiple atherosclerotic risk factors and the idea that atherosclerosis is a multifactorial disease. The Framingham study, which has taught us all so much, introduced the concept of "risk factors" and fostered the view that the greater the number of risk factors present, the greater the chance of atherosclerotic events (12). As a consequence, "elevated cholesterol" became just one of several risk factors and was perceived as essentially having no more influence than elevated systolic blood pressure, diabetes mellitus ("glucose intolerance"), cigarette smoking, abdominal obesity, lack of regular physical activity, family history, or left ventricular hypertrophy except in the younger patients (13). The view that atherosclerosis is a multifactorial disease has muddled the waters in my view. This is not to say that cigarette smoking, elevated blood pressure, diabetes mellitus, obesity, and inactivity are not harmful—of course they are— *but* if the serum LDL cholesterol is <60 mg/dL or the serum total cholesterol is <150 mg/dL, there is no evidence (with extremely rare exceptions [14]) in my view that these other "risk factors" cause atherosclerosis.

A second factor is the introduction and propagation of the thesis that atherosclerosis is an inflammatory disease (15). Yes, a few mononuclear cells are regularly seen in experimentally produced atherosclerotic plaques but not commonly in plaques of patients with fatal coronary disease or in plaques excised by endarterectomy (16, 17). And, yes, some blood inflammatory markers are commonly elevated in persons with atherosclerotic events. But, many patients have atherosclerotic events when the high-sensitivity (hs) C-reactive protein (CRP) is normal (<1 mg/dL), and patients with the highest levels of hs-CRP (e.g., rheumatoid arthritis, systemic lupus erythematosus) have only a slightly higher frequency of atherosclerotic events than do others of similar age and sex with normal or near-normal hs-CRP levels. The same principle, however, does not apply to cholesterol. The patients with the highest serum levels of total and LDL cholesterol, namely those patients with homozygous familial hypercholesterolemia, have an incredibly high frequency of atherosclerotic events, and they have them at very young ages—teenage years (18). And patients with the next highest serum LDL cholesterol levels, namely those with heterozygous familial hypercholesterolemia, have atherosclerotic events often in their 30s and 40s.

A third factor preventing acceptance of the causal relation between abnormal serum LDL cholesterol and atherosclerosis has been the observation that among adults with nonfamilial hypercholesterolemia but similar levels of serum LDL cholesterol, some develop atherosclerotic events and others do not. It is in this group particularly in my view that the other "risk factors" as well as high-density lipoprotein (HDL) cholesterol levels come into play. Of two people of similar age and sex and similar serum LDL cholesterol levels, say 130 mg/dL, the patient whose systolic systemic blood pressure is 170 mm Hg versus the other patient with a systolic pressure of 115 mm Hg is at much greater risk of an atherosclerotic event. And cigarette smoking may work in a similar fashion. Nevertheless, if the serum LDL cholesterol is <60 mg/dL, maybe <50 mg/dL, irrespective of the degree of blood pressure elevation or the number of cigarettes smoked daily, atherosclerotic plaques do not develop.

Another factor may be the use of multiple atherosclerotic risk factors in the guidelines for whom to treat and whom not to treat with lipid-lowering drugs. Although the guidelines do focus on the serum LDL cholesterol level, the number of other "risk factors" present plays a prominent role in this therapeutic decision (19). If no other nonlipid risk factors are present or if only one non-LDL cholesterol risk factor is present and there have been no previous atherosclerotic events and diabetes mellitus is not present, the magical drug treatment number is an LDL cholesterol level >190 mg/dL. Refraining from drug intervention until this very high LDL cholesterol level is reached plays down or even nullifies the importance of cholesterol in preventing events. (It is important to realize that the lipid-lowering drug guidelines [1988, 1993, 2001, and 2004] have to do only with reducing atherosclerotic events. They do not concern themselves with preventing atherosclerotic plaques in the first place. Of course, if atherosclerotic plaques are prevented, atherosclerotic events do not occur!)

Such high guideline drug treatment levels keep, in my view, many persons deserving of lipid-lowering drug therapy from receiving these magical agents (20). The danger of high cholesterol levels to longevity was recognized by the life insurance companies in the 1930s but not by physicians. The normal range of serum total cholesterol in laboratory reports for decades was listed as 150 to 300 mg/dL. In 1972, one of the world's most prominent lipidologists reported that his total cholesterol "worry level" for patients was a value >300 mg/dL. If the expert uses such high numbers, what importance can be placed on cholesterol by the nonexpert community? Incidentally, for the first several decades of the Framingham study, an "elevated cholesterol" was defined as a serum total cholesterol >250 mg/dL. At this level, it is easy to understand how this "risk factor" did not separate itself from the others.

It is time to move on from a goal "to decrease risk" to a goal "to prevent plaques" (21). To do so requires much lower levels of LDL cholesterol than advocated by the guideline publications. My goal for all individuals worldwide is a serum LDL cholesterol at least <100 mg/dL and ideally <60 mg/dL. The beauty of the JUPITER trial is that it dramatically demonstrates what incredible reductions in events can be produced in a short period of time (<2 years) by reducing the LDL cholesterol by 50% even when starting from a level considered by many to be normal (<130 mg). The mean level (108 mg/dL) might be considered "good" or even "great" by many physicians, but lowering it to 55 mg/dL (by rosuvastatin 20 mg/dL) decreased all events by >40%, indeed nearly 50%, including a reduction in stroke by 48%! This trial beautifully shows that we can drastically reduce or even prevent atherosclerotic events and expensive procedures by taking a single pill every day and do it safely. Most Americans will not reach the JUPITER treatment levels (LDL cholesterol 55 mg/dL) by diet alone. The statin drugs have been ingested by humans now for nearly 30 years, and their safety and thus benefit/risk ratio may be the best of any proven useful medication. The toxicity resides mainly in atherosclerosis, not in the drug.

I consider it unfortunate that there continues to be so much criticism of statin drugs, which I consider to be the *best cardiovascular drug ever created.* * These drugs can prevent first and subsequent atherosclerotic events, they can reduce cardiovascular and all-cause mortality rates, they have the capacity to reduce the quantity of atherosclerotic plaques already present, and by decreasing the frequency of myocardial infarcts they reduce the frequency of heart failure and malignant ventricular arrhythmias. Their ability to reduce the serum levels of CRP may have benefits not yet fully appreciated. The discoverer of the first statin drug (Akira Endo, PhD) is deserving of the Nobel Prize for medicine!

The lower the LDL cholesterol the better, and this principle has been established repeatedly despite the voices of the anticholesterol, antistatin fallacy mongers! *It's the cholesterol, stupid!*

US LIPID LEVELS, 1996–2006

Data from the second, third, and fourth National Health and Nutrition Examination Surveys (NHANES) (1976–1980, 1988–1994, and 1999–2006) were examined to assess trends in our serum lipid levels, lipid-lowering medication use, and body weight (22). During the 30-year period, the mean age fell from 50 to 45 years; the percentage with total cholesterol levels ≥240 mg/dL fell from 25% to 16% and those with levels <200 rose from 45% to 52%; the percentage with LDL cholesterol levels ≥160 fell from 20% to 12% and those with levels <100 rose from 17% to 31%; the percentage with HDL cholesterol levels <40 was unchanged (21% and 19%) and those with levels ≥60 rose from 18% to 28%; the percentage with triglyceride levels ≥200 was unchanged (16% and 18%)

*I have no investments in pharmaceutical or device companies, I receive no grants from them, and I am on no advisory boards of industry. I have, however, in the past given talks sponsored by pharmaceutical companies. This editorial was originally published in the *American Journal of Cardiology* (2010;106:1364–1366) and is reprinted with permission from Elsevier.

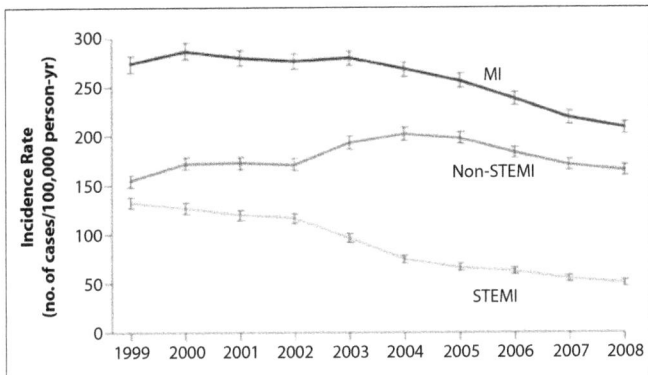

Figure. Age- and sex-adjusted incidence rates of acute myocardial infarction, 1999 to 2008. I bars represent 95% confidence intervals. MI indicates myocardial infarction; STEMI, ST-segment elevation myocardial infarction. Reprinted with permission from Yeh RW et al., *N Engl J Med* (23). Copyright Massachusetts Medical Society.

and those with levels <150 mg/dL also were unchanged (67% and 67%). The percentage of those who were obese (body mass index ≥30 kg/m²) increased from 15% to 34%. During the 30 years, the mean total cholesterol fell from 209 to 200; LDL cholesterol in men fell from 135 to 120 and in women from 132 to 117; HDL cholesterol in men was unchanged (45 and 47) and in women rose from 54 to 58; triglyceride levels in men rose from 153 to 161 and in women from 121 to 131 mg/dL. Thus, this report provides both good and bad news. The lowering of total cholesterol and LDL cholesterol levels is obviously good, but the increased obesity and triglyceride levels are not good. The mean body mass index increased from 26 to 29 kg/m² during the 30 years.

HEART ATTACKS DECREASING

Yeh and colleagues (23) from several US medical centers identified 46,086 hospitalizations for myocardial infarction during 18,691,131 person-years of follow-up from 1999 to 2008. During the 9-year follow-up, the age- and sex-adjusted incidence of myocardial infarction decreased from 274 to 208 cases per 100,000 person-years, representing a 24% relative decrease over the 9-year study (*Figure*). During the period, the incidence of non-ST-elevation myocardial infarction actually increased, and the incidence of ST-elevation myocardial infarction dramatically decreased (from 133 to 50 cases per 100,000 person-years). Thirty-day mortality also decreased significantly during the 9-year period of study. This is good news, of course!

STAYING WELL

Gene Stone authored *The Secrets of People Who Never Get Sick,* which appeared in 2010 (24). The book tells the stories of 25 people who each possess a different secret of excellent health. The following are some "secrets" described in this superb book.

Luigi Cornaro. He was a wealthy Venetian nobleman born to a prosperous family around 1460. Like his peers in Renaissance Italy, Cornaro lived extravagantly, and that included eating whatever and whenever he wanted. He consumed four or five

massive meals a day. In the 1490s, as he was approaching his 40th birthday, he fell ill. His doctors informed him that if he wanted to survive, he would have to moderate his diet. Cornaro designed himself a new diet, cutting back drastically on the quantity of food he consumed. Each day, he limited himself to 12 ounces of solid food and 14 ounces of wine (the water of the day). His plan worked almost immediately. His health improved so dramatically that he continued his plan until age 68 when his doctors worried that his food intake was too meager and insisted he eat and drink more generously. He complied but soon began feeling badly and promptly returned to his lighter menu, which he maintained for the rest of his life, until age 102. Cornaro wrote about his plan in his four-volume book, often translated as *Discourses on a Temperate Life*, in which he articulated his philosophy that people should eat less as they grow older. Cornaro not only lived a very long time but he remained healthy until just before his death. As he noted, "A long life full of disease and misery is worse than no life at all."

George Burns. His real name was Nathan Birnbaum. He picked up alias George Burns when he entered show business. One of 12 children, Burns started singing when he was a child, quitting school in the fourth grade to make it a profession. He was doing a solo vaudeville act—singing, dancing, and telling jokes—when he met Grace Ethel Cecile Rosalie Allen, a young Irish-Catholic singer. Soon afterwards, the two realized they worked better together than on their own and became Burns and Allen, one of the most famous comedy teams of the 20th century. Gracie died in 1964 at age 69, and Burns scaled back for a while but then became a major success in several movies. He once remarked, "I get a standing ovation just standing." Burns also was the author of 10 bestselling books. Even when Burns was approaching 90 he looked remarkably healthy. After lunch, he would play cards, take a nap, go about his day, and meet friends for dinner. He was asked by one of his friends when he was nearly 100, "How do you stay so fit and healthy? What is your advice?" Burns took a puff from his ever-present cigar, exhaled, and said in his gravelly voice, "Eat half."

No question: caloric reduction is a lifespan extender. Luigi Cornaro may have been the first person to write about eating less for better health. In the early 20th century, a Newburgh, New York, physician, William Jones, reported that a fasting spider will live longer than one that eats a normal diet. In the 1930s, studies at Cornell University showed that rats on a limited diet lived twice as long as other rats. Similar results were found in mice.

Thomas Edison stated:

I keep my health by dieting. People gorge themselves with rich foods, use up their time, ruin their digestion, and poison themselves. . . . If the doctors would prescribe dieting instead of drugs, the ailments of normal man would disappear. Half the people are food drunk all the time. That is the secret of my health.

In his 1983 book, *How to Live to Be a Hundred—or More,* George Burns wrote on his supposed diet. Breakfast: one small glass of orange juice, a bowl of bran cereal with milk, and

2 cups of black coffee. *Lunch:* a bowl of canned salmon with white vinegar and lemon, half an English muffin toasted, and one cup of black coffee. *Dinner:* a bowl of soup, a mixed green salad, broiled fish, 2 vegetables, one slice of bread, one cup of black coffee, and ice cream.

Stone's book went on to discuss cold showers, detoxification, eating dirt, the importance of friends, garlic, germ avoidance, herbal remedies, hydrogen peroxide, lifting weights, napping, positive attitude, probiotics, and several other topics.

I was particularly intrigued by Stone's comment on sleeping. According to research by sleep specialist Neil Stanley, MD, of the University of Surrey, UK, sharing a bed with a partner is not necessarily a healthy idea for either party. Between restless limbs, snoring, and disagreements over what time to set the alarm, couples suffered an average of 50% more sleep disturbances if they shared a bed than if they slept solo, according to one study. The tradition of sharing a marital bed is relatively new, dating from the Industrial Revolution, when population growth meant more people with less furniture. In ancient Rome, for example, the marital bed was used only for sex, not sleeping. Robert Meadows, PhD, another researcher at the University of Surrey, demonstrated that when couples share a bed and one of them moves in his or her sleep, there is a 50% chance that the partner will be disturbed. Scientists appear to have concluded that if you are successfully sleeping with someone, fine; if not, there is no shame, and much to gain, in sleeping apart.

ROAD ACCIDENTS AND TRAVELING ABROAD

According to a *USA Today* analysis of the past 7½ years of State Department data, about 1800 Americans—almost a third of all Americans who died of nonnatural causes while abroad—were killed in road accidents in foreign countries from January 1, 2003, through June 2010 (25, 26). On average, one American traveler dies on a foreign road every 36 hours. Almost 40% of the deaths occurred in Mexico, followed by Thailand, the Dominican Republic, Germany, and Spain. The lethal cocktail of killer roads, unsafe vehicles, dangerous driving, and disoriented travelers is killing an estimated 25,000 travelers to foreign countries each year.

The number of tourist deaths is dwarfed by the total number of road fatalities worldwide. Nearly 1.3 million people die and up to 50 million people are injured each year, according to the World Health Organization estimates. About half of the fatalities are occupants of four-wheel motor vehicles; the other half are bicyclists, motorcyclists, and pedestrians. More than 90% of the world's road fatalities occur in low-income and middle-income countries, which have nearly half of the world's registered vehicles. The fatality rates on their roads are nearly double those of high-income countries. Mexico is the most common foreign country visited by Americans, followed by Canada. A total of 682 American travelers died in Mexico from January 2003 through June 2010; Canada registered 31 road deaths of US citizens.

Why so many deaths in low- and middle-income countries? Many of these countries have roads that were designed poorly and lack safety features such as barriers. Many roads are shared by motorists, pedestrians, cyclists, and animal-drawn carts and lack safe zones for the more vulnerable road users. Many countries lack or fail to enforce laws for speeding, drunken driving, and other traffic hazards. Many also lack or fail to enforce laws for wearing seatbelts and motorcycle helmets and using child restraints. The most recent World Health Organization statistic shows that two middle-income countries, China and India, have the most road deaths. In 2007, nearly 221,000 people were killed in China and about 196,000 in India. Every 6 seconds someone is killed or injured on the world's roads.

For safety on foreign roads, travelers might consider the following: read foreign country road travel reports on the State Department's website, http://travelstate.gov. The Road Safety Overseas page links to many road-safety resources. Consider hiring a well-trained driver instead of driving a car in low-income and some middle-income countries. Drive or ride in vehicles only with an accessible seatbelt. Learn how to use all controls and signals on a rental vehicle in the parking lot before getting on a road. Practice driving in a less populated area before driving in heavy traffic, especially if you are in a country where drivers drive on the left side of the road. Become familiar with the local road culture and road regulations. Learn about seasonal hazards and local holidays when road crashes are particularly high. Avoid night road travel in countries with poor safety records or mountainous terrain. Avoid lightweight minivans, motorcycles, scooters, and mopeds. If you travel on a motorcycle, scooter, or moped, wear a helmet that meets safety regulations. Pedestrians are at most risk, so be aware of local traffic patterns, cross roads only at crosswalks, and wear reflective clothing at night.

MORE ON THE NATIONAL DEBT

As of October 2010, the Obama administration has borrowed $3 trillion according to the US Treasury Department (27). It took from 1776, when the USA became an independent country, until 1990, the year after the Berlin Wall fell, for the federal government to accumulate a total of $3 trillion in debt. It took only from January 2009, the day President Barack Obama was inaugurated, until October 15, 2010, for the Obama administration to add $3 trillion to the federal debt! The overall debt of the federal government, according to the Treasury Department, is now $13.666 trillion. Each business day the Treasury Department's Bureau of the Public Debt publishes the exact amount, to the penny, of total federal debt as of the close of the previous business day. At the close of business on January 20, 2009, the total debt of the federal government was $10,626,877,048,912.08. On October 15, 2010, the federal government borrowed an additional $58,15,979,549,154.06, bringing the total federal debt at the close of business to $13,665,926,643,255.96, an increase of $3,039,049,594,342.88 since President Obama's inauguration.

COSTS OF OBAMACARE

Dr. Mark Siegel, an associate professor of medicine at New York University Langone Medical Center, discussed the new health care reform law in a piece in *USA Today*, October 2010 (28). According to Siegel, the new health care law mandates and extends the kind of insurance that breeds overuse, thereby driving up costs and premiums. The medical system is about to be overwhelmed because there are no disincentives for overuse. The new bill covers all Americans with preexisting conditions. That's not the issue, says Dr. Siegel. We are going to get into trouble because of the kinds of coverage that the new law mandates. There are no breaks on the system. Copays and deductibles will be kept low and preventive services will have no copays at all. Without at least a pause to consider necessity and/or costs, expect waiting times to increase, emergency rooms to be clogged, and lead times to be longer for appointments. Patients with new Medicaid who can't find a physician will go to emergency rooms. The escalating costs of these visits (both the necessary and unnecessary ones) will be transferred directly to the American public, both in the form of taxes as well as escalating insurance premiums.

Beginning in 2014, insurance exchanges will be set up in every state so that individuals can choose a health insurance plan. But don't expect to find individually tailored plans or those with higher deductibles or copays. They won't be there because they can't receive the government's stamp of approval. In the new system, patients can go to their physician as often as they like. But will they get the same level of care? Almost certainly no, says Dr. Siegel. He anticipates that expensive chemotherapy, coronary procedures, and organ transplants will have a tougher time being approved, as is already the case in Canada.

The new Independent Payment Advisory Board, established by the health reform law to "recommend proposals to limit Medicare spending growth," will advise Medicare that some treatments are more essential and more cost effective than others. These value judgments will reduce the options of practicing physicians, and private insurers will follow suit.

Although President Obama indicated that we would be able to keep our current insurance plans, the new private markets will have to remake their plans, meaning that the cost will rise and the plan we were told we could "keep" is in all likelihood no longer available.

Private health insurance is a low-profit industry with profit margins of about 4%. With the additional costs of no lifetime caps and no exclusion for preexisting conditions, these companies will be compelled to raise their premiums to stay in business. The increased numbers of Medicaid participants are supposed to preserve profits but that seems unlikely, says Dr. Siegel, with all the new regulations.

Dr. Siegel provided this analogy: Imagine if your car insurance covered every scratch or dent. Wouldn't you expect your premiums to rise to meet the expanded coverage? And wouldn't you expect your auto repair shops to become clogged with cars that really didn't need to be repaired, competing for time and space with other cars with broken transmissions or burnt-out motors?

If we want lower insurance premiums, we will need to return to a system that favors high-deductible, high-copay catastrophic-type insurance with a built-in disincentive for overuse. Patients could pay for office visits from health savings accounts or other flexible spending tax shelters. More than 10 million Americans already have such accounts. Unfortunately, the new law takes away the kind of insurance that compels patients to pay more themselves. As a result, medical care will cost more and be inferior to that provided today. Dr. Siegel concludes that the kind of insurance the new law mandates will, over the years, wear out the health care system.

TODAY'S PRACTICES DESTINED TO FUTURE CONDEMNATION

William Osler stated, "The philosophies of one age have become the absurdities of the next, and the foolishness of yesterday has become the wisdom of tomorrow." Kwame Anthony Appiah (29) has suggested four contenders for future moral condemnation.

The US prison system. Roughly 1% of adults in the USA are incarcerated. The USA has 4% of the world's population but 25% of its prisoners. No other nation has as large a proportion of its population in prison. China's rate is less than half that of the USA. Most of our prisoners are nonviolent offenders, many detained on drug charges. More than 100,000 inmates suffer sexual abuse, including rape, each year; some contract HIV. Our country holds at least 25,000 prisoners in isolation ("super max" facilities) under conditions that many psychologists say amount to torture.

Industrial meat production. Of the nearly 100 million cattle in the USA, at least 10 million at any time are packed into feedlots, saved from the inevitable diseases of overcrowding only by regular doses of antibiotics, surrounded by their own feces, their nostrils filled with the smell of their own urine. In the European Union, many of the most inhumane conditions we allow are already illegal or, like the sow stalls into which pregnant pigs are often crammed in the USA, will be illegal soon.

Institutionalized and isolated elderly. Nearly 2 million of America's elderly are in nursing homes, out of sight, and, to some extent, out of mind. Nearly 10,000 for-profit facilities have arisen in the USA in recent decades to hold them. Other elderly Americans may live independently but often are isolated and cut off from their families. Keeping aging parents close to their children is a challenge, particularly in a society where almost everybody has a job outside the home. Nevertheless, many old people, despite having many living relatives, suffer growing isolation.

Abuse of the environment. Our wasteful attitude toward the planet's natural resources and ecology is obvious everywhere. Desertification, which is primarily the result of destructive land-management practices, threatens a third of the earth's surface. Tens of thousands of Chinese villages have been overrun by sand drifts in recent decades. Vast expanses of portions of Russia, which decades earlier were a lush and verdant landscape, are now vast expanses of parched badlands. We know the harm done by deforestation, wetland destruction, pollution, overfishing, and greenhouse gas emissions. When our descendants inherit this devastated earth, they are unlikely to have the luxury of such recklessness.

We should all have our own suspicions about which practices will someday prompt people to ask in dismay: "What were they thinking?"

MICHAEL MILKEN ON OUR CHALLENGES

In his forthcoming book *Where is Sputnik?*, Mr. Milken lists six challenging areas in the USA (30).

Housing. Investors have suffered some $1 trillion in losses on supposedly safe mortgage-backed assets. Mr. Milken opines that we consider how many more jobs small businesses would have created if they had enjoyed the same terms we gave homeowners—easy access to 30-year, government-guaranteed loans at near-prime rates with no prepayment penalties. Those terms encouraged larger houses. The average size doubled in a generation to 2500 square feet, even as family size shrank. This required more land further from cities, and we bought bigger cars for longer, energy-wasting commutes. It was a great allocation of resources spurred by government policy and individual choices. We justified it on the theory that homeownership is a social good that builds personal responsibility and contributes to stable communities. But these ill-conceived policies produced the opposite: excessive consumer debt, irresponsible lending, mortgage defaults, unemployment, and declining neighborhoods. Ironically, a larger share of the population owns homes in many other countries where borrowers do not have a mortgage interest tax deduction and put up far more equity. American policymakers got it backwards. In the long run, jobs support housing, not the other way around.

Entitlement. Unrealistic promises of overgenerous health and retirement benefits forced General Motors, once the world's largest company, into bankruptcy. Unfortunately, the simple math of the GM situation applies to many institutions, including state and local governments that face massive pension commitments. And, looming even larger are the federal government's long-term obligations to recipients of Social Security and other entitlements. The problem is rooted in unrealistic assumptions about rates of return on assets; a falling ratio of current workers to retirees; workers who pay into the system for too few years; and pensioners who live longer than the original planners assumed. An important first step would be to periodically adjust the minimum retirement age to 85% of average life expectancy. Higher wage taxes and lower real benefits might follow.

Education. The Milken Family Foundation in 1982 began studying which factors have the greatest impact on student achievement. What they found was that teacher quality was far and away the most important school-related factor. We must hire and keep the highest-quality teachers possible. That requires powerful, embedded professional development, transparent and fair teacher evaluation, and performance-based pay.

Health. Out of every $10 the USA collects in taxes, the government invests only a few pennies in research. We need more publicly supported research! We also should require more self-responsibility for our health. The Milken Institute's 2007 study, "An Unhealthy America," found that 70% of health costs (more than $2 trillion a year) are related to lifestyle. Government programs are no substitute for personal responsibility in reducing the costs that flow from smoking, poor diets, and inadequate exercise.

Immigration. While the public debates center on undocumented low-skill workers, we should be equally focused on high-skilled professionals whom we have often shut out. More than half of Silicon Valley's science and engineering workforce is foreign born. Canada, the United Kingdom, and Australia encourage immigrant investors. China, Russia, Israel, and Singapore encourage the importation of smart entrepreneurs and scientists. Milken indicates that any nation that fails to welcome them will fall behind. Milken favors expanded visa programs for skilled workers and substantial investors who purchase property or create jobs. He believes we should grant permanent residency to graduates from accredited science and engineering programs.

Energy. In 1970, the USA imported about 36% of its oil. We now import 60% of our oil. Energy security is at least as important as cotton and tobacco, whose prices we support. Oil needs similar support to avoid a repeat of the 1980s when many financial institutions and investors who responded to the call for energy independence were devastated by plunging prices. Lack of that support will discourage new investments and sustainable energy sources. Regrettably, the political hurdle is high because people want lower prices at the gas pump. We forget that we also pay for energy security with aircraft carriers, antiterrorism measures, environmental degradation, and, most tragically, military and civilian lives. Our competitors are directing increasing resources to human capital development and energy security. We have the capacity to match them, but do we have the will?

TOO MUCH MONEY

Mumbai (Bombay), India, is one of the largest and poorest cities in the world. But, Mumbai also has some very rich people. One is Mukesh Ambani, whose $27 billion fortune ranks him among the richest people in the world (31). He has just built a 27-floor tower which will be the residence for his family, including his wife and their three children. Six of the 27 floors are a parking garage. Three helipads are on the roof. There are terraces upon terraces, airborne swimming pools, and hanging gardens. The tower reportedly cost $1 billion. For decades, the Ambani family has been India's most famous corporate soap opera. The father, Dhirubhai Ambani, was a rags-to-riches tycoon who established Reliance Industries after rising out of the city's tenements. Today, Reliance is the world's largest producer of polyester fibers and yarns and accounts for almost 15% of India's exports. The two sons, Mukesh and Anil, inherited and divided the empire and spent years feuding. Of Mumbai's 20 million population, 62% live in slums. High rises are considered inevitable and necessary given the peninsula city's limited land and swollen population. Something is wrong with all of this.

HENRIETTA LACKS AND HER IMMORTAL CELLS

In 1951 at the age of 30, Henrietta Lacks, a descendant of freed slaves, was diagnosed with an aggressive form of cervical cancer (32). Her doctor took a small tissue sample without her knowledge or consent. A scientist put the sample into a test tube and, though Henrietta died 8 months later, her cells— known worldwide as HeLa—are still alive today. They became the first immortal human cell line ever grown in culture and one of the most important tools in medicine. Research on HeLa cells was vital to the development of the polio vaccine as well as drugs for treatment of herpes simplex, leukemia, influenza, hemophilia, and Parkinson's disease; it helped uncover some secrets of cancer and the effects of the atom bomb and led to important advances like cloning, in vitro fertilization, and gene mapping. Since 2001, five Nobel Prizes have been awarded on research involving HeLa cells. No one knows exactly how many of Henrietta's cells are alive today. One scientist estimates that if you could pile all the HeLa cells ever grown onto a scale, they would weigh >50 million metric tons—the equivalent of at least 100 Empire State Buildings.

Today, nearly 60 years after Henrietta's death, her body lies in an unmarked grave in Clover, Virginia. But her cells are still among the most widely used in labs worldwide—bought and sold by the billions. Those cells have done wonders for science. Henrietta, whose legacy involves the birth of bioethics and the history of experimentation on African Americans, is all but forgotten.

BOTOX AND MIGRAINE

In October 2010 the Food and Drug Administration (FDA) approved Botox, the antiwrinkle shot from Allergan, as a treatment to prevent chronic migraines, a little more than a month after the company agreed to pay $600 million to settle all allegations that it had illegally marketed the drug for unapproved uses like headaches for years (33). The agency's decision endorses use of Botox to treat patients with a severe form of migraine headaches occurring at least 15 days a month. Britain's drug agency approved Botox for the same use in 2010.

Botox had worldwide sales in 2009 of about $1.3 billion, divided equally between medical and cosmetic uses. The producer said sales of Botox for chronic migraines and other medical uses would soon eclipse sales of the drug as a wrinkle smoother. Allergan is also studying the drug for a variety of new medical uses, including overactive bladder. A Botox migraine treatment generally involves a total of 31 injections in the forehead, temples, back of head, neck, and shoulders. To treat the chronic condition, injections are given about every 3 months. It is estimated that the migraine treatment would cost $1000 to $2000, depending on the amount of drug used and the physician's fee. Some private insurers are likely to cover the migraine treatment now that it has received FDA approval. Some physicians are a bit leery of using Botox for chronic migraines, suggesting that it has only a marginal effect on headaches compared with a placebo.

NOBEL PRIZE AND IN VITRO FERTILIZATION

Robert Edwards of Britain won the 2010 Nobel Prize in medicine for developing in vitro fertilization (34). Edwards, an 85-year-old professor emeritus at the University of Cambridge, started working on in vitro fertilization in the 1950s.

He developed the technique in which eggs are removed from a woman, fertilized outside her body, and then implanted into the womb. He worked with British gynecologist Patrick Steptoe, who died in 1988. On July 25, 1978, Louise Brown in Britain became the first baby born through the groundbreaking procedure, marking a revolution in fertility treatment. Since then some 4 million have been born using the technique, a rate that is up to about 300,000 babies worldwide each year. Ms. Brown, now 32, gave birth to her first child in 2007. The boy was conceived naturally.

MARRIED ADULTS VS UNMARRIED ADULTS

For the first time since the USA began tallying marriages, more Americans of prime marrying age (25–34 years) have stayed single rather than marry (35). High divorce rates, rising cohabitation, and a tendency to delay marriage are the main factors. Although marriage rates among young adults have been dropping for decades, data released by the Census Bureau in September 2010 show that for the first time the proportion of people between the ages of 25 and 34 who have never been married exceeded those who were married in 2009 (46% vs. 45%). The remainder is a mix of those who have lost spouses and divorcees who, if combined with the unmarried group, tilt the balance even further. The long-term slide in marriage rates has pushed the proportion of married adults of all ages to 52% in 2009. In contrast, in 1960, 72% of adults over age 18 were married. (The USA began tracking marriage statistics in 1880.)

The cities with the highest percentage of adults aged 25 to 34 who are married are Fort Worth, 52%; El Paso, 51%; Colorado Springs, 50%; Las Vegas, 47%; and Tulsa, 46%. The cities with the highest percentage of adults aged 25 to 34 who have never married are San Francisco, 82%; Boston, 82%; Detroit, 80%; Atlanta, 80%; and Cleveland, 80%. The change in marriage habits has been most pronounced among those with less education. Between 2000 and 2010 the share of young adults who are married dropped 10 percentage points to 44% among those who didn't attend college. Marriage rates among those in the same age group who hold bachelor's or more advanced degrees, meanwhile, fell 4% over that time to 52%. This is a departure from past trends. In the past, college graduates were much more likely to postpone matrimony to focus on their career or further education. Now, a higher proportion of those without 4-year degrees are postponing marriage.

GRANDPARENTS RAISING GRANDKIDS

Roughly 7 million children live in households that include one grandparent, according to the most recent Census Bureau data from 2008 (36). Of that number, nearly 3 million were being raised by their grandparents, up 16% from 2000. Reasons for grandparents' taking over childrearing duties are many and include a single parent who becomes overwhelmed with financial problems, is incarcerated, succumbs to illness or substance abuse, or dies. High rates of divorce and teen pregnancies fuel the phenomenon, as do long overseas deployments confronting some parents in the military. The American Academy of Child and Adolescent Psychiatry notes that many children living with grandparents enter that arrangement with preexisting problems (abuse, neglect, prenatal exposure to drugs and alcohol, and loss of their parents).

PROHIBITION

The 18th amendment to the Constitution was ratified on January 16, 1919. It reads as follows:

> After one year from the ratification of this article the manufacture, sale, or transportation of intoxicating liquors within, the importation thereof into, or the exportation thereof from the United States and all territory subject to the jurisdiction thereof for beverage purposes is hereby prohibited. The Congress and the several States shall have concurrent power to enforce this article by appropriate legislation. This article shall be inoperative unless it shall have been ratified as an amendment to the Constitution by the legislatures of the several States, as provided in the Constitution, within seven years from the date of the submission hereof to the States by the Congress.

How did a freedom-loving people decide to give up a private right that had been freely exercised by millions since the first European colonists arrived in the New World? How did they condemn to extinction what was, at the very moment of its death, the fifth largest industry in the nation? With a single previous exception, the original Constitution and its first 17 amendments limited the activities of the government, not of citizens. Now there were two exceptions: you could not own slaves and you could not buy alcohol. Prohibition changed the way we lived, and it fundamentally redefined the role of the federal government. How in the world did it happen?

The answer comes in a wonderful book entitled *Last Call: The Rise and Fall of Prohibition* by Daniel Okrent (37). What follows was taken entirely from his 468-page book.

Alcohol in 19th-century America. America had been awash in alcohol almost from the start. In 1839, an English traveler described the role liquor played in American life:

> I am sure the Americans can fix nothing without a drink. If you meet, you drink; if you part, you drink; if you make acquaintance, you drink; if you close a bargain, you drink; they quarrel in their drink, and they make up with a drink. They drink because it is hot; they drink because it is cold. If successful in elections, they drink and rejoice; if not, they drink and swear; they begin to drink early in the morning, they leave off late at night; they commence it early in life and continue it, until they soon drop into the grave.

Virtually every homestead in America had an orchard from which thousands of gallons of cider were made every year. In the cities, it was widely understood that common workers would fail to come to work on Mondays, staying home to wrestle with the aftershocks of a weekend binge. By 1830, the tolling of a town bell at 11:00 AM and again at 4:00 PM marked "grog time." Soldiers in the US Army received 4 ounces of whiskey as part of their daily ration since 1782. And the propertied classes

drank heavily also. George Washington kept a stile on his farm, John Adams began each day with a tankard of hard liquor, and Thomas Jefferson had his renowned collection of wines and rye whiskey made from his own crops. James Madison consumed a pint of whiskey daily.

By 1830, American adults were guzzling per capita 7 gallons of pure alcohol a year. In modern terms, those 7 gallons would be equivalent to 1.7 bottles of standard 80-proof liquor per person per week—nearly 90 bottles a year for every adult in the nation—even with abstainers factored in, and there were millions of them. If what Americans drank today was multiplied by three, that would give an idea of what much of the 19th century in the USA was like.

The beginnings of the temperance movement. The first prominent American temperance advocate was the Philadelphia physician *Benjamin Rush*, who encouraged the whiskey-riddled to consider a transitional beverage: wine mixed with opium or laudanum. (The word *temperance* at first meant moderation and later meant abstinence.)

The nation's first large-scale expression of antialcohol sentiment began in a barroom in Baltimore in 1840 when six habitual drinkers pledged their commitment to total abstinence. (It was later known as "*the Washingtonian movement*.") They abdicated no changes in the law; they refused to pin blame for their circumstances on tavern operators or distillers; they asked habitual drinkers only to sign a pledge of abstinence. In the same speech in which he condemned the ubiquity of alcoholic beverages, Abraham Lincoln, who thought mandatory prohibition a bad idea, praised the Washingtonian movement for its reliance on kind persuasion.

Neal Dow, a prosperous businessman from Portland, Maine, led a group of Portland employers who denied their workers their daily "eleveners"—grog time. Elected mayor in 1851, he immediately persuaded the Maine legislature to enact the nation's first statewide prohibitory law, mandating fines for those convicted of selling liquor and imprisonment for those engaged in its manufacture. *The Maine Law*, as it came to be known, enabled the antiliquor forces who had been stirred by the Washingtonians to use this template to pass similar laws in a dozen other states. By the end of the 1850s, however, states that had enacted versions of the Maine Law had repealed them, Maine included.

The movement reappeared in the 1870s after Dr. Dioclesian Lewis spoke in December 1873 in Hillsboro, Ohio, a town of 5000 about 50 miles east of Cincinnati. Dio, as he was called, was not a physician—his MD was an honorary one granted by a College of Homeopathy—but he was an educator, physical culturist, health food advocate, bestselling author, and one of the more compelling platform speakers of his day. In his lecture on alcohol he urged the women of Hillsboro to use the power of prayer to rid the town of its saloons, not only praying for the liquor sellers but praying with them. The next morning 75 Hillsboro women emerged in an orderly two-by-two column from a meeting at the Presbyterian church. At their head was *Eliza Jane Tremble Thompson*, the daughter of an Ohio governor, the wife of a well-known judge, and mother of eight. She was 57 and a devout Methodist. On that Christmas Eve and for 10 days afterwards, Thompson led her band to the town's saloons, hotels, and drugstores (many of which sold liquor by the glass). At each one, they fell to their knees and prayed for the soul of the owner. The women worked in 6-hour shifts, running relays from their homes to the next establishment on their list, praying, singing, reading from the Bible, and generally creating the largest stir in the town's history. If they were allowed inside, they would kneel on a sawdust floor that had been defiled by years of spilled drinks and the expectorations of men who had missed, or never tried for, the spittoon. If not, they remained outside singing and praying in the winter cold. In 11 days, Thompson and her sisters persuaded the proprietors of nine of the town's 13 drinking places to close their doors. By February 1874, federal liquor tax collections were off by more than $300,000 in just two revenue districts. The events in Hillsboro launched a crusade that spread across the Midwest into New York and onto New England. In more than 110 cities and towns, every establishment selling liquor yielded to the hurricane set loose by Eliza Thompson. But, within a few months, this hurricane was spent.

Nevertheless, Mother Thompson, as she was referred to, set other women agitating against alcohol. Soon the new movement led by Susan B. Anthony and Elizabeth Cady Stanton also gave rise to the suffrage movement, which was a direct consequence of the widespread prohibition sentiment. The most urgent reasons for women to want to vote in the 1800s were alcohol related: they wanted the saloons closed down or at least regulated. They wanted the right to own property, to shield their families' financial security from the profligacy of drunken husbands, to divorce those men and have them arrested for wife beating, and to protect their children from being terrorized by them. To do these things they needed to change the laws that consigned married women to the status of chattel. And to change the laws, they needed the vote. But the universal vote was decades away. Some women in the 1840s banded together to threaten sexual abstinence if their husbands could not achieve alcohol abstinence. Many rural and small-town women had to endure the dire ravages of the early saloon: the wallet emptied into a bottle; the job loss or the farm work left undone; and a scourge that late in the century was identified by physicians as "syphilis of the innocent" contracted by the wives of drink-sodden husbands who had found something more than liquor lurking in the saloons.

The Woman's Christian Temperance Union. Twenty years after Mother Thompson's crusade had subsided, the Woman's Christian Temperance Union (WCTU) was launched by Frances Willard (my daughter's married name). At age 35, Willard was among a small group of women who in 1874 founded the WCTU, and for the rest of her life she was field general, propagandist, chief theoretician, and nearly a deity to a 250,000-member army, undoubtedly the nation's most effective political action group in the last decades of the 19th century. Willard was raised on a farm in Janesville, Wisconsin. At 16, she asked her parents to sign a pledge she had pasted in the family Bible: "A pledge we make, no wine to take, nor brandy red that turns the head . . . so we pledge perpetual hate to all that can intoxicate." A few years later Willard moved to Evanston, Illinois, with her family. The town was dominated by New College (later Northwestern University) founded by a legal proscription against the sale of alcoholic beverages within 4 miles of its campus and buttressed by the creation of a similarly liquor-loathing women's school that opened nearby. Willard graduated from Northwestern Female College as valedictorian and became its president a decade later. The two schools merged in 1873. In 1874 on a trip east, Willard found herself on her knees in a saloon on Market Street in Pittsburgh singing "Rock of Ages." A few weeks later, she walked away from her academic career so she could give her life to the temperance cause.

Willard made temperance a woman's issue. She further believed that temperance was not enough. Only some form of legal prohibition could crush the liquor demon, and no prohibition would ever be enacted without the votes of women. In 1876, she told a WCTU audience that women should have the right to vote on matters relating to liquor. Willard urged her followers to agitate for a set of goals that stretched far beyond the liquor issue. She campaigned for suffrage; prison reform; free kindergarten; vocational schools; an 8-hour work day; workers' rights; government ownership of utilities, railroads, factories, and theaters; vegetarianism; cremation; less restrictive women's clothing; and alcohol-free, tobacco-free, lust-free marriages. Her determination to connect prohibition (the legislated imposition of teetotalism on the unwilling) to other reforms also was being propagated by the Prohibition Party in its first national campaign, which was in 1872. The party endorsed universal suffrage, public education, and the elimination of the electoral college, among other issues.

Frances Willard invited *Mary Hanchett Hunt*, a former chemistry teacher from Massachusetts, to speak at the WCTU Convention in 1879. Hunt believed it her mission to reach the nation's children, to saturate them in facts—as she perceived them—that would make young people despise alcohol as much as she did. Through them, Hunt enlisted the WCTU's battalions in an assault on the nation's school boards with a program of "scientific temperance instruction," which she intended to introduce into every American schoolroom. With Willard's support, Hunt sought to have two or more monitors from every WCTU chapter lay siege on their local school boards. From there, she targeted state legislatures, beginning in 1881. She became known as the "queen of the lobby." Vermont in 1882 was the first state to pass a compulsory temperance education law, followed later by many other states. By 1901, when the population of the entire country was about 80 million, compulsory temperance education was on the books of every state in the nation, and all 22 million American children and teenagers had three weekly lessons on temperance. In Boston, Hunt also created the "Scientific Temperance Museum." *Professor Charles H. Stowell* of the University of Michigan Medical School, a stalwart antialcohol man, authored a series of health and anatomy books supported fully by Hunt. In his textbook for high school students, he described alcohol as "a narcotic poison with the power to deaden or paralyze the brain."

Carry Amelia Moore Gloyd Nation, 6 feet tall with the biceps of a stevedore, was the next of the major prohibition leaders. The hatchet made her famous, and she used it to destroy a saloon. The hatchet soon transformed itself from weapon to symbol to calling card for her career as a platform speaker. Through her prohibition lectures, which she delivered on the vaudeville circuit, she had a major impact.

Saloons and breweries. By the end of the 19th century, production and consumption of whiskey and other distilled spirits had declined substantially, to a per capita figure not radically dissimilar from what it would be 100 years later. In 1850, Americans annually averaged drinking 36 million gallons of beer; by 1890, annual consumption of beer had increased to 855 million gallons. During that 4-decade span, while the population tripled, that population's capacity for beer had increased 24-fold. Immigration was the main reason. Those coming from Ireland and Germany loved the "liquid bread." And of course the settlement of the West provided numerous more saloons. The number of saloons in the USA increased from 100,000 in 1870 to nearly 300,000 by 1900. In Leadville, South Dakota, population 20,000, there was one saloon for every 100 inhabitants—women, children, and abstainers included. San Francisco in 1890 had one saloon for every 96 residents. In Manhattan there were 4000 saloons for every 100 churches.

The typical saloon featured more than just drink and companionship, particularly in urban immigrant districts and in the mining and lumber settlements. In these places, where customers' ties to a neighborhood might be new and tenuous, saloon keepers cashed checks, extended credit, and supplied a mailing address or a message drop for men who had not yet found a permanent home. And in some instances, saloons provided sleeping space at 5¢ a night. Some saloon keepers were labor contractors for dock workers. Many saloons had the only public toilets or washing facilities in the neighborhood. By the 1890s, most saloon keepers had complimentary spreads to lure customers and promote the sale of beer. These saloons had nice paintings (Custer's *Last Fight* was the most popular) or large mirrors, nice furniture, brass foot rails, iron and porcelain spittoons, and nice glassware.

These ornaments were provided by the breweries. The surest way a brewer could secure his piece of the local action was through the "tied house." If a saloon operator would agree to serve only one brand of beer, the brewer would provide cash, loans, and whatever other emoluments were necessary to furnish the place, stock the lunch table, meet the license fee, and when necessary line the pockets of politicians. By 1909, 70% of American saloons were owned by, in debt to, or otherwise indentured to the breweries.

The antiprohibition campaigns, of course, were levied by the brewers, the most prominent of whom was *Adolphus Busch*, the youngest of 21 children of a prosperous Rhineland merchant. Busch immigrated to the USA in 1857, went into the brewery supply business, and in 1861, at age 22, married Lilly Anheuser, the daughter of one of his customers. Adolphus' brother, Ulrich, married Lilly's sister, Anna. Adolphus soon took over the management of his father-in-law's company and in time appended his surname to it. Busch also built glass factories and ice plants and acquired railroad companies to ferry coal from mines to the vast Anheuser-Busch factory complex in St. Louis. Busch got into the manufacture of refrigerated railcars and truck bodies that could be used not just by breweries but also by customers such as meat-packing companies. He got exclusive US rights to a novel engine technology developed by his countryman, Rudolph Diesel. In 1875, Busch produced 35,000 barrels of beer; by 1900 his annual output surpassed a million barrels. In 1903, he helped craft an agreement essentially signed by nine breweries to fund a committee "promoting antiprohibition matters in Texas" such as paying poll taxes of black and Mexican Americans who were expected to vote for legal beer. He purchased the editorial support of newspapers. Busch died at the age of 74 from cirrhosis of the liver.

The Anti-Saloon League. The Anti-Saloon League (ASL) was founded by *Howard Hide Russell*, who in his early 20s was a prosperous lawyer in Iowa but at age 28 entered the Theology School of Oberlin College in Ohio. The Oberlin community possessed deep convictions, and at one point dietary restrictions were so severe at the college that in addition to alcohol, tea, coffee, and meat, the list of proscribed foods included pepper, gravy, and butter. Ordained at age 31, Russell occupied ever larger pulpits and at age 36 founded the ASL. Driven by focus and intimidation, the league declared war on alcohol *and only on alcohol*—only one target, a direct rebuke to the unfocused efforts of both the WCTU and the Prohibition Party. Frances Willard's "do everything" policy had been distracting. The ASL cared only about alcohol and about freeing the nation from its grip. There would be one big question mark before the name of every candidate for public office: "Is he right on this question?"

To gather support needed to fund the group's effort, Russell and his colleagues mobilized the nation's Protestant churches and their congregations. The ASL slogan read: "The church in action against the saloon." The leadership, the staff, and the directorates of the ASL and its affiliate organizations were overwhelmingly Methodist and Baptist. The clergymen occupied a minimum of 70% of the board seats of any state branch. It set out to reach the hundreds of thousands of churchgoers in church and through their pastors. Once the ASL had established its network of churches, it did not take long for it to replace the WCTU at the head of the prohibitionist movement.

In 1908, the *Reverend Purley A. Baker*, a fearsome Methodist preacher from Columbus, succeeded Howard Russell as the ASL's national superintendent. Baker was the one who hired *Wayne Bidwell Wheeler*, an Oberlin College graduate, who was penniless when he arrived there in 1890. (He died in 1927 at age 57.) He was 65 inches tall and, at the peak of his power, looked more like a clerk in an insurance office than a man who, as described by the *Cincinnati Enquirer*, "made great men his puppets." Wheeler was one of ASL's first full-time employees. One classmate had described him as a "locomotive in trousers." While attending Western Reserve Law School, he worked full-time for the ASL. After earning his law degree in 1898, he took over the Ohio ASL legal office. His productivity accelerated, and his responsibilities steadily increased. By 1901, the Ohio ASL had 31 full-time paid staff members coordinating a legion of zealous pastors. John D. Rockefeller, a lifelong teetotaler as well as America's wealthiest Baptist, financially gave 10% of whatever the league was able to raise from other sources. Wheeler was described by one of his associates as the figure who

> controlled six Congresses, dictated to two presidents, directed legislation for the most important elective state and federal offices, held the balance of power in both Republican and Democratic parties, distributed more patronage than any dozen other men, supervised a federal bureau from the outside without official authority and was recognized by friend and foe alike as the most masterful and powerful single individual in the United States.

By 1909, the ASL had over 800 business offices and at least 500 men and women on regular salary. Additionally, it employed large numbers of speakers on contract, from the governor of Indiana down to the local pastor of the Methodist church.

Political issues and taxes related to prohibition. Just as the urban saloon served as mail drop, hiring hall, and social center for the immigrant masses, so too was it birthplace, incubator, and academy for the potent political machines that captured control of the big cities of the East and Midwest in the last quarter of the 19th century. In New York in 1884, 12 of the 24 members of the board of alderman owned saloons, and four others owed their post to saloon backing. The same was true in Detroit, Chicago, and other big cities.

For prohibition to become the law of the land, it had to connect with certain other groups who were pushing other issues. Tax on alcohol made up a large portion of federal revenues. A tax on alcohol maintained our revolutionary army against the British. This tax lapsed in 1802, was reimposed by James Madison to pay for the War of 1812, was suspended in 1817, and was brought back by Abraham Lincoln in 1862 to finance the Civil War. After that, the tax did not fade away when the war ended. It had spawned an underground tax-free trade in an illegal substance that would forever be known as "moonshine" and a collection apparatus staffed by men from the Bureau of Internal Revenue, known as "revenuers." For most of the 30 years the imposte on alcohol annually provided at least 20% of all federal revenue; in some years, it provided more than 40%. By the time the excise was doubled to cover the cost of the Spanish-American War, the brewers had finally realized that the tax might be their salvation, and they patriotically declared that they had financed 40% of the war's cost. By 1910, the federal government received more than $200 million a year from the bottle and the keg—71% of all internal revenue and more than 30% of all federal revenue. Only the tariff provided a larger share of the federal budget.

Thus, for prohibition to become law, the USA needed to create a tax on income. No one was better equipped to yoke these two causes together than *William Jennings Bryan*, the dominant leader of the Democratic Party from 1896 until 1912. Bryan was devoutly religious and avoided alcohol his entire life. To the devoted admirers that backed him in his three failed presidential campaigns, he was the peerless leader and later "the great commoner." Between 1913 and 1919, amendments establishing income tax, direct election of senators, prohibition, and women's suffrage were engraved in the nation's Constitution, and Bryan was in the forefront in the campaign for each. Imposition of an income tax was an absolutely necessary step for the prohibitionists if they were going to break the federal addiction to the alcohol excise tax. By the time Congress voted to approve a constitutional amendment authorizing income tax (1913), the Anti-Liquor Caucus and the Pro-Tax Caucus were fully together.

The movement toward a constitutional amendment. Until 1913, the ASL had focused on state-by-state prohibition laws, but in that year, Congress overrode a veto by William Howard Taft of the Webb Kenyon Act, a measure outlawing the importation of alcoholic beverages into a dry state. The passage moved the ASL's new goal to national prohibition and the adoption of a constitutional amendment. Each month thereafter, more than 40 tons of prohibitionist propaganda was published each month by ASL. The policy statement announcing ASL's commitment to the amendment strategy was entitled "The Next and Final Step." By delivering his voters to one candidate or another in a close race, Wayne Wheeler controlled elections. "We'll vote against all the men in office who won't support our bills. We will vote for candidates who will promise to." A constitutional amendment required legislative majorities in 36 states as well as the two-thirds majorities in both houses of Congress. Acquiring these numbers required all the talents of Wayne Wheeler, and he had them. The adoption of the tax amendment and subsequent passage of the Revenue Act of 1913 confirmed the virtual collaboration with other interest groups, but the ASL's partnership with women who backed a suffrage amendment proved the most important collaboration. The suffrage movement brought the prohibition movement to the brink of success. A congressional resolution calling for a prohibition amendment to the Constitution had been introduced in every Congress since 1876, but none had ever emerged from committee. In 1914, both the prohibition amendment and the universal suffrage amendment were reported out of committee on the same day. They had become welded to each other. Jack London, who both drank to excess and maybe wrote to excess, believed that "the moment women get the vote in any community, the first thing they proceed to do is close the saloons" and, therefore, "when no one else drinks, and when no drink is obtainable," he would finally be able to stop drinking. London wanted the suffrages to vote him into sobriety. In 1916, the ASL formally endorsed woman's suffrage—the only time in its history it violated its single-issue pledge.

A key member of the prohibition movement was *Richmond Hobson*, who had won renown as a Spanish-American war hero for his bravery while commanding a failed mission aboard the USS *Merrimack* in Cuba. After that he began a lecture tour, and it was apparent that his auscultatory skill matched his military powers. He was an irresistible orator. He entered the House of Representatives in 1906 and not only did he oppose alcohol, he opposed the tariff, sought to break up the industrial trusts, introduced the resolution calling for the abolition of the electoral college, and supported both the income tax and women's suffrage. His defining issue, however, the one that made him one of the most popular platform speakers of the day, was the elimination of the trade in alcoholic beverages. Hobson became the floor manager of the constitutional amendment for prohibition. He argued that his amendment forbade only the use, manufacture, and transportation of alcohol "for sale." It was not coercive; it would not prevent men and women from making and drinking their own. He stressed that he was not asking members to vote for or against alcohol, only to allow the state legislatures the opportunity to pass judgment on the amendment. Therefore, he insisted, any congressman who voted against the resolution would be wrong "to deny the states their right, a referendum." The final vote on the Hobson Amendment was 197 for, 190 against—not the two-thirds majority the Constitution required, but an astonishing result nevertheless. That was December 22, 1914.

The 1915 ASL Convention took place shortly after the symbolic triumph of the Hobson Amendment warmed old campaigners and drew new ones. John L. Sullivan, the heavyweight champion, spoke on behalf of the cause. Dr. J. H. Kellogg, the famous physician from Battle Creek who had placed cornflakes on the American breakfast table, came to speak. Booker T. Washington was another speaker. One speaker quoted British Prime Minister David Lloyd George, whose country had been at war for a year: "We are fighting the Germans, the Austrians, and drink. And the deadliest of these is drink." Although Lloyd George never tried to institute actual prohibition in Britain, he did increase the excise taxes 7-fold on alcohol, and the imposition of the peculiar schedule of pub closing hours was not revoked until 2005. Other countries, including France, Sweden, Germany, Iceland, Spain, Norway, Finland, Russia, and Canada (save for Catholic Quebec), all instituted some kind of prohibition laws during World War I.

Just 5 days before the Hobson Amendment's failure, Congress had enacted a much more modest measure called the Harrison Narcotics Tax Act. The law empowered the Internal Revenue Service to tax, and thus to regulate, opiates, coca derivatives, and other drugs. The Harrison Act conferred on the federal government powers on matters of personal behavior. This act was the logical precedent for federal regulation of the liquor traffic.

By 1916, the ASL's printing machine was pouring out more than 10 tons of printed paper daily. In addition, the league had a massive speakers operation, with more than 20,000 trained lecturers ready to deliver the ASL gospel and to reap the ASL tithe. The league's honorarium men—the highly paid speakers who drew the largest audiences and could raise the largest sums—were generally the driest of the congressional drys. But the biggest draws were two men no longer in public office, William Cullen Bryan and Richmond Hobson. In a single week in 1915, delivering an average of 10 speeches a day, Bryan addressed more than 250,000 Ohioans. In Ann Arbor, 5000 students turned out to hear him; in Philadelphia, he had 20,000 listeners and begged the assembled on his knees to pledge total

abstinence. The "Great Destroyer," Richmond Hobson, gave 83 speeches for the ASL in a single summer. By November 1916, election day, the ASL's leadership, its publicists, and its 50,000 lecturers, fundraisers, and vote counters on the front lines had completed their work. The ASL had made it safe for candidates to be dry. The dry laws were now on the books in 23 of the 48 US states.

After the 1916 election, prohibitionism attracted still more allies, including Asa Candler, founder of the Coca-Cola Company (a very close friend of my father's father), and Lee Schubert, the owner of several of Broadway's theaters and bars. The only wets left were the "Stand Pat" Republicans in Congress who generally opposed the income tax, the vote for women, child labor legislation, and anything else that transferred an ounce of power to the federal government. With few respectable allies, the brewers, distillers, wholesalers, and dealers for a time attempted to recast their own image but failed.

Back in 1912, when the formal push for the prohibition amendment was launched, before the ratification of the 16th (income tax) and 17th (direct election of senators) amendments, ASL's leaders were setting themselves a historically daunting task. Except for the three amendments enacted during the aftershocks of the Civil War, the Constitution had been amended only twice in the preceding 118 years. It was one of those Civil War amendments that opposed the last roadblock to congressional approval of constitutional prohibition.

The South may have been the part of the country with the most intense antiliquor sentiment and the widest range of state liquor laws. In Alabama, for example, liquor advertisements of any kind were forbidden, even in out-of-state newspapers that circulated within the state. But despite the white South's general sympathy for the dry cause, its distinctive politics—particularly its wide attachment to the concept of state rights—compelled the ASL to devise a distinctive lobbying approach. It also required a distinctive lobbyist to carry it out, and that was *Reverend James Cannon*, "the dry messiah." He was a Methodist minister in Virginia, and by his early 40s he had become one of the most dominant individuals in the public life of the state. He was the principal of Blackstone Female Institute, a 2-year college in the south central part of the state. He engineered in 1914 the Temperance Forces in the Commonwealth to a successful statewide dry vote. After that, the ASL came calling. In contrast to the "dry-drys," the "wet-drys" were especially abundant in southern Democratic politics. As Wayne Wheeler had said, "Wet-drys are men who vote as they pray rather than as they drink." The worry for the ASL was that southern Democrats had a higher loyalty to state rights than they did to prohibition, and the pending prohibition amendment would logically require them to accept the validity of an amendment already in the Constitution—the 15th, affirming the voting rights of all men, black and white. In the end, though, when the 18th amendment was brought to a vote in the House of Representatives in December 1917, James Cannon and his colleagues were able to pry from the wet column nine southern and border state House Democrats who had voted against the Hobson Amendment in 1914, and they lost none going the other direction. Although the final vote of 218 to 128 seemed a landslide, in requiring a two-thirds majority, the Constitution demanded a landslide; without the nine who had migrated from "wet" to "dry" the resolution that had passed the Senate with ease would have died in the House. The promising young Sam Rayburn of Texas was among those who made the switch. (Rayburn would remain in Congress another 44 years, for 17 of them as speaker of the house.)

As it traveled its path from the Hobson Amendment of 1914 to another one in 1917, prohibition leapt ahead of universal suffrage in the reform queue. It also underwent substantial legislative tinkering. The debate was not about prohibition, the drys tried to say, it was only about "submission" of the amendment to the states where two-third majorities in both houses of Congress were needed so the states would have a chance to decide for themselves in the ratification process. The Senate Judiciary Committee did not even bother with hearings; neither had its House counterpart. Floor debate in the Senate was largely given over to an argument over timing. The House crammed its discussion of the resolution into a single afternoon. The real debate had been taking place for more than 60 years.

In addition to the congressional wets, a few moderate drys whose votes were still somewhat in question wanted to provide compensation to the distillers and brewers, much of whose property was about to become worthless. In 1917, 13 million gallons of bourbon were aging in Kentucky warehouses alone. Nationwide, the liquor and beer industries represented nearly $1 billion in invested capital, by that measure making the combination the nation's fifth largest industry! The no-compensation argument eventually prevailed. One of the conciliatory drys who had supported the idea of compensation was *William G. Harding*, the junior senator from Ohio. Harding was about as moist as a dry could get, both in his attitude and in his personal life (he favored scotch and soda and owned stock in a brewery). Harding not only believed that the liquor interest deserved compensation, but also felt that there should be a cap on how much time the states were allowed for ratification, a constraint that had never been applied to previous amendments. Harding suggested 5 years but Wheeler stretched it to 7. In exchange, Harding and the other moderates got a new opening clause to the amendment, stipulating that its provisions would not take effect until 1 year after its ratification. This gave a 12-month grace for the brewers and distillers, the wholesalers, the saloon owners, the bartenders, the barrel makers, the bottlers, the teamsters, the ice dealers, and all the other people dependent on the American taste for alcoholic beverages. This grace period was a facsimile of compensation.

One of the major players in making the prohibition amendment possible was *William Ashley Sunday (Billy Sunday)*. He played baseball for the Philadelphia Phillies until 1890 when he put away his glove, bat, and spikes. He had just completed a season in which he had stolen 84 bases and earned $3500, roughly nine times the wages of the average American industrial worker at the time. But he loved Christ and he hated alcohol and he decided to turn away from the sporting life and preach. He became an evangelist and the most successful American preacher of his era, perhaps the most successful one ever. It is said that Billy Sunday preached to more than 100 million people in his 40 years in the pulpit. Sunday's speeches were devoted first to his fundamentalist view of Jesus; his fanatic opposition to the beer and liquor interest came a close second. To Billy Sunday, liquor was "God's worst enemy" and "hell's best friend," and he considered those who profited from the alcohol trade earthly satans. He said, "I will fight them till hell freezes over." The liquor interest hated Billy Sunday. A magazine poll in 1914 attempted to determine who was "the greatest man in the United States." Sunday placed eighth, tied with Andrew Carnegie. He gave as many as 250 speeches a year, addressing the enormous audiences he could command in the late 1910s. Sunday gave shape to the new attitude—increasingly ferocious, even vengeful—that characterized the prohibition forces as they stood at the edge of victory.

Prohibition efforts and World War I. After the 18th amendment was ratified, resentful wets frequently expressed the belief that World War I, which exploded in Europe in 1914 and which the USA entered in 1917, was especially great for the ASL and its allies. Although a myth, the wets attributed the amendment's adoption to the absence of 2 million soldiers from American shores and voting booths. Further, the series of War Revenue Acts that Congress passed at Woodrow Wilson's request, which increased liquor taxes to help finance the war effort, in effect made the purchase of alcohol beverages in the early days of World War I a patriotic act. The populist, antibusiness, Bryan-led wing of the dry coalition, capitalizing on the looming disappearance of liquor tax revenues, used the war crisis to usher in sharply progressive income tax rates. (By the time prohibition took effect, the highest bracket had been jacked up past 70%, more than six times the prewar level.)

The month the USA entered the war (April) the distinguished Yale economist Irving Fisher assembled a group of famous Americans, few of them previously associated with the movement, to endorse the need for national prohibition. The lineup included novelists Upton Sinclair and Booth Tarkington, aviation pioneer Orville Wright, and the chairman of US Steel. Fisher parlayed his renown by issuing an analysis of the damage being done to the war effort by the wanton waste of food resources. The same amount of barley used in American breweries could instead yield 11 million loaves of bread a day. Bryan later said, "How could we justify the making of any part of our bread stuff into intoxicating liquors when they could nourish the army and feed the starving Belgians?"

Between April 1917 and November 1918—the length of US involvement in World War I—a series of "for-the-duration" laws, proclamations, and executive orders first outlawed the sale of alcohol to soldiers and then proscribed the importation of distilled spirits and forbade their manufacture. Dry zones were established around naval bases and around coal mines, shipyards, and munitions plants. In the name of the war effort, food administrator Herbert Hoover ordered the amount of grain available to the brewery industry reduced by 30%. Legal beer was limited to 2.75% alcohol by weight. The war emergency handed proponents of government activism essentially a hunting license to "seize railroads, requisition factories, take over mines, fix prices, put an embargo on all exports, commandeer all ships, standardize all loafs of bread, punish all careless use of fuel, draft men for an army, and send that army to a war in France." Compared to all that, the closing down of distilleries and breweries didn't seem too dire after all. The war also produced an anti-German hysteria in the USA. All the large breweries in the USA had German-American heads: Pabst, Schlitz, Blitz, and Miller. Germanism meant anti-Americanism, and by Wheeler's conflation it also meant "wet."

Ratification of the amendment. As 1917 drew to a close, submission had been accomplished. Ratification seemed a more daunting prospect. By this time, 23 states had dry laws of one form or another, although few were as "bone dry" as the 18th amendment. Looming ahead was the trench warfare of the state-by-state ratification in which the drys would need to win a minimum of 36 separate battles to reach the three-quarters requirement. In the end, ratification proceeded with astonishing speed. The income tax had made a prohibition amendment fiscally feasible. The social revolution wrought by the suffragists had made it politically plausible. The war was the final tool the drys needed to wage the amendment into the Constitution.

On January 8, 1918, the 33 members of the Mississippi State Senate and the 96 members of the State House gathered in Jackson to vote on the 18th amendment to the Constitution. The vote, which proceeded without debate, took exactly 15 minutes, passing 28 to 5 in the upper house and 93 to 3 in the lower one. Mississippi was much more agreeable to this second constitutional amendment ever to place limits on individual behavior than it was to the first one. It didn't get around to ratifying that one—the 13th, abolishing slavery—until 1995!

The universal malapportionment of state legislatures was helpful in the ratification process. In New York, for example, the legislature was configured so that an urban assemblyman might represent seven times as many people as the rural representative. But, the vote of a farmer from upstate Preston Hollow—more likely native born, Republican, and dry—was equivalent to the vote of seven Democratic, Irish American wets from Hell's Kitchen in Manhattan. In New Jersey, where each member of the state senate represented a single county irrespective of its population, the man from Cape May County served just 20,000 constituents while his colleague from Essex County represented 650,000. The farmers and fisherman who controlled Maryland's legislature had conspired to avoid any redistricting since 1867. In the intervening decades, while the population of urban ethnic Baltimore had jumped 175%, the population in the rest of the state had only increased 46%. By 1918, democracy in Maryland had been imprisoned for half a century. That same type of distribution occurred in numerous other states at the time.

The state legislators had the authority to enact constitutional prohibition, and with their rural domination they did so with the speed of an epidemic, immune from referenda or gubernatorial vetoes. More than 80% of the nation's state legislators voted dry. The more rural the state, the more arid the vote. Among the six states whose legislators were unanimous for ratification were Idaho, Kansas, South Dakota, Utah, and Wyoming.

On January 16, 1919, when Nebraska's lower house went 98 to 0 for prohibition, the 18th amendment was embedded in the US Constitution. From that moment of submission, it had taken 394 days to meet the approval of 36 state legislators—less than half as long as it had taken 11 of the first 14 states to approve the Bill of Rights.

Life after prohibition. The opening clause of the 18th amendment—"After one year from the ratification of this article"—meant that life in the USA was no different on January 17, 1919, from what it had been on January 16. Immediately after ratification, H. L. Mencken sold his 1915 Studebaker and told a friend that he "invested the proceeds in alcohol." Harry S Truman, fighting in Europe, wrote to Bess Wallace: "It looks to me like the moonshine business is going to be pretty good in the Land of the Liberty Loans and Green Trading Stamps and some of us want to get in on the ground floor. At least we want to get there in time to lay in a supply for future consumption." He was on target. The experience of states that had already gone dry suggested there was a large and liquid gulf between how people voted and how they drank. William Howard Taft, serving in the interval between his presidency and his chief justiceship of the Supreme Court, said, "The business of manufacturing alcohol, liquor and beer will go out of the hands of law-abiding members of the community and will be transferred to the quasi-criminal class." As Daniel Okrent stated, "The only ill chosen word in that sentence was 'quasi.'"

The man whose legislative skills were called upon to prevent the realization of Taft's prediction was *Andrew John Volstead*, whose name would forever be attached to prohibition. Webster's recent unabridged dictionary defined *Volsteadism* as "the doctrine of or adherence to prohibition." He was the one who sponsored the legislation required to enforce the 18th amendment. He had been in the House 16 years before assuming the chairmanship of the Judiciary Committee and therefore was responsible for the National Prohibition Act, which was the formal name of the legislation that would turn the 18th amendment's declaration into a code of enforcement.

The Volstead Act eventually had 67 separate sections. The final bill covered everything from the definition of "intoxicating" (its single most crucial sentence) to whether dealcoholized beer could still be called beer or "near beer," to whether a foreign ship would be allowed to pass through the Panama Canal. Volstead (and Wheeler) spent several months crafting a measure so tight that not one of its provisions was ever deemed unconstitutional. What was carefully kept out of the criminal code was any specific prescription against drinking or buying alcohol; savage drys knew that without this enormous carveout no user would ever testify against his supplier. The phrase "intoxicating liquors" won out over "alcoholic beverages" in the amendment itself. This conscious dodge had enabled fence sitters, conflict avoiders, and wishful thinkers to support the amendment in the hope that the eventual definition would leave room for some of the milder forms of stimulation.

To pass the Volstead Act, only a majority was needed in each House of Congress, rather than two thirds of each House plus three quarters of the state legislatures. The word "intoxicating" was defined as anything ingestible that contained more than 0.5% alcohol content. This proscribed the lightest of wines and the most diluted forms of beer, but exceptions were placed in the Volstead Act to render it less than absolute. The orthodox Jews and the Catholics came away with continued access to sacramental wines for their congregations. Many hardline drys wanted to deny physicians the right to prescribe alcohol, but this too wasn't worth the fight. No one questioned the need for the continued production of industrial alcohol for its many critical and/or popular uses. In a nod to those who had invested in their personal cellars (including various dry senators and representatives), the act allowed individuals to continue to own and to drink in their own homes any alcohol that was purchased before the 18th amendment's effective date.

The Volstead Act specifically exempted cider and other "fruit juices" that just might happen to acquire an alcoholic tinge through the natural processes of fermentation. They were not subject to the 0.5% ceiling. The law made home manufacture of hard cider perfectly acceptable. No husband-man would be denied the barrel by the homestead door, the jug stashed in a corner of the field, the comforting warmth on cold country nights. Alvin Barker of Kentucky, who later became vice president, noted that if it was legal to transfer the juice of the apple into something stronger, then "why not corn juice?"

The Volstead Act failed to provide a judicial procedure other than trial jury for anyone accused of any violation, dooming the federal court system to an unremitting 14-year flood of petty cases. The army of federal agents hired to enforce the act would not be part of the civil service because Andrew Volstead, among others, feared that civil service protection would guarantee "the offices would be filled with wets that we could not get rid of." The total initial appropriation for federal enforcement of this radical and far-reaching new law amounted to $2.1 million.

By the time the Volstead Act had become law, the drys had become giddy in their political dominance and confident they would retain power sufficient to correct any errors or omissions. The prohibition amendment was the culmination of 50 years of continuous effort by the drys. In contrast, the wets were disorganized, dysfunctional, and disbelieving. But now they had to adjust. In 1921, Andrew J. Volstead told his House colleague, John Garner, that although "we will gradually work out the machinery that will, with the cooperation of the states, make the country dry, we cannot hope that this law can be enforced so as not to be violated. All laws will be violated." The product of 80 years of marching, praying, arm twisting, vote trading, and law drafting would be subjected to a plague of trials, among them hypocrisy, greed, murderous criminality, of-

ficial corruption, and the unreformable impulses of human desire. The drys had their law, and the wets would have their liquor.

The liquor industry was not dead. The new version was illegal, underground, and nearly ubiquitous. But many Americans began to drink less. A significant proportion of the population either felt duty bound to take the constitutional strictures seriously or found the procedural roadblocks elected by the Volstead Act too daunting. Alcohol-related deaths fell in 1920, as did arrests for public drunkenness. Welch's Grape Juice began to set new sales records. Diminished criminal behavior occurred in several cities. Many neighborhoods registered a general lack of street disorders and of family quarrels. Songwriter Albert von Tilzer, who had taken America out to the ballgame in 1908, had a new song, "I Never Knew I Had a Wonderful Wife Until the Town Went Dry." But in the decade after the arrival of the 18th amendment, alcohol consumption in the USA dropped only 30%!

So why did prohibition fail? It encouraged criminality and institutionalized hypocrisy. It deprived the government of money. It imposed profound limitations on individual rights. It fostered a culture of bribery, blackmail, and official corruption. It also maimed and murdered. But in one critical respect, prohibition was an unquestioned success. As a direct result of its 14-year reign, Americans drank less, and they continued to drink less for decades afterward. Back in the first years of the 20th century, before most state laws limiting access to alcohol were enacted, average consumption of pure alcohol ran to 2.6 gallons per adult per year—the rough equivalent of 32 fifths of 80-proof liquor or 520 bottles of 12-ounce beer. Judging by the most carefully assembled evidence, that quantity was slashed by more than 70% during the first few years of national prohibition. It started to climb as American thirst adjusted to the new regime. But even repeal did not open the spigots: the preprohibition per capita peak of 2.6 gallons was not again obtained until 1973. (It stayed that high only until the mid-1980s, when it began to drop again to current levels of roughly 2.2 gallons per person per year.)

Repeal of prohibition. In the surprisingly slow growth of postprohibition drinking lay the central irony of repeal: the 21st amendment made it harder, not easier, to get a drink! During the latter stages of prohibition, especially in the big cities or near the coasts or adjacent to the Canadian border, little effort was required to obtain a drink, a bottle, or in some places even a shipment of contraband. What was formerly illegal was necessarily unregulated. Repeal changed that, replacing the almost-anything-goes ethos with a series of state-by-state codes, regulations, and enforcement procedures. Now there were closing hours, age limits, and Sunday Blue Laws and a collection of geographic proscriptions that kept bars or stores distant from schools, churches, or hospitals. State licensing requirements forced legal sellers to live by the code, and in many instances statutes created penalties for buyers as well. Just as prohibition did not prohibit making drink legal, its repeal did not make drink entirely available.

The 21st amendment to the US Constitution, enacted in 1933, reads as follows:

The eighteenth article of amendment to the Constitution of the United States is hereby repealed. The transportation or importation into any State, Territory, or possession of the United States for delivery or use therein of intoxicating liquors, in violation of the laws thereof, is hereby prohibited. The article shall be inoperative unless it shall have been ratified as an amendment to the Constitution by conventions in the several States, as provided in the Constitution, within seven years from the date of the submission hereof to the States by the Congress.

FREE COLLEGE

Al Neuharth, the founder of *USA Today*, supports making tuition free in public colleges and universities (38). These are his reasons. Families spend an average of $64 billion in tuition a year to send 13.9 million students to public colleges and universities. For the last 10 years, $1.1 trillion has been spent on the wars in Iraq and Afghanistan, an average of more than $110 billion annually. Sixty-four billion dollars annually for higher education and $110 billion annually for wars! The two wars have also cost approximately 5700 military lives, and many of those killed in the wars were college-aged men and women. The war costs are paid for through present taxes but mostly debts piled up for future generations. The college costs are paid for by parents and/or long-time debts for graduating students. As Neuharth questions: "Can you think of any reason why anybody should not want to substitute higher education for our young men and women to ensure their future rather than military service and the futile nation-building efforts abroad?"

William C Roberts

—WILLIAM CLIFFORD ROBERTS, MD
17 November 2010

1. Green LA. Cholesterol-lowering therapy for primary prevention: still much we don't know. *Arch Intern Med* 2010;170(12):1007–1008.
2. Ray KK, Seshasai SR, Erqou S, Sever P, Jukema JW, Ford I, Sattar N. Statins and all-cause mortality in high-risk primary prevention: a meta-analysis of 11 randomized controlled trials involving 65,229 participants. *Arch Intern Med* 2010;170(12):1024–1031.
3. de Lorgeril M, Salen P, Abramson J, Dodin S, Hamazaki T, Kostucki W, Okuyama H, Pavy B, Rabaeus M. Cholesterol lowering, cardiovascular diseases, and the rosuvastatin-JUPITER controversy: a critical reappraisal. *Arch Intern Med* 2010;170(12):1032–1036.
4. Roberts WC. Atherosclerotic risk factors—are there ten or is there only one? *Am J Cardiol* 1989;64(8):552–554.
5. Roberts WC. Atherosclerosis: its cause and its prevention. *Am J Cardiol* 2006;98(11):1550–1555.
6. Steinberg D. *The Cholesterol Wars: The Skeptics vs. the Preponderance of Evidence.* Amsterdam, the Netherlands: Elsevier, 2007 (227 pp.).
7. Truswell AS. *Cholesterol and Beyond: The Research on Diet and Coronary Heart Disease, 1900–2000.* Sydney, Australia: Springer, 2010 (227 pp.).
8. Keys A. *Seven Countries: A Multivariate Analysis of Death and Coronary Heart Disease.* Cambridge, MA: Harvard University Press, 1980 (381 pp.).
9. Verschuren WM, Jacobs DR, Bloemberg BP, Kromhout D, Menotti A, Aravanis C, Blackburn H, Buzina R, Dontas AS, Fidanza F, Karvonen MJ, Nedelijkovi S, Nissinen A, Toshima H. Serum total cholesterol and long-term coronary heart disease mortality in different cultures. Twenty-five-year follow-up of the Seven Countries study. *JAMA* 1995;274(2):131–136.
10. Kromhout D, Menotti A, Blackburn H, eds. *The Seven Countries Study: A Scientific Adventure in Cardiovascular Disease Epidemiology.* Bilthoven, the Netherlands: Marjan Nijssen-Kramer, 1993 (219 pp.).
11. Anitschkow NN. A history of experimentation on arterial atherosclerosis in animals. In Blumenthal HT, ed. *Cowdry's Arteriosclerosis: A Survey of the Problem*, 2nd ed. Springfield, IL: Charles C. Thomas, 1967:21–44.
12. Kannel WB, Dawber TR, Kagan A, Revotskie N, Stokes J 3rd. Factors of risk in the development of coronary heart disease—six year follow-up experience. The Framingham Study. *Ann Intern Med* 1961;55:33–50.
13. Kannel WB, Castelli WP, Gordon T. Cholesterol in the prediction of atherosclerotic disease. New perspectives based on the Framingham study. *Ann Intern Med* 1979;90(1):85–91.
14. Mautner SL, Sanchez JA, Rader DJ, Mautner GC, Ferrans VJ, Fredrickson DS, Brewer HB Jr, Roberts WC. The heart in Tangier disease. Severe coronary atherosclerosis with near absence of high-density lipoprotein cholesterol. *Am J Clin Pathol* 1992;98(2):191–198.
15. Libby P, Ridker PM, Maseri A. Inflammation and atherosclerosis. *Circulation* 2002;105(9):1135–1143.
16. Roberts WC. Qualitative and quantitative comparison of amounts of narrowing by atherosclerotic plaques in the major epicardial coronary arteries at necropsy in sudden coronary death, transmural acute myocardial infarction, transmural healed myocardial infarction and unstable angina pectoris. *Am J Cardiol* 1989;64(5):324–328.
17. Roberts WC, Turnage TA 2nd, Whiddon LL. Quantitative comparison of amounts of cross-sectional area narrowing in coronary endarterectomy specimens in patients having coronary artery bypass grafting to amounts of narrowing in the same artery in patients with fatal coronary artery disease studied at necropsy. *Am J Cardiol* 2007;99(5):588–592.
18. Sprecher DL, Schaefer EJ, Kent KM, Gregg RE, Zech LA, Hoeg JM, McManus B, Roberts WC, Brewer HB Jr. Cardiovascular features of homozygous familial hypercholesterolemia: analysis of 16 patients. *Am J Cardiol* 1984;54(1):20–30.
19. Grundy SM, Cleeman JI, Merz CN, Brewer HB Jr, Clark LT, Hunninghake DB, Pasternak RC, Smith SC Jr, Stone NJ; National Heart, Lung, and Blood Institute; American College of Cardiology Foundation; American Heart Association. Implications of recent clinical trials for the National Cholesterol Education Program Adult Treatment Panel III guidelines. *Circulation* 2004;110(2):227–239.
20. Roberts WC. The underused miracle drugs: the statin drugs are to atherosclerosis what penicillin was to infectious disease. *Am J Cardiol* 1996;78(3):377–378.
21. Roberts WC. Shifting from decreasing risk to actually preventing and arresting atherosclerosis. *Am J Cardiol* 1999;83(5):816–817.
22. Cohen JD, Cziraky MJ, Cai Q, Wallace A, Wasser T, Crouse JR, Jacobson TA. 30-year trends in serum lipids among United States adults: results from the National Health and Nutrition Examination Surveys II, III, and 1999–2006. *Am J Cardiol* 2010;106(7):969–975.
23. Yeh RW, Sidney S, Chandra M, Sorel M, Selby JV, Go AS. Population trends in the incidence and outcomes of acute myocardial infarction. *N Engl J Med* 2010;362(23):2155–2165.
24. Stone G. *The Secrets of People Who Never Get Sick.* New York: Workman Publishing, 2010 (212 pp.).
25. Stoller G. Traveling abroad's top risk: roads. *USA Today*, October 21, 2010.

26. Stoller G. U.N. program urges global road safety. U.S. traveler dies on foreign road every 36 hours on average. *USA Today*, October 21, 2010.

27. Jeffrey TP. It's official: Obama has now borrowed $3 trillion. CSN News. Available at http://www.cnsnews.com/news/article/it-s-official-obama-has-now-borrowed-3-t; accessed October 18, 2010.

28. Siegel M. Why ObamaCare will clog the system. *USA Today*, October 19, 2010.

29. Appiah KA. Accepted now, unforgivable later. *Dallas Morning News*, October 17, 2010.

30. Milken M. Toward a new American century. *Wall Street Journal*, October 7, 2010.

31. 27 floors just right for family of five. *Dallas Morning News*, October 30, 2010.

32. Henrietta Lacks. In Wikipedia. Available at http://en.wikipedia.org/wiki/Henrietta_Lacks; accessed November 17, 2010.

33. Singer N. Botox ok'd as migraine treatment. *Dallas Morning News*, October 17, 2010.

34. Ritter K, Rising M. In vitro pioneer wins Nobel in medicine. *Dallas Morning News*, October 5, 2010.

35. Dougherty C. New vow: I don't take thee. *Wall Street Journal*, September 29, 2010.

36. Associated Press. Grandparents raising kids: rising numbers, rising stress. *Dallas Morning News*, September 11, 2010.

37. Okrent D. *Last Call: The Rise and Fall of Prohibition*. New York: Scribner, 2010 (468 pp).

38. Neuharth A. Should free college be a part of education? *USA Today*, November 12, 2010.

Chapter 2

April 2011

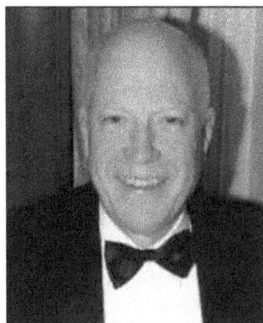

William C. Roberts, MD

THE X-RAY MACHINE AND THE ELECTROCARDIOGRAM IN HOSPITALS

Although today we accept machines as a desirable part of medical practice, that was not always the case (1). Medical technology has been widely used only since the 20th century. The machines that had the greatest impact were the x-ray and the electrocardiogram. Roentgen's description of x-rays in 1895 shocked the Western world. The ability to see within the human body had a profound impact on both lay and professional communities, and the x-ray machine quickly came to symbolize the most advanced, scientific approach to medicine. According to a splendid article by Howell (1), the Pennsylvania Hospital in 1897, like many other hospitals, purchased its first x-ray machine. Although trauma accounted for 4 of the 5 common surgical diagnoses at the Pennsylvania Hospital at the turn of the century, there is no mention of x-ray use in 1897. In 1902, the x-ray machine was still rarely used.

The person responsible for taking the x-ray films changed during the first 15 years. From 1897 to 1909, the chief resident operated the x-ray machine, one of his many duties, which also included running the operating room, sterilizing room, and photography room as well as being responsible for the maintenance and care of "all apparatus and instruments." X-ray equipment eventually assumed more time, and in both 1910 and 1911 the former chief resident stayed on for a year to run the x-ray machine.

The year 1912 marked a turning point in the operation of the x-ray machine. In that year, responsibility for running the machine shifted from a yearly succession of chief residents to a single physician who devoted his career to roentgenology. The first head of radiology at the Pennsylvania Hospital was David Bowen. After graduating in 1894 from Jefferson Medical College, he was a country general practitioner until 1906 when he came across some discarded x-ray equipment that he was able to repair. The following year he studied roentgenology for 2 weeks in Cincinnati and attended the annual meeting of the new American Roentgen Ray Society. He received further training from 1911 through 1920 in the radiology department of Jefferson Hospital Philadelphia, published several articles, and became an editor for *The American Journal of Roentgenology and Radium Therapy*. From 1907 on, Bowen attempted to limit his practice to taking and interpreting roentgenograms.

The terms of Bowen's employment differed significantly from those of his predecessors. As compensation for devoting 50% of his time to the x-ray department, Bowen received a salary of $1500 per year. In addition, his income included 75% of all fees generated by taking x-ray films of paying patients. The hospital retained 25%. By 1917, roentgenograms had become routine for patients with kidney stones and limb fractures. Those with suspected broken legs often had examinations performed on admission, not 2½ weeks later, as in 1902. Physicians made diagnoses of tuberculosis, renal stones, and fractures solely on the basis of radiologic evidence.

World War I encouraged the use of x-ray machines in two ways. First, many nurses and physicians from the Philadelphia Hospital staffed base hospital tents in France. While caring for the many casualties, they witnessed the value of x-ray films for diagnosing fractures and foreign bodies. Second, World War I stimulated advances in x-ray technique. X-ray pictures were originally taken on glass plates imported from Belgium. After 1914, these plates became difficult to obtain, and manufacturers switched to film to record x-ray pictures. After World War I, the Pennsylvania Hospital's x-ray department expanded rapidly. In 1920, Bowen went from part-time to full-time radiographer, a year in which 4005 patients were examined by x-ray film. A portable unit also was purchased.

Unlike the sudden discovery of x-rays, the development of the electrocardiograph followed many earlier attempts to record the electrical action of the heart. After Einthoven described the electrocardiogram in 1902, hospitals did not rush to buy one as rapidly as they had purchased x-ray machines in 1897. When the Pennsylvania Hospital finally purchased an electrocardiograph in 1921, the board of managers quickly approved the same 75%-25% split of fees for the "electrocardiographer" as they had earlier for the radiographer. Electrocardiograph reports appeared on patient charts within the year, usually on patients with irregular heartbeats. A separate room was set aside to house the electrocardiograph. By 1927, although not used as widely as the x-ray machine, the electrocardiograph was on its way to becoming a routine part of patient care. A part-time technician was employed by the electrocardiograph laboratory. A special heart clinic attracted large numbers of patients, and a fellowship in cardiac diseases was established.

By 1927, there was an even more significant transformation than the increased number of patients receiving an x-ray or electrocardiographic examination. For the first time, patient records indicate that individuals entered the hospital specifically to use the complex diagnostic machinery. By 1927, however, a combination of new tubes, improved power supplies, and a moving grid had greatly improved the quality of x-ray pictures and made the x-ray a more useful clinical tool. In contrast, the electrocardiogram was of very little clinical value in the 1920s.

In 1897, patient charts contained no pictures, no separate forms, few numbers, and no graphs save the temperature chart. The intern wrote the entire document by hand. By 1912, urinalysis results appeared on a small printed slip of paper laid into the chart. The form defines specific examinations made on each urine specimen. Also in 1912, interns started to illustrate their physical examinations by drawing pictures of the patient's body. By 1917, laboratory results, including urinalysis, results of blood examinations, and pathological findings, were summarized on a single full-size pink sheet rather than being scattered on the earlier patchwork of pieces of paper pasted into the record. Also, no longer handwritten by the intern, a formal official x-ray film reading was reported on a separate standard form signed by the radiologist.

In 1917, the American College of Surgeons began a national drive for standardization of hospital records. Electrocardiographic reports written in precise, numerical terms appeared on patients' charts by 1922, along with handwritten diet charts recording diabetic patients' intake of fat, protein, and carbohydrates in grams. The radiology department introduced forms for reporting results of gastrointestinal x-ray examinations on which the interpreting radiologist needed only to circle the appropriate description for each anatomic portion, thus limiting the descriptions of each to a few phrases.

Technology has become a ubiquitous feature of 20th-century medicine. Technology, of course, has transformed the American hospital, but before medical technology could be incorporated into hospital medicine, the hospital itself had to be transformed into an institution more hospitable to the place of machines in medicine.

HEALTH CARE INVESTMENT, LONGEVITY, AND THE ECONOMY

Michael Milken, who made millions on Wall Street and now chairs FasterCures, a Washington-based center of the Milken Institute, has written several pieces on means to improve our health and our lives. He indicates in a February 9 piece in the *Wall Street Journal* that since 1820, world per-capita income has risen >8-fold, thanks in part to the spread of democracy, open trading markets, and the rule of law (2). He indicates that improvements to health, which have given us longer and more productive lives, have produced as much as half the increase

in the global economy over the past 2 centuries. It would be logical to assume, he suggests, that companies whose products make us healthier would be among the most valued enterprises on the planet, but this assumption is wrong. The stock market presently values companies that make cosmetics, beer, soft drinks, and detergents far above pharmaceutical companies! Contributing to the lower evaluations, of course, are patent expirations, regulatory complexity, litigation exposure, and high US taxes on repatriated foreign income. These factors undoubtedly influenced the decision by Procter & Gamble to leave the pharmaceutical business in 2009 and concentrate on consumer products. Procter & Gamble simply responded to market signals that discouraged development of life-saving drugs. Milken suggests ways to remove some of the barriers to growth in medical research:

1. *Match the inducements of other countries.* Many nations offer generous tax incentives, easier recruitment of clinical-trial subjects, strong government partnerships, and far less litigation.

2. *Recognize the return on investment in federal health research.* Although we clearly need spending restraint in Washington, DC, the economic gains that come from longer, healthier life spans and the savings from improved therapies more than make up for the investment. One study in 2006 showed that life-expectancy gains since 1970 added $3.2 trillion per year to America's national wealth. A mere 1% reduction in cancer deaths would be worth $500 billion, and the present value to future generations of a full cure of cancer is nearly $50 trillion, more than three times today's gross domestic product. Congress doubled the budget of the National Institutes of Health (NIH) between 1998 and 2003. It was money well spent: 39 new cancer drugs have been approved since 2004. Progress is accelerating on a range of diseases as traction is gained by using rapidly evolving technology and by investigators collaborating across disciplines. But, the prospects for continuing this discovery bonanza have been threatened. NIH funding has trended down in real terms since 2003, and current budget realities portend severe future cuts that will cause some younger medical scientists to either change careers or take their work to places like Singapore that put out the welcome mat for promising researchers.

3. *Support prevention.* The single best way, of course, to contain rising health care costs is to keep people from getting sick in the first place. That starts with recognizing that lifestyles, not genes, are the biggest contributors to disease! Programs aimed at even slight reductions in obesity, tobacco use, and other damaging behaviors pay large social and economic dividends.

4. *Give the Food and Drug Administration (FDA) adequate resources.* Imports of products subject to FDA inspection have increased from 6 to 20 million shipments in the last 10 years. An estimated 25% of the US economy is affected by FDA oversight. And the new food safety legislation that Congress passed in December 2010 further expands the agency's responsibilities. The FDA, as a result, soon will not

be able to keep up with the pace of innovation in areas such as medical device development and regenerative medicine. The result will be a further slowing of the movement of effective drugs and devices from laboratories to patients.

Although the USA ranked first in previous studies, a 2009 study by the Information Technology and Innovation Foundation indicated that the USA now ranks sixth out of 40 nations. We are slipping and making the slowest progress toward what the report characterizes as a knowledge-driven, high-innovation economy.

Milken concludes that improved public health translates directly into greater national productivity, which underpins all economic growth.

WALKING SPEED AND LONGEVITY

Studenski and 18 colleagues from several medical centers described an analysis of 9 studies involving nearly 34,500 people aged 65 or older, and faster walking speeds were associated with longer lives (3, 4). Predicted years of remaining life for each age and both sexes increased as gait speed increased. The most significant gains were after age 75. For example:

- The probability that an 80-year-old will live to age 90 is only 10% for men and 23% for women with a walking speed of 1 mph but increases to 84% and 86%, respectively, among those with a walking speed of 3.5 mph.
- The median life expectancy for an 80-year-old is only 4 years for men and 7 for women with a walking speed of 1 mph but increases to 14 and 17 years, respectively, among those with a walking speed of 3.5 mph.

The investigators found that predicting survival in these older people based on gait speed was as accurate as predictions based on age, sex, chronic conditions, smoking history, blood pressure, body mass index, and hospitalization frequency! The investigators indicated that walking is a reliable tool to measure well-being because it requires body support, timing, and power, and it places demands on the brain, spinal cord, muscles, joints, heart, and lungs. Slowing down is associated with aging. By age 80, gait speed usually is 10% to 20% slower than in younger adults.

In the study, gait speed was calculated using meters in seconds. All subjects were told to walk at their usual pace from a standing start. Average speed was 3 feet a second (about 2 miles an hour). During the 14-year course of the study, there were 17,528 deaths. Those who walked slower than 2 feet a second (about 1.36 miles an hour) had an increased risk of dying. Those who walked 3.3 feet a second (about 2.25 miles per hour) or faster survived longer than would be expected by age or sex alone.

Walk, walk, walk!

CHOLESTEROL IN EGGS

According to the US Department of Agriculture, a large egg today has about 185 mg of cholesterol, down from 215 mg in 2002 (5). Researchers collected large eggs from 12 locations around the country and sent them to a laboratory for testing. The drop in cholesterol may be because of changes in hens' diets, the way the animals are bred, or other factors. The government's latest dietary guidelines indicate that eating one egg a day is okay. A large egg, according to the US Department of Agriculture's Agricultural Research Service, contains the following: 70 calories; 185 mg of cholesterol; 6 g of protein; 4.7 g of fat, including 1.6 g of saturated fat; 41 international units of vitamin D; and 71 mg of sodium. That amount of vitamin D is only about 7% of the 600 international units recommended. Certainly an egg is more healthful than bacon or sausage.

RED LIGHT CAMERAS

Researchers for the Insurance Institute for Highway Safety looked at 14 US cities that used red light cameras from 2004 to 2008 but not from 1992 to 1996 (6). They found that cities with red light cameras had fewer fatal accidents caused by red light runners than cities without them. In 2000, 25 US cities employed red light cameras. Today, 500 do. Garland, Texas, saw a 25% decrease in the number of fatal accidents involving red light runners at intersections with cameras. Now 41 cities in Texas use cameras, including Dallas, Fort Worth, Richardson, Irving, and Plano. In Dallas, 60 cameras are situated at 49 intersections. According to July 2010 data provided by the city, accidents caused by red light running decreased 61% in the 3 years after the cameras were installed. Keep the red light cameras on.

DOGS DISTRACTING DRIVERS

Man's best friend may not be a driver's best friend. While lawmakers have been banning drivers from texting or using cell phones, many motorists are riding around with another dangerous risk: their dogs (7). An unrestrained dog—whether curled up on a lap, hanging out the window, or resting its paws on the steering wheel—can be deadly. Although no solid numbers are available, thousands of car accidents are believed to be caused every year by unrestrained pets. The issue is drawing attention in some state legislatures. Hawaii is the only state that specifically forbids drivers from operating a vehicle with a pet on their lap. Oregon lawmakers are considering fining drivers who hold their pets.

According to the National Highway Traffic Safety Administration, in 2009, 5474 people were killed and 448,000 injured in crashes caused by distracted drivers in the USA. Cell phones, of course, were the top distraction—the cause of 18% of the fatalities and 5% of the injury crashes. Although the agency does not track accidents caused by pets, the latter are counted among "other distractions" such as disruptive passengers, misbehaving children, or drivers who try to put on makeup or read.

In a crash, an unrestrained pet can turn into a deadly projectile. A harness or carrier to secure the pets in the middle of the back seat is recommended. That keeps dogs from getting hurt or hurting others. This all makes me feel guilty because when I drove from Washington, DC, to Dallas, Texas, in 1993, about 1300 miles, my wonderful Pembroke Welsh Corgi sat in the passenger seat next to me. Additionally bad, I had my right paw on his body for a good number of those miles. I know better now.

HOT-CAR DEATHS IN CHILDREN

Meteorologist Jan Null has been keeping track of children who died of heat stroke while trapped in a hot car, truck, van, or SUV (8). Null indicates that at least 494 children have died since 1998 from heat stroke (hyperthermia) in vehicles in the USA, averaging 38 children per year. The year 2010 was the deadliest year since records began in 1998: 49 children died in hot vehicles. Cars transform essentially into ovens when direct sunlight heats objects inside. Temperatures can soar to 120° or 130° even when the outdoor temperature is only in the 80s. People can lose consciousness. The body's natural cooling methods, like sweating, can shut down once the core body temperature reaches 104°. Death usually occurs at 107°. Children are particularly vulnerable because they have difficulty escaping from a hot vehicle on their own and their respiratory and circulatory systems cannot handle heat as well as adults. The obvious lesson is that children should never be left alone in vehicles for any period of time.

PEDESTRIAN TEXTING

About 95% of American adults have cell phones (9). Nearly one third of those are smart phones. We all know that texting while driving is dangerous, but according to David Bauder, who watched pedestrians in New York City for 2 months, about 1 in 10 pedestrians text while walking. It is not a good idea.

AIRLINE SAFETY

US commercial airlines did not have a single fatality in 2010 (10). Indeed, it was the third time in the past 4 years that there were no deaths. Last year also marked the first time that there were no passenger fatalities on any airline based in developed nations. In 2010, US carriers flew >10 million flights and carried >700 million passengers. Only 14 people suffered serious injuries, and there were no major accidents. The last fatal accident occurred on February 12, 2009, when a crash in a Buffalo, NY, neighborhood killed 49 people on board and one on the ground.

PROFESSIONAL FOOTBALL AND INJURIES

There are presently 32 teams in the National Football League (NFL) in the USA. Each team has 16 regular season games, and each team has 22 starters, 11 on offense and 11 on defense, or 352 starters in the 16 regular-season games. For these 352 starters, the average number of games lost was 42.3; the average number of starters per team who finished the season on injured reserve was 3.0 (11).

The Green Bay Packers, who won the Super Bowl on February 6, 2011, had a league high of 91 games lost by starters because of injuries this season! Green Bay's 2010 season began with half their defensive backfield in sick bay with holdover injures from 2009. In all, 13 Green Bay starters missed time with injuries this season, including quarterback Aaron Rodgers and Pro Bowl pass rusher Clay Matthews. Only 3 NFL teams since 2000 lost more games by starters because of injuries than

the 2010 Packers. None of those 3 teams won >6 games, but the 2010 Packers won 10 of 16 regular season games to claim a wild-card playoff spot. The Packers finished ninth in the NFL in offense in 2010 despite losing 44 games by offensive starters. They finished fifth in defense despite losing 47 games by starters on that side of the ball.

The Atlanta Falcons were the healthiest team in the NFL this season, losing only 9 games by starters because of injuries. The Falcons parlayed their good health into the best record in the NFL (13-3) and a top playoff seed. In total, 1354 games were lost by starters because of injury, down 148 from a year earlier.

The Tampa Bay Buccaneers led the NFL with 8 starters on injured reserve. In all, 95 starters were placed on injured reserve in 2010, down 5 from 2009. The Cowboys had 13 players start all 16 games, tops in the NFL. The Philadelphia Eagles had only one player start all 16 games, the league low. There were 278 players who were 16-game starters, up 30 from 2009.

I prefer baseball, tennis, and golf.

TUCSON, GABRIELLE GIFFORDS, AND GUNS

In 2008, the Supreme Court ruled that local governments could not impose strict gun-control provisions (12). In Arizona, Jared Lee Loughner could simply walk into a gun store, buy his Glock, and carry it concealed without a permit. He could carry it into a bar or a church. He carried it into a political rally and used it. In 15 seconds he fired 31 bullets, killing 6 and injuring 13. One of the victims, of course, was Congresswoman Gabrielle Giffords.

Michael Grunwald appears to be a numbers man, and here are some of his figures (13). In the USA in 1 year, 31,224 people die from gun violence; 12,632 people are murdered; 17,352 people kill themselves; 3067 children and teens die from gun violence; and 351 are killed by police intervention. All together, >100,000 people in the USA are shot annually in murders, assaults, suicides, accidents, or by police intervention. A total of 66,768 survive gun injuries. To put it another way, in one day 8 children and teens die from gun violence and 268 people in the USA are shot in murders, assaults, suicides, accidents, or by police interventions, of whom 86 people die, including 35 who are murdered. These numbers are by far the worst in the world.

Arizona has been on the forefront of the gun-rights movement. Last year it passed a law making it the third state, after predominantly rural Vermont and Alaska, to allow citizens to carry concealed weapons without a permit. Another law allows Arizonians to carry guns in bars, as long as they are not drinking alcohol.

Gun control laws in the USA are strongest in California and in the Northeast and weakest in Utah, which has no gun control law. Gun ownership rates tend to be higher where gun laws are looser. In Montana, Idaho, Wyoming, West Virginia, Alabama, Louisiana, and Missouri, just over 65% of households own a firearm. In Hawaii, only 10% do. The highest death rate from guns is in Louisiana (with 20 gun deaths per 100,000 people), but Mississippi and Alabama are close. The lowest is in

Hawaii, with 3 per 100,000. When the Constitution was passed, the USA had a population of 5 million people. Today that population is about 310 million and growing—and a population with 310 million has a number of crazy people in it, such as Jared Lee Loughner.

Although I favor strict gun control and the elimination of household pistols, my father, who died in 1941, had a rifle gun rack, and my boys own guns. I have never had a gun. I side with the conservative stalwart Judge Robert Bork who in 1989 stated: "The Constitution's Second Amendment guaranteed the right of states to form militias, not for individuals to bear arms," but the National Rifle Association is powerful and lobbies for the right of individuals to bear arms in this country.

DALLAS CRIME

Dallas reported 73,286 offenses in 2010 (14). That seems like a lot to me, but it is a 36% reduction in crime over the last 7 years. Violent crime has fallen nearly 50% in the last 9 years. Dallas crimes between 2009 and 2010 decreased as follows: business robberies, 31%; auto thefts, 20%; and violent crimes, 10%. Public surveillance cameras, special crime-reduction operations, and the addition of 750 officers since 2004 probably accounted for the reduction. All this is good news, I guess, but over 73,000 crimes in a single city as wonderful as Dallas is a bit scary.

In 2010, there were 158 murders in Dallas. According to Tanya Eiserer, the last time fewer people were murdered in Dallas was 1967, when there were 133, and that year Dallas had 500,000 fewer residents (15). The city's murder toll has declined about 40% since 2004, and 2010 was the third consecutive year of declines. No one knows exactly what is behind the decline. Better emergency treatment for trauma victims and a larger police presence are possible contributing factors. The Dallas Police Department has grown from about 2900 officers in 2004 to nearly 3700 today.

ARMY SUICIDES

Overall in 2010, the US Army reported 323 suicides of soldiers, army civilians, and family members, 69 more than in 2009, according to the Department of Defense (16). Twenty-two of those suicides in 2010 were at Fort Hood.

ILLNESSES ABOARD CRUISE SHIPS

The number of outbreaks of gastrointestinal illnesses on cruise ships sailing from US ports dropped again in 2010 (17). The US Centers for Disease Control and Prevention (CDC) recorded just 14 outbreaks of illnesses such as Norovirus on ships operating out of US ports in 2010, lower than in any year since 2001, when there were just 4 outbreaks. The number was down from 15 in 2009, 21 in 2007, and 34 in 2006. The decline came even as the number of people cruising continued to rise. The industry in 2010 carried 15 million passengers, up from 13 million in 2009. Cruise ships arriving in US ports must report all cases of gastrointestinal illnesses treated by on-board medical staff to the CDC's Vessel Sanitation Program Division, and a separate notification is required when the number of cases exceeds 2% of passengers and crew. When cases exceed 3% of passengers and crew, the CDC issues a public report.

Eight of the 14 outbreaks in 2010 were due to Norovirus, a common stomach bug. The causes of the 6 other illnesses are unknown. Sometimes called the "24-hour flu," even though it is unrelated to influenza, Norovirus is the most common cause of gastrointestinal illness in the USA, accounting for about half of all cases, according to the CDC. It breaks out in schools, hospitals, offices, and other places people congregate.

MORE FROM THE US CENSUS BUREAU

Since 2000 both the death rates and the tax rates in the USA have declined (18). We marry less and divorce more. The 130th edition of the *Statistical Abstract of the United States,* the annual profile of the country, was published on January 6, 2011, by the US Census Bureau. The number of individuals reporting income of ≥$1 million rose to 392,000 in 2007 from 240,000 in 2000. Most Americans of Armenian ancestry live in the West! Since 2000 there are more atheists and Wiccans, fewer Unitarians and Jews. The consumption of fresh fruit declined. There are more pigs than people in five states (Minnesota, Iowa, Nebraska, North Carolina, and South Dakota), and twice as many young adults bowl as ride bicycles. We eat less red meat, 108 pounds per person in 2008, down 5.4 pounds since 2000. We are eating fewer vegetables too: 393 pounds per person, down more than 30 pounds. The marriage rate is lowest since 1970, 7.3 per 1000 people, and the divorce rate is similar to 1970 levels at 3.6 per 1000 people. There were 4.8 million acres of organic farmland in 2008, a 170% increase since 2000. The proportion of developed land reached a new high: 5.6% of all land in the continental USA. And a record 41% of all live births were to unmarried women, up 22% since 1980. In 2008, 26% of men and 30% of women had 14 or more days a month when they didn't get enough sleep. The number of pharmacies increased: 42,300 in 2007, up 500 from the year before. But there were 400 fewer bookstores than in 2000: 10,600. In 2008, 7.3 million adults were in jail, on probation, or on parole, the highest number ever. In 2007, airport screeners confiscated 1.1 million knives, 11,908 box cutters, and 1416 guns. These numbers may be more than you ever wanted to know.

SUPERCENTENARIAN

The oldest person on planet Earth now is Besse Cooper, who was born in 1896 (19). She lived alone until she was 105. She attributes her longevity to minding her own business and avoiding junk food. That's good advice for all of us. The Gerontology Research Group in Los Angeles keeps track of the planet's supercentenarians (those ≥110 years old).

CORONARY STENTS

Khouzam and colleagues (20) from New York described a 56-year-old man with angina pectoris who had 67 stents in one or more coronary arteries! During a 10-year period, he had 28 cardiac catheterizations with stents placed in his native coronary arteries as well as in 3 aortocoronary bypass grafts. All stents were placed to relieve angina pectoris. I've never heard of

Table 1. Standard of living in 1980 compared to 2011 in the USA*

Variable	1980	2011
Personal income	$24,080	$40,450
Housing	$3,260	$6,130
Health care	$1,800	$5,440
Recreation	$910	$2,310
Vehicles, gas	$2,015	$2,270
Clothing	$1,080	$1,090
Airline miles per person	960	1,900
New house size (ft²)	1,740	2,440
Wireless phones (millions)	0	293
Vehicles/100 driving-age people	92	104
2.5 gigabytes of computer power	$214,000	$7
Life expectancy at age 50 (years)	78	81
Violent crimes/1000 people	17	5
Carbon dioxide emission, from energy (metric tons/person)	21	18

*Data from *USA Today* (21).

a patient having close to that number. With each stent costing approximately $1100, it adds up.

LIVING STANDARDS IN THE USA, 1980 VS 2011

Table 1 shows how much richer the average American is in 2011 compared with 1980 (21). The dollar figures in both columns in the table are adjusted for inflation. The biggest change is the cost of health care.

LEARNING IN COLLEGE

According to the book *Academically Adrift: Limited Learning on College Campuses*—based on transcripts and surveys of >3000 full-time traditional-aged students on 29 campuses nationwide and on their results on the Collegiate Learning Assessment, a standardized test that gauges students' critical thinking, analytical reasoning, and writing skills—college students in a 168-hour (7-day) week spend their time as follows: socializing, recreating, other, 51%; sleeping, 24%; working, volunteering, student clubs, 9%; attending class/labs, 9%; studying, 7% (22). Authors Richard Arum and Josipa Roksa noted that students in the study, on average, earned a 3.2 grade-point average. Thirty-five percent of the students reported spending 5 or fewer hours per week studying alone. That fact reminds me of the comment by Johann von Goethe: "Talents are best nurtured in solitude; character is best formed in the stormy billows of the world." Whether character is being substituted for talent in colleges remains to be seen. The book also indicated that students who studied in groups tended to have lower gains in learning than those who studied in solitude. Fifty percent of the students surveyed said they never took a class where they wrote >20 pages; 32% never took a course where they read >40 pages a week. No wonder the Chinese and Indians and Europeans are smiling a bit at us in the USA.

CHINESE MOTHERS

Amy Chua (23) asks how Chinese parents raise such successful kids. What do these parents do to produce so many math whizzes and music prodigies? Here are some things Ms. Chua's two daughters were never allowed to do: attend a sleepover; have a play date; be in a school play; complain about not being in a school play; watch TV or play computer games; choose their own extracurricular activities; get any grade less than an A; not be the top student in every subject except gym and drama; play any instrument other than the piano or violin; and not play the piano or violin. She used the term "Chinese mother," knowing that some Korean, Indian, Jamaican, Irish, and Ghanaian parents also would qualify. Even when Western parents think they are being strict, they usually don't come close to being Chinese mothers. Some strict Western parents consider themselves strict when they make their children practice their instruments 30 minutes or at most 60 minutes every day. For Chinese mothers, their children practice 2 and 3 hours daily.

In one study of 50 Western mothers and 48 Chinese immigrant mothers, almost 70% of the Western mothers said either that "stressing academic success is not good for children" or that "parents need to foster the idea that learning is fun." By contrast, roughly zero of the Chinese mothers felt the same way. Instead, most Chinese mothers said they believe their children can be "the best" students, that "academic achievement reflects successful parenting," and that if children did not excel at school then there was "a problem" and parents "were not doing their job." Other studies indicate that compared to Western parents, Chinese parents spend approximately 10 times as long every day in academic activities with their children. By contrast, Western kids are more likely to participate in sports.

Ms. Chua indicates that what Chinese parents understand is that nothing is fun until you get good at it. To get good at anything you have to work! And children on their own never want to work, which is why it is crucial to override their preferences. This often requires fortitude on the part of the parents because children resist. Things are always hardest at the beginning, which is when Western parents tend to give up. Tenacious practice, practice, practice is crucial for excellence. Repetition is underrated in the USA. Once a child starts to excel at something, he or she gets praise, admiration, and satisfaction. This builds confidence and makes the once not-fun activity fun. This in turn makes it easier for the parent to get the child to work even more.

Parenting advice in China has long stressed discipline and authority. Among the character-building exercises parents use was having children hold ice cubes in their hands for long stretches. In recent years, books that encourage parents to nurture their children's independence and confidence, as opposed to focusing exclusively on high academic achievement, have grown increasingly popular. These books reflect a quiet shift in the parenting style of middle-class families, especially in China's growing cities. The current bestselling parenting book in China is titled *A Good Mom Is Better than a Good Teacher*. The book has sold >2 million copies since it was published in 2009. Its author, Yin Jianli, advocates listening to kids and developing their potential without forcing them to obey authority.

BEEF FAT CLOGS HOUSTON SHIP CHANNEL

About 15,000 gallons of animal fat poured into the Houston Ship Channel in early January 2011 through a storm drain after an onshore storage tank leaked 250,000 gallons of the greasy substance (24). Unlike oil, beef fat doesn't create a colorful sheen on the surface of the water that can be skimmed off. When it hits the water it instantly thickens. It turns into a thick patty. Workers cleaned it up using fish nets to corral the fat and then pitchforks to lift 1 × 1-ft chunks of the cream-colored debris. Animal fat, of course, is used in cosmetics, soaps, pet food, and a variety of other products. It seems better to me to let the cows move on the surface of the planet and then this would not happen.

OUT OF WORK AND OUT OF JOBS

It is clear that the greater the amount of education, the less the likelihood of being out of work (25). Unemployment rates for selected groups in November 2010 in the USA were as follows: bachelor's degree or higher, 5.1%; Asians, 7.6%; some college, 8.7%; women, 8.9%; whites, 8.9%; high school grad (no college), 10.0%; men, 10.6%; Hispanics, 13.2%; less than high school diploma, 15.7%; and blacks, 16.0%. The national average was 9.8%. The decline in jobs is a result of megatrends including the growth of technology and the rise of globalization, writes Zachary Karabell. Neither of these trends is going away.

US companies have become more profitable in the past 2 years, even as unemployment has grown. That's because they've been able to tap an emerging global middle-class in China, Brazil, India, and elsewhere, both as consumers and lower-cost workers. This, along with the hyper-efficiencies produced by technology, has allowed businesses to generate record revenue and profits while shedding record numbers of workers. Company after company is hiring outside the USA and firing in the USA. IBM now has more workers outside the USA than it has in the USA, and that won't change. These structural issues will not go away simply because the government pumps more money into the financial system or Washington spends more in the form of tax cuts or stimulus. The manufacturing jobs that have been lost are gone forever. The USA can manage high unemployment only if it focuses on building a new economy with cutting-edge infrastructure and education that rivals that found elsewhere in the world.

Among the happiest people around will be those working in the technology sector; network system analysts and data analysts are the fastest growing occupations in the USA after biomedical engineers. This is no surprise, since companies have been ramping up their spending on software and computer services. For technology companies, it seems, the most recent recession did not occur.

STATES FOR RETIREMENT

According to John Brady, president of the website *Top Retirements.com,* the best states for retirees are Florida, Texas, Arizona, and the Carolinas (26). The worst 10 are Illinois, California, New York, Rhode Island, New Jersey, Ohio, Wisconsin, Massachusetts, Connecticut, and Nevada. The bad ones tend to have high taxes, bad climate, high crime, poor recreation facilities, poor transportation, inadequate health care, and high costs of living.

STATE DEFICITS

In the January/February 2011 issue of *AARP Bulletin,* a figure was provided showing the percentage of shortfall in state and national budgets for fiscal year 2011 (27). Forty-seven states and the District of Columbia spent more than they received, and the shortfall ranged from 1.7% in the District of Columbia to 54% in Nevada. Illinois, the home of the president, had a shortfall of 41.5%. The four states in the black were Alaska, Arkansas, Montana, and North Dakota. Neither the US government nor states nor individuals can save more than they spend. California had a shortfall of 21.6%; New York, 15.3%; and Texas, 10.2%. We must all work harder to keep the money in our purses and wallets, and if we don't we will all sink.

THE EGYPTIAN ECONOMY

Hernando de Soto's organization, the Institute for Liberty and Democracy, was hired by the Egyptian government in 1997, with financial support from the US Agency for International Development, to learn how much of the Egyptian economy operated "extralegally," that is, without the protections of property rights or access to normal business tools, such as credit (28). The objective was to remove the legal impediments holding back people and their businesses.

After years of field work and analysis—involving over 120 Egyptian and Peruvian technicians with the participation of 300 local Egyptian leaders and interviews with thousands of ordinary people—Hernando de Soto's organization in 2004 presented a 1000-page report and a 20-point action plan to the 11-member economic cabinet of Egypt. The report was championed by the minister of finance at the time, and the Egyptian cabinet approved its policy recommendations. Shortly thereafter, the minister of finance was fired, a cabinet shakeup occurred, and the crucial elements of the reforms were blocked.

Hernando de Soto's investigation uncovered three key facts:

1. Egypt's underground economy was the nation's biggest employer. The legal private sector employed 6.8 million people; the public sector, 5.9 million; and the extralegal sector, 9.6 million.
2. Only 8% of Egyptians held their property with a normal legal title.
3. All extralegal businesses and property, rural and urban, amounted to $248 billion, 30 times greater than the market value of the companies registered on the Cairo Stock Exchange and 55 times greater than the value of foreign direct investment in Egypt since Napoleon invaded, including the financing of the Suez Canal and the Aswan Dam. (Those same extralegal assets would be worth more than $400 billion in today's US dollars.)

The entrepreneurs who operate outside the legal system do not have access to the business organizational forms (partnerships, joint stock companies, corporations, etc.) that would enable them to grow the way legal enterprises do. Because such enterprises are not tied to contractual and enforcement rules, outsiders cannot trust that their owners can be held to their promises or contracts. This makes it difficult or impossible to employ the best technicians and professional managers, and the owners of these businesses cannot issue bonds or IOUs to obtain credit. Nor can such enterprises benefit from the economies of scale available to those who can operate in the legal Egyptian market. The owners of extralegal enterprises are limited to employing their kin to produce for confined circles of customers.

Without clear legal title to their assets and real estate, the entrepreneur-owned property cannot be leveraged as collateral for loans to obtain investment capital, or as security for long-term contractual deals. Thus, most Egyptian enterprises remain small and relatively poor. The only thing that can emancipate them is legal reform, and only the political leadership of Egypt can do it. Emancipating people from bad law and devising strategy to overcome the inertia of the status quo is a major challenge in Egypt.

Most Egyptians choose to remain outside the legal economy because Egypt's legal institutions fail most people. Due to burdensome, discriminatory, and bad laws, it is impossible for most people to legalize their properties and businesses, no matter how well intentioned they might be. To open a small bakery, de Soto's investigation found, would take >500 days to get legal title to a vacant piece of land and >10 years of dealing with red tape. To do business in Egypt, an aspiring poor entrepreneur would have to deal with 56 governmental agencies and repetitive government inspections.

All of this helps explain why so many Egyptians have been smoldering for decades. Despite hard work and savings, they can do little to improve their lives. Bringing most of Egypt's people into an open legal system is what is needed. Empowering the poor begins with the legal system's awarding clear property rights to the $400 billion-plus assets they had created. This would unlock an amount of capital hundreds of times greater than foreign direct investment and what Egypt receives in foreign aid. Unless its existing legal institutions are reformed to allow economic growth from the bottom up, the aspirations for a better life that motivated the recent street demonstration will remain unfulfilled.

SOUTHERN AND WESTERN MIGRATION

Today one of every 12 Americans lives in Texas, the same proportion that lived in New York City in 1930. Michael Barone, the presidential scholar, recently compared Census results in 1970 to those in 2010, a 40-year interval (29) *(Table 2)*. The year 1970 was, as Barone called it, "a flex point," as high-tech and high-finance were replacing big government, big business, and big labor in the USA. The decades-long farm-to-factory migration also drew to a close, and the unanticipated major immigration from Latin America and Asia began. It was also

Table 2. US population changes in the past 80 years*

Variable	1930–1970	1970–2010
US population increase (millions)	80 (65%)	105 (52%)
Location of population increase:		
Megalopolis (New York to DC)	69%	19%
Northeast + North Central	49%	13%
Pacific states	208%	88%
South Atlantic states	102%	114%
Rocky Mountain states	124%	166%
Great Plains	23%	26%
Interior South	26%	39%

*Data from Barone (29).

the time that lavish welfare spending and lax crime control really began. In the 40-year period of 1930 to 1970, the US population increased by 80 million (65%), and in the period of 1970 to 2010, it increased by 105 million (52%). During the 1930–1970 period, the population increased mainly in the Northeast, centering in New York City and ending in Washington, DC. But as taxes in New York increased to record levels and as local governments squeezed out much of private industry, New York City lost 1 million people in the 1970s, and growth in the region has been sluggish since with immigrant inflow balanced by native outflow. Overall, the region grew just 19% in 1970–2010, far below the national average of 52%. Faring even worse was the North Central area from upstate New York and Pennsylvania west to the Great Lakes and the Mississippi River. Population there increased 49% in 1930–1970, fed by farm-to-factory migration and the movement of a third of American Blacks from the rural South to the urban North in 1940 to 1965. In the last 40 years, unionized factories and high urban crime rates have wrecked huge cities like Detroit. People in the North Central areas have been outmigrating since 1970, and the region's net population increased only 13% from 1970 to 2010, the lowest rate of any region in the nation.

The population of the Pacific states, including California, Oregon, Alaska, and Hawaii, tripled (up 208%) in the 1930–1970 period, but growth since has slowed. High tax and slow growth policies that raised housing prices are factors. Latino immigrants have been streaming in, but almost as many native-born citizens have been moving out. The Pacific states grew 88% in 1970–2010, well above the national average but far slower than in 1930–1970 and slower than in the South Atlantic states, Virginia, North and South Carolina, Georgia, and Florida. The population in those five states doubled (up 102%) in 1930–1970, but growth accelerated in the 1970–2010 period. Black outmigration halted in the late 1960s, and businesses were attracted by favorable public policies including right-to-work laws and low tax rates. The population of the South Atlantic states increased 114% in the 1970–2010 period, and the 2010 census shows they have overtaken the five Pacific states in population, 51 million vs. 50 million.

The Rocky Mountain States started off from a low base but had a 124% population gain in the 1930–1970 period and a 166% increase in the 1970–2010 period, greater than any other region. Phoenix, Denver, and Las Vegas have become nationally significant metropolitan areas. The Great Plains, which languished in the 1930–1970 period with only 23% population growth as farmers emptied out, picked up at a 26% increase in 1970–2010. The interior South, the southern states west of the South Atlantic and east and north of Texas, grew 26% in 1930–1970, nearly 40 points below the national average, but they have grown 39% in the 1970–2010 period, only 12 points below the national average.

And then there is Texas. In 1930, the Lone Star State had 6 million people versus 13 million in New York. In 1970, there were 11 million in Texas and 18 million in New York. Each had grown by about 5 million. But in 2010, there were 25 million in Texas and 19 million in New York! People like Texas with its low tax rates, light regulation, and openness to new business and enterprises, rather than the New York version of bigger government, higher taxes, and more unions. Metropolitan Dallas and metropolitan Houston, with about 6 million people each, today threaten to overtake our fourth largest metro area, San Francisco (population about 7 million) in the next decade.

In 1930, half of all Americans lived in New England and in the northern states stretching to the Mississippi River. Now, only one third of Americans live in those regions, the same proportion as live in the South Atlantic, interior South, and Texas. I suspect these trends will continue.

—William Clifford Roberts, MD
15 February 2011

1. Howell JD. Early use of x-ray machines and electrocardiographs at the Pennsylvania Hospital 1897 through 1927. *JAMA* 1986;255(17):2320–2323.
2. Milken M. Health-care investment—the hidden crisis. *Wall Street Journal*, February 9, 2011.
3. Studenski S, Perera S, Patel K, Rosano C, Faulkner K, Inzitari M, Brach J, Chandler J, Cawthon P, Connor EB, Nevitt M, Visser M, Kritchevsky S, Badinelli S, Harris T, Newman AB, Cauley J, Ferrucci L, Guralnik J. Gait speed and survival in older adults. *JAMA* 2011;305(1):50–58.
4. Lloyd J. Study: Walking speed appears to predict longevity in seniors. *USA Today*, January 4, 2011.
5. Hellmich N. An egg a day gets the OK as cholesterol declines: shifts in hen diet, breeding may be factors. *USA Today*, February 9, 2011.
6. Huisman M. Red-light cameras save lives, study says. *Dallas Morning News*, February 2, 2011.
7. Manning S. Man's best friend distracting in autos. *Dallas Morning News*, January 22, 2011.
8. Rice D. Hot-car deaths rise for kids in 2010. Trapped succumb to heatstroke. *USA Today*, January 5, 2011.
9. Bauder D. Pedestrians' eyes glued to phones, not road. *Dallas Morning News*, January 22, 2011.
10. Levin A. No U.S. airline fatalities in 2010: experts credit years of safety advances. *USA Today*, January 23, 2011.
11. Gosselin R. Wounded Packers don't pack: coach's experience helps Green Bay thrive despite rash of injuries. *Dallas Morning News*, January 15, 2011.
12. O'Connell V, Fields G. Many mentally ill can buy guns. *Wall Street Journal*, January 12, 2011.
13. Grunwald M. Fire away: you might think attacks like the one in Tucson would lead to tougher gun restrictions, but you'd be dead wrong. *Time*, January 14, 2011.
14. Eiserer T. Dallas crime falls again, by 10%. *Dallas Morning News*, January 8, 2011.
15. Eiserer T. Murders drop for third year. City's larger police presence, improvements in trauma care are possible factors in trend. *Dallas Morning News*, January 7, 2011.
16. Wire reports. Fort Hood seeks help to stop soldier suicides. *Dallas Morning News*, February 2, 2011.
17. Sloan G. Illnesses aboard cruise ships decline again in 2010. *USA Today*, January 24, 2011.
18. New York Times staff. U.S. Census Bureau: who, what, huh? We marry less, divorce more and, in 5 states, pigs outnumber us. *Dallas Morning News*, January 16, 2011.
19. Brumback K. Woman, 114, is world's new oldest person. *Dallas Morning News*, February 2, 2011.
20. Khouzam RN, Dahiya R, Schwartz R. A heart with 67 stents. *J Am Coll Cardiol* 2010;56(19):1605.
21. Cauchon D. Our standard of living: is it better than ever? *USA Today*, February 3, 2011.
22. Arum R, Roksa J. *Academically Adrift: Limiting Learning on College Campuses.* Chicago: University of Chicago Press, 2011 (272 pp.).
23. Chua A. Why Chinese mothers are superior. Can a regimen of no playdates, no TV, no computer games and hours of music practice create happy kids? And what happens when they fight back? *Wall Street Journal*, January 8–9, 2011.
24. Plushnick-Masti R. Workers fish beef fat from waterway. *Dallas Morning News*, January 6, 2011.
25. Karabell Z. Where the jobs aren't. Jobs are finally being created, but many of the positions we lost are never coming back. *Time*, January 17, 2011.
26. Powell R. 10 worst states for golden years. Perilous fiscal health, high taxes, poor climate are turnoffs. *Dallas Morning News*, December 18, 2010.
27. Currie D. State news. Pushing for prudent budgets and choices in long-term care. *AARP.org/bulletin*, January-February 2011.
28. de Soto H. Egypt's economic apartheid. *Wall Street Journal*, February 3, 2011.
29. Barone M. The great Lone Star migration. *Wall Street Journal*, January 8–9, 2011.

Chapter 3

July 2011

HOTTER DAYS

My son Charles sent me "The Hot Zone" by Linda Marsa from a recent issue of *Discover* (1). She quoted a British scientist writing in the *Lancet* in 2010 that "climate change is the biggest global health threat of the 21st century." Climate change brings back some "old" diseases. There is dengue in Texas, malaria in New York, hypertoxic pollen in Baltimore.

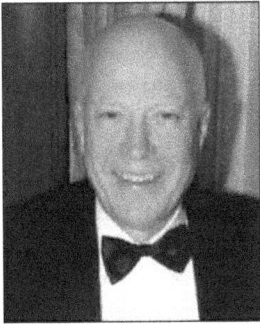

William C. Roberts, MD

Long thought eradicated in the USA, dengue is back. There had been prior cases of the disease's milder cousin, classic dengue fever, in Brownsville, Texas, but now the more serious form of dengue infection, hemorrhagic fever, appeared in a patient in Brownsville, Texas, in 2005. From 1995 to 2005, some 10,000 cases were reported in the USA, including the Texas-Mexico border region. The Centers for Disease Control and Prevention (CDC) suggested that many cases are never counted, so these figures may be large underestimates.

Several factors influence the spread of the dengue virus, but rising global temperatures may be the most important. Like many tropical diseases, dengue is spread by mosquito bites, and mosquitoes are exquisitely sensitive to climate. Frost kills both adult mosquitoes and larvae, which is why the disease hasn't previously been able to get a foothold in the US. But with the advent of warmer winters, there is nothing holding the insects back. The two species of mosquitoes capable of transmitting dengue fever, casually known as the Asian tiger mosquito, have substantially expanded their habitat range since the middle of the 20th century. They are now in 28 US states, even as far north as New York and New Hampshire. Hotter, more humid weather shortens mosquito breeding cycles. Heat speeds up the incubation of the dengue virus, making it infectious much sooner and for more of the insects' lifespan. Female mosquitoes bite more frequently when the temperature rises. Climate change is likely to usher in an era of more extreme weather, including the heavy rains and flooding that create ideal mosquito breeding grounds, and dengue is far from the only risk. Ticks, mice, and other carriers are also surviving milder winters and fanning out across the country, spreading other pathogens: Lyme disease, Rocky Mountain spotted fever, equine encephalitis, St. Louis encephalitis, anaplasmosis, and babesiosis, a once uncommon malaria-like infection.

Despite the 1000 who have been stricken, most Americans are not aware of dengue. Epidemic outbreaks have occurred throughout Latin America—in Brazil, Mexico, Honduras, Paraguay, Costa Rica, Bolivia, and Cuba—and they now hit nearly 1 million people annually. And the virus is affecting people now in many northern states including Maine, Minnesota, and Washington. The aggressive Asian tiger mosquito transmits not only dengue but also Chikungunya fever, a particularly nasty infection that causes excruciating joint pain.

The increased mobility of the modern world also makes the situation worse. The most virulent form of Lyme disease may have reached the USA from Europe by ship. Infected individuals ("parasitic hitchhikers") can now go anywhere in the world in <24 hours and deliver reservoirs of malaria, dengue, or Chikungunya fever. The warmer temperatures, extreme weather (both wet and dry), and increased mobility enabled the West Nile virus to become entrenched in North America. The deadly pathogen first emerged in Uganda in 1937 and then laid dormant for about 20 years before appearing again in Israel in the 1950s and in Romania in 1996. Each of those outbreaks occurred after an unusually dry hot spell, creating the perfect incubator for *Culex pupiens,* a common house mosquito that transmits West Nile. In 1999, the virus was identified in New York City. Once again, that summer was unusually hot and dry. Stagnant pools of water teaming with mosquitoes lured birds and they became infected, transmitting the West Nile virus.

Infectious disease is not the only consequence of the rising temperatures. An average increase in the USA of 2°F over the past 50 years worsens pollution and urban crowding. Cities are particularly affected due to air pollution and what are now called "urban heat islands," created as asphalt, pavement, and buildings concentrate heat. People are moving to these giant urban slums without adequate sanitation, creating perfect mosquito breeding grounds.

Noninfectious diseases like allergies and asthma, already epidemic in the USA, are also likely to gain a boost from rising temperatures. Indeed, at least 50 million Americans suffer from these ailments: asthma affects about 10% of American adults and children. Their incidences are climbing. Both air pollution and pollen, two of the chief culprits behind asthma and allergies, intensify as temperatures increase. Ozone smog is created when sunlight cooks pollutants in the atmosphere. When the air heats up, more ozone is produced. Pollens released into the air by flowering plants, trees, and grasses appear earlier and for longer periods of time under warmer conditions. Hotter temperatures coupled with higher concentrations of carbon dioxide in the air prompt flowering plants to produce pollen that is far more noxious than pollen of the past. US Department of Agriculture scientists grew weeds in three sites: on an organic farm in western Maryland, in a park in a suburb of Baltimore, and in downtown Baltimore, which is cooked with smog and about 3° to 4° warmer than the surrounding countryside because of the urban heat island effect. The weeds in the hotter CO_2-enriched environment grew to nearly twice the size of plants on the farm—up to 12 feet versus 6 to 8 feet in the country—and generated more pollen, specifically, more allergenic pollen.

Intense heat waves will become more common over the next few decades according to a 2009 report released jointly by the National Wildlife Federation and Physicians for Social Responsibility. That increase will elevate the risk of heat-related deaths. Heat waves swept across Europe in 2003 and 2005 and killed >70,000 people. The 2003 event was one of the deadliest climate-related disasters in Western history.

In the summer of 2010, Russia wilted under the worst heat waves in 130 years of recordkeeping there, with daily highs in Moscow exceeding 100° compared with the normal summer average of 85°. In the countryside, severe drought ignited wildfires that smothered the city in poisonous smog for 6 straight days. The combination of unprecedented heat, dryness, and suffocating haze doubled death rates to an average of 700 people a day. People stated that they were hardly able to see more than a block away. People walked around with surgical masks on and kept the windows of their apartments tightly shut. Oscillating fans, which normally sold for about $10, that summer sold for $100.

This is what is on the horizon. Over the next century, global temperature will probably increase another 2° to 12° on average according to a 2009 report from the US Global Change Research Program. This shift will mean more extremely hot summer days. By 2080, it could be above 90° some 120 days a year in Kansas. Much of Florida and Texas could be above 90° for half the year, and many parts of the country, especially the Sunbelt, could have >2 months each year with 100° weather. Temperatures in the 110° to 120° range could soon become commonplace. The sizzling weather in Chicago in 1995, which claimed >700 lives, was possibly a prelude to what will happen in the future. Chronic illnesses could also be aggravated if weather-related national calamities, like fires, floods, and severe storms, overwhelm public services.

The migration to the South may be reversed in coming decades.

WATER GREED

Some predict that water will be more expensive than oil in the decades to come. Although our planet is called Planet Earth, it more appropriately might be called Planet Water since 70% of the surface is covered by water. Nevertheless, many land areas on Earth are enormously short of water. Kim and McCann (2) had a piece recently illustrating water consumption in selected Texas cities in gallons per day in 2008, the most recent statistics available. Highland Park leads the list with an average of 360 gallons per capita per day, followed by Southlake, Texarkana, Frisco, Plano, Richardson, and Dallas (non-Highland Park). Residents of Houston use one third the water per capita that is used in Highland Park. North Texas communities consumed almost 500 billion gallons of water in 2010. That is the largest quantity consumed by any region in Texas. With the huge droughts in Texas, we all need to be more conservative with our water use. A long shower is nice but it's greedy. Leaving the faucet running while we brush our teeth is greedy. Clearly the Dallas–Fort Worth area is a drain on Texas' water supplies.

DALLAS TREES

Trees absorb air pollutants. Their shade lowers temperatures and can reduce energy use. By easing water runoff, they improve water quality and diminish the potential for flooding. They can enhance property values, soften noise, and provide wildlife habitat. They also grow up, get sick or injured, get old or cleared away. To protect and preserve them, trees need to be nurtured and their number and species known. With the help of Dr. Fang Qui, an associate professor at the University of Texas at Dallas, some of his students and an airplane equipped with remote-sensing laser devices determined the location, height, foliage spread, and species of >316,000 trees in two areas of Dallas covering 20 square miles (3). Images collected along Turtle Creek North into the Park Cities identified 92,540 trees with heights ranging from 5 to 29 feet (average, 12). The second area, near and north of White Rock Creek, had 223,788 trees ranging in height from 5 to 39 feet (average, 13). In both areas, cedar elms, pecans, live oaks, and the invasive tree of heaven were most prevalent. Projecting the count across the city's 385 square miles gave an estimate of >6 million trees, almost 5 per person.

Having such specific information and keeping it updated can help foresters, arborists, property owners, government officials, and others to monitor and manage wooded areas. It can help track tree diseases, the health of selected species, and the spread of invasive ones. It can provide evidence of illegal cutting and help guide tree planting and maintenance efforts. Let's try to increase that number to 10 trees per Dallas resident.

WORKING HOURS AND CORONARY HEART DISEASE

Kivimäki and colleagues (4) from United Kingdom, Finland, and France examined 7095 adults (2109 women and 4986 men) aged 39 to 62 years working full-time without evidence of coronary heart disease at baseline (1991–1993) and followed them for evidence of coronary heart disease until 2004. A total of 192 participants developed clinical evidence of coronary heart disease during a median 12.3-year follow-up. After adjustment for their Framingham risk score, participants working ≥11 hours per day had a 1.67-fold increased risk for coronary heart disease compared with participants working 7 to 8 hours per day. Thus, information on working hours appears to improve risk prediction for coronary heart disease in low-risk working populations.

LOWERING CHOLESTEROL MORE

The JUPITER trial, which I consider the best of the lipid-lowering drug trials, included 11,001 men aged ≥50 years and 6801 women aged ≥60 years with low-density lipoprotein (LDL) cholesterol <130 mg/dL, high-sensitivity C-reactive protein (hsCRP) ≥2.0 mg/L, and no history of cardiovascular disease or diabetes mellitus. The trial was published in 2008. The trial was stopped because the event rates were reduced so much in the 20-mg rosuvastatin group compared with the placebo group. The current paper by Hsia and colleagues (5) divided the JUPITER trial participants into those who had their LDL cholesterol lowered to <50 mg/dL and those in whom the LDL cholesterol never got below 50 mg/dL. (In the initial trial of 17,000+ patients, the mean LDL cholesterol at baseline was 109 and nearly 2 years into the trial the mean LDL cholesterol had fallen to 55 mg/dL.) In the recent analysis, there were 4000 patients in whom the LDL never got below 50 and 4156 patients in whom the LDL was <50 mg/dL. There were 8150 patients in the placebo group. The average age of all groups was 66 years, and almost 40% in each group were women. After a median follow-up of 2 years in the rosuvastatin-allocated subjects without and with LDL cholesterol levels <50 mg/dL, baseline and 1-year cholesterol levels (median) were 109 and 110 mg/dL in the placebo group; 113 and 70 mg/dL in the rosuvastatin-allocated subjects with no LDL cholesterol <50; and 103 and 44 mg/dL in the rosuvastatin-allocated patients with LDL <50 mg/dL.

In the previously reported trial, rosuvastatin reduced the primary study endpoint, a composite of cardiovascular death, myocardial infarction, stroke, arterial revascularization, and unstable angina pectoris, by 44%. This treatment effect was consistent regardless of baseline LDL cholesterol level. The magnitude of clinical benefit was directly related to the obtained LDL cholesterol level. Compared with the placebo group, rosuvastatin-allocated patients with no LDL cholesterol <50 had a smaller risk reduction for the primary endpoint. Subjects whose LDL cholesterol was lowered to <50 mg/dL had a 65% reduction in major cardiovascular events compared with those whose LDL was never lowered to that level. Similarly, all-cause mortality was reduced by 20% for the entire 17,000+ patients and by 46% in the patients obtaining an LDL <50 mg/dL.

Rosuvastatin reduced major cardiovascular events by 44% compared with placebo for the entire JUPITER subjects and by 65% among those attaining LDL cholesterol <50 mg/dL. Similarly, all-cause mortality was reduced by 20% for the entire cohort and by 46% among patients attaining LDL cholesterol <50 mg/dL. With regard to adverse events, myalgia and diabetes mellitus were somewhat more common among participants attaining LDL cholesterol <50, but these rates were not significantly different from rates of those not attaining LDL cholesterol <50 mg/dL. Rates for other adverse events, including muscle weakness, myopathy, neuropsychiatric events, renal dysfunction, hemorrhagic stroke, and cancer, were not higher among patients allocated to rosuvastatin than among patients allocated to placebo, regardless of attained LDL cholesterol level.

A major strength of this analysis is its large sample size. The number of JUPITER study participants with an LDL <50 mg/dL was greater than the entire active treatment group of many placebo-controlled statin trials. This study provides further evidence that the lower the LDL cholesterol, the better. This study suggests that the LDL cholesterol threshold, if it exists, may be <50 mg/dL. I am going for <50 mg/dL from here on.

CALORIE POSTINGS ON MENUS

The calorie labeling provision was part of President Barack Obama's 2010 health overhaul law. The rule, expected to take effect in 2012, provides details on eateries with 20 outlets or more and on vending machines (6). Convenience stores, supermarket eateries, pastry and retail confectionary stores, coffee shops, snack bars, and ice cream bars will be required to post calorie counts. The new law requires the posting of calorie counts of foods and drinks on menu boards. Movie theaters, airplanes, bowling centers, amusement parks, hotels, and other establishments where the sale of food is not the primary business are excluded from having to post calorie labeling. The regulation will apply to establishments where more than 50% of the total floor area is used for the sale of food. Bars and restaurants will not have to post calorie labels on beer, wine, and other alcoholic beverages, which come under the Alcohol and Tobacco Tax and Trade Bureau rather than the Food and Drug Administration (FDA). The FDA estimates that the proposed regulations would apply to just under 280,000 establishments out of an estimated 600,000 restaurants nationwide. These calorie postings are done of course to decrease the average calories per transaction.

HEART ATTACK GRILL

John Basso started Heart Attack Grill in Chandler, Arizona, and now he is bringing it to Dallas' West End (7). Pretend-doctors flip massive burgers and charred-in-lard fries, served by naughty nurses and washed down by Jolt cola. A 2-lb hamburger is served free to anyone weighing >350 pounds. It consists of 4 half-pound beef patties and 8 slices of cheese served in a lard-coated bun. Also available are maximum-density butterfat shakes. Fortunately for its patrons, the grill will be relatively close to Baylor University Medical Center at Dallas.

APPENDICITIS—EMERGENCY SURGERY OR NOT?

Should appendectomy for appendicitis be done in the middle of the night or should it wait until the next morning after putting these patients on antibiotics and pain medications? A 2010 report on 309 appendicitis patients at a New Haven, Connecticut, hospital found those who had surgery within 12 hours of arriving at the emergency room fared no better than those who waited up to 24 hours for their appendectomy (8). Angela Ingraham, a general surgery resident at the University of Cincinnati, analyzed nearly 33,000 US appendectomy patients and found that timing <6, 6–12, or >12 hours after hospital admission made no significant difference in their condition 30 days afterwards. It also made no difference in the length of their operation or hospital stay. No matter when the appendix is removed, people seem none the worse without it. That led Charles Darwin to conclude that it is a useless evolutionary leftover. William Parker at Duke believes the appendix is there to store friendly bacteria that could get wiped out in the gut by severe diarrhea. Appendicitis was pretty much unheard of in Western countries when diarrhea was common. It's still apparently rare where diarrhea from contaminated drinking water is common. "Let's do it in the morning."

PRESCRIPTION PAIN MEDICATIONS

The deadliest drugs in the USA are not heroin or cocaine. The larger problem is abuse of drugs that are perfectly legal: prescription pain medications. According to a piece in *USA Today*, they kill an estimated 2 people every hour and send 40 more to emergency rooms with life-threatening overdoses (9). Powerful drugs such as OxyContin, Dilaudid, and Vicodin are obviously blessings to people with severe pain. But by themselves or in combination with antidepressants and muscle relaxers, they have become a scourge that kills >18,000 people a year, according to estimates by the Prescription Monitoring Program Center of Excellence at Brandeis University. The administration's prescription monitoring programs routinely enter prescriptions for certain drugs in a database that physicians can consult when prescribing powerful painkillers. More than 40 states have created these databases and >30 have them up and running. Physicians can consult these databases before writing prescriptions for painkillers. According to the *USA Today* editorial, most people who abuse painkillers get them from friends and family, sometimes innocently, sometimes by theft. A pernicious problem is unscrupulous physicians who deliberately overprescribe painkillers. Florida is said to be the home to numerous "pill mills," where it's so easy to get painkillers that people routinely flock from other states along the "OxyContin Highway." Florida's decision to open a pharmacy database might help deter these predators.

Prescription-monitoring programs may sound like a good idea, but they are not supported by all individuals or all states (10). That's why such proposals have been defeated several times in the past and why some proposals face substantial opposition. First of all, privacy advocates are concerned about creating another online database full of sensitive personal information with every doctor, pharmacist, and health care provider in the state accessing it. Cost also is a major issue, particularly in low-tax states. Federal grants are allegedly available to pay the start-up costs, but expenses are a burden in a number of states. The costs are not equitably spread. Chain pharmacies already have the hardware needed to comply with such programs, but independent neighborhood pharmacies will need to purchase the hardware and train their staff. The entire burden of the program falls on pharmacists to input the data and maintain the system. It's optional for physicians. Considering that one intention of the program is to prevent physician shopping, exempting physicians from checking the database before prescribing seems inappropriate. Some are also concerned about "mission creep." With the program not yet in place, advocates are already talking about expanding it to more types of medications—eventually to every prescription medication liable to be abused. They also want to extend the time for which records are kept, from the initial 100 days to maybe years.

Finally, one claimed benefit of a monitoring program is that physicians reassured that their patients are not abusing prescription drugs will be able to treat pain without fear of being targeted by the Drug Enforcement Administration for "overprescribing." Creating a new government program to fix problems with an existing program is a formula for ever-expanding government.

CESAREAN SECTIONS

According to Jason Roberson (11), one third of 4.2 million babies born in the USA in 2008 were delivered by cesarean section, and C-sections make the recovery period from childbirth longer and the cost higher. In 1997, about a fifth of deliveries were performed via C-section. In Texas, C-section charges are about 60% higher than vaginal birth charges. It is said that every 1% decrease in the nation's C-section rate could save more than $300 million in maternity charges. In Texas, the median charge for a C-section birth without complications in 2009 was $13,198, and for a vaginal delivery, $8288. In Dallas County, hospitals charged $10,424 for a C-section compared with $7421 for a vaginal delivery.

LIFE EXPECTANCY AND INFANT MORTALITY RATES

The CDC issued a report in March 2011 on health and well-being across American society (12). Some observations: life expectancy in the US rose from 78.0 in 2008 to 78.2 in 2009. Life expectancy is one of the best measures of socioeconomic progress because it captures improvements in living standards, health care, safety, nutrition, and the environment. Ten years have been added to American life spans since 1950, and 30 years since 1910. Furthermore, Americans are living healthier and more active lives at every age.

Infant mortality rates hit an all-time low of 6.42 per 1000 live births, as did death rates for children under the age of 5. There is less chance of losing a child to early death now than at any time in history. In 2010, the death rate fell 4.2% for those <1, 7.7% for those aged 1 to 4, and 6.7% for those aged 15 to 24. In 1950, a child was nearly 4 times more likely to die before the age of 5 than he or she is today.

The overall age-adjusted death rate (the probability of dying at any particular age) fell to 741 from 759 per 100,000 in 2009, the 10th consecutive year the death rate has fallen. All of this progress took place over a decade when lack of health insurance was supposedly dooming many Americans to inadequate care. Advances in medical treatments matter far more to overall health progress than do insurance coverage rates.

The age-adjusted death rate also decreased significantly for 10 of the 15 leading causes of death: heart disease, cancer, various chronic diseases of the liver or respiratory system, influenza, and pneumonia. Death rates from accidents and homicide also fell significantly. Today, the 5-year US survival from cancer is 66%, the highest rate in the world, and up from 50% in 1975. The death rate from heart attacks and strokes is now one half to one third the age-adjusted rate of 50 years ago.

There also is some bad news: the incidence of obesity and diabetes mellitus has increased. These, of course, are less the result of medical care inadequacies than of lifestyle decisions, particularly quantity of consumed calories and caloric choices. The major health gains in 2009 were achieved by every race except blacks. This reverses the trend of recent decades when the "health gap" between African Americans and European Americans has been narrowing.

These numbers show that average Americans have not seen their living standards fall over the last 30 years, as is often claimed by those who focus only on wage data. Medical breakthroughs are available to the rich, the middle class, and the poor alike. A poor person in America today has access to much better health care than did a billionaire or a prince in the 1950s! Yes, American health care is expensive, but the CDC report shows that its benefits include longer and better lives.

CRIB DEATHS

Sudden infant death syndrome (SIDS) is officially any death of a baby <1 year of age that remains unexplained after a thorough investigation. About 2500 babies die from SIDS each year, down from about 4000 per year in 1992, in part due to campaigns urging parents to put infants to sleep on their backs (13). Infant fatalities attributed to accidental suffocation and strangulation in bed quadrupled between 1984 and 2004, according to the CDC. A study in *Pediatrics* in March 2011 indicated that on average, 26 babies <2 years old are injured every day in the USA in a crib, bassinet, or playpen.

The use of bumpers, which line the inside of the crib, is controversial (14). The Consumer Products Safety Commission and the American Academy of Pediatrics have urged parents not to use the puffy bumpers—the kind that a baby's face could sink into—but both have stopped short of advising against any bumpers at all, as some consumer groups urge.

Other concerns focus on the cribs themselves. Starting in June 2011, it will be illegal to make, sell, or resell any crib in the US that doesn't meet tough new federal standards. Drop-down sides, linked to 32 infant deaths since 2000, will be prohibited. The new rules also require stronger slates, mattress supports, and hardware that can withstand vigorous shaking by toddlers. Most cribs on the market now do meet these new standards, according to the Juvenile Products Manufacturers Association. Tags with the code 16 CFR 1219 for full-sized cribs and 16 CFR 1220 for compact-sized cribs indicate that cribs meet the standards. The Juvenile Products Manufacturers Association estimated that the new rules will add 10% to 15% to the cost of the new cribs, which can range from $150 to over $1000. Yet millions of old cribs will remain in circulation, many of which are handed down through families or passed along to friends.

Experts and manufacturers agree that pillows, blankets, comforters, and piles of stuffed animals should not be placed in cribs with children <12 months of age. Loose fabric and soft cushions can block a baby's nose and mouth, and sleeping babies may not wake up sufficiently to fight for air, leading to SIDS.

Some baby products marketed as "making babies safer" have ended up posing more hazards. Positioning pillows designed to keep babies from rolling onto their sides or stomachs have been involved in at least 13 infant deaths since 1997. Experts have long warned against having babies sleeping in parents' beds, given the risk of suffocating in bedding or being crushed by a sleeping adult. The safest sleeping arrangement is to have the baby sleep in the parents' room for the first 6 months but in a separate bassinet or crib.

THE CONGENITALLY BICUSPID AORTIC VALVE

It appears that 99% of us have three-cuspid aortic valves and 1%, a bicuspid aortic valve. Fifty years ago (in April 1961), Dr. Jesse E. Edwards published an editorial entitled "The Congenital Bicuspid Aortic Valve" (15). At the time, Dr. Edwards was the world's foremost student of the aortic valve. In that editorial he asked a simple question, "How does a congenitally bicuspid valve open and close during the two phases of the cardiac cycle?" To my knowledge, that question had never been asked previously. Dr. Edwards preceded his answer to the question by describing how the normal three-cuspid aortic valve opens and closes. He demonstrated that the latter does so because the distance between any two commissures (lateral attachments of each independent cusp) along their free margins is greater than a straight line. The greater-than-a-straight-line distance allows each cusp to move to the center of the aortic lumen during ventricular diastole, thus closing the orifice, and move near the wall of the aorta during ventricular systole, thus opening the orifice maximally or nearly so.

So how does a congenitally bicuspid aortic valve open if theoretically the distance between the two commissures across the aortic orifice is a straight line? Dr. Edwards demonstrated that the length of at least one of the two cusps along its free margin is not a straight line but indeed is greater than a straight line. This fact is both its savior and its defeater. It is a "savior" because if at least one of the two cusps was not longer than a straight line, the valve could not open during ventricular systole. That the length of at least one cusp along its free margin is greater than a straight line is also its "defeater" because the elongation allows each cusp to contact the other during ventricular diastole in a traumatic fashion, and that trauma over many years causes the cusps to thicken and eventually to calcify, leading to stenosis. If the cusps do not calcify, pure regurgitation is the usual hemodynamic consequence. Rarely does a congenitally bicuspid valve function normally or near normally during an entire lifetime.

Dr. Edwards also pointed out that a congenitally bicuspid aortic valve was rarely if ever stenotic from birth. The aortic valves that are stenotic from birth are nearly always unicuspid, mainly unicommissural. His publication 50 years ago was a great step forward in our understanding of the congenitally bicuspid aortic valve.

EARLY PUBERTY

According to a study of 1239 girls published in *Pediatrics* in 2010, about 15% of American girls now begin puberty by age 7 (16). One in 10 white girls begin developing breasts by that age—twice the rate seen in a 1997 study. Among black girls, 23% hit puberty by age 7. During the last 30 years, the childhood of girls has been shortened by about 18 months. According to one investigator, girls are being catapulted into adolescence long before their brains are ready for the change, a phenomenon that may pose risk to their health.

Why the age of puberty is falling is unclear. There is no evidence that boys are maturing any earlier. Girls once matured much later than today, probably because poor diets and infectious diseases left them relatively thin. Girls' lack of body fat may have sent a message to their bodies that they weren't yet ready to carry a pregnancy. In the 1840s, for example, girls in Scandinavia did not begin menstruating until age 16 or 17, according to Paul Kaplowitz, the author of *Early Puberty in Girls.* As nutrition and living conditions improved, the age at first menstruation occurred 2 to 3 months earlier each decade. By 1900, American girls were getting their periods at age 14. Although the age at which girls get their first period has continued to fall slowly since then, the age at which girls begin developing breasts has declined much more dramatically. Early puberty increases girls' odds of depression, alcohol use, illicit drug use, eating disorders, behavioral problems, and attempted suicide. When these girls grow up they apparently face a higher risk of breast and uterine cancers, likely because they are exposed to estrogen for a longer period of time.

In only a generation, children have become less connected to nature and in many ways less free. Today's children rarely, if ever, are permitted to roam wild or play outdoors alone out of sight of watchful parents. Schools are eliminating recess as vending machines are installed in school cafeterias. This generation of children is heavier, less active, and more prone to chronic disease and hormonal changes.

The clearest influence on the age of puberty seems to be obesity. In general, obese girls are much more likely to develop earlier than thin ones. And the number of heavy girls is growing. According to the CDC, 30% of children are overweight, many being obese. Obesity raises the level of key hormones, such as insulin, which helps regulate blood sugar, and leptin, a hormone made in fat cells that helps regulate appetite. While leptin may not trigger it, puberty cannot start without it. Prematurity, which has increased 18% since 1990, also may contribute to early puberty. Babies born early or who are very small for their gestational age tend to experience "catch-up growth" that can lead to overweight. Another factor may be environmental chemicals, found in everything from pesticides to flame-retardants and perfume, which can interfere with the hormonal system. Chemicals used to soften plastic called phthalates can act like hormones. Bisphenol A (BPA), which is found in hard plastics, the linings of metal cans, and many other consumer products, causes early puberty in animals. Its role in humans is less clear, but 90% of Americans have BPA in their bodies.

CONSEQUENCES OF REQUESTING "DISPENSE AS WRITTEN"

All US states have adopted generic substitution laws to reduce medication costs. Physicians may override these regulations, however, by prescribing branded drugs and requesting that they be "dispensed as written." Patients also can make these requests. Little is known about the frequency and correlates of "dispense-as-written" requests or their association with medication filling. Shrank and colleagues (17) examined 5.6 million prescriptions for >2 million patients in January 2009. Approximately 2.7% were designated as "dispense as written" by physicians, and 2.0% by patients. Substantial variations in "dispense-as-written" requests were seen by medication class, patient and physician age, and geographic region. The odds of requesting "dispense as written" was 78.5% greater for specialists than for generalists. When chronic prescriptions were initiated, physician "dispense as written" and patient "dispense as written" was associated with greater odds that patients did not fill the prescription. Thus, "dispense as written" requests are common and are associated with decreased rates of prescription filling. Reducing rates of "dispense as written" requests may reduce costs and improve medication adherence.

HIGHWAY DEATHS

Highway deaths have plummeted to their lowest levels in >60 years, helped by more people wearing seatbelts, better safety equipment in cars, and efforts to curb drunken driving (18). The Transportation Department estimated that 32,788 people were killed on US roads in 2010, a decrease of 3% from 2009. It is the lowest number of deaths since 1949 when >30,000 people were killed on US roads. Traffic deaths typically decline during an economic downturn because many motorists cut back on discretionary travel. The number of miles traveled by American drivers in 2010 increased by 20.5 billion or 0.7% compared with 2009, according to the Federal Highway Administration. Separately, the rate of deaths per 100 million miles traveled is estimated to hit a record low of 1.09 in 2010, the lowest since 1949.

WINNING CLOSE CRUCIAL GAMES AND AUTOMOBILE FATALITIES

Researchers from North Carolina and the University of South Carolina found that traffic deaths rise in the hometowns of winning teams on game days, and also that the closer a game is the greater the chance of automobile fatalities (19). The researchers examined data from 271 professional and collegiate football and basketball games from 2001 to 2008, focusing on highly anticipated events such as playoff and rivalry games. They found that the closer the game, the more automobile fatalities there were. The increase in number of fatalities only happened in locations with high numbers of winning fans (game sites and winning hometowns). Prior research has shown that winning fans exhibited sharp increases in testosterone at the end of games while losers exhibited sharp decreases. Increases in testosterone are associated with increased aggressive behavior in both men and women. The researchers found that "going from a blowout to nail-biter" increased fatalities by 133%. They found that the

MOTORCYCLIST DEATHS

In 2010 motorcycle deaths fell for the second straight year to about 4376, according to the Governors Highway Safety Association (20). The decline, however, was much smaller than 2009's 16% drop. The 2010 decline was concentrated in the early months when fewer bikers were on the road, and the death rate rose in the later months. The use of helmets approved by the Department of Transportation dropped 16%. Motorcycle ridership appears to be growing as the economy improves. Thus, there is concern that these fatalities will increase in 2011.

The Governors Highway Safety Association recommends that states take measures to further lower motorcyclist deaths. 1) Increase helmet use, which has been shown to help prevent fatal injuries. (In 2008, 42% of fatally injured bikers were not wearing helmets; 30 states do not require helmets for all motorcyclists.) 2) Reduce impaired driving. (In 2009, 29% of motorcyclists killed in crashes had blood alcohol levels above the legal limit for operating a motorized vehicle.) 3) Reduce speeding, a factor in 35% of motorcycle crashes in 2008, compared with 23% for passenger vehicles and 19% for light trucks. 4) Provide training to all bikers who need or seek it.

These two-wheelers are not for me.

JAPAN—A BEAUTIFUL EXAMPLE

Lee Kuan Yew (21), the former minister of Singapore, described some consequences of the March 11, 2011, earthquake centering on Fukushima and the tsunami that hit the coast of Sendai. The city and neighboring countryside were destroyed. The nuclear meltdown of the Fukushima Daiichi Power Plant followed, causing radiation leaks and contamination. These consequences have severely tested the people of Japan. The Fukushima quake measured 9.0 on the Richter scale. But the Japanese have seen this before. In 1923, an earthquake measuring 7.0 on the Richter scale hit Japan near Kanto, devastating hundreds of miles of coastline, and towns were washed away by mudslides and trains were carried out to sea. Three weeks after the disaster, 260,000 households had no running water and 170,000 had no electricity.

The Fukushima power plant has six reactors, whose cooling systems were interrupted and damaged. Efforts to bring the reactors under control have had some success, but it may take months to bring the reactors to a stable cold shutdown. Building new cooling systems is also expected to take several months.

Northeastern Japan, where the tsunami hit, is also where the ports, steel mills, oil refineries, nuclear power plants, and manufacturers of electronic components are situated. Many of these businesses have been damaged, and nationwide power shortages have decreased auto and electronic production, causing many automobile plants in key production centers to be closed. Global companies, from the makers of semiconductors to shipbuilders, face disruptions to their operations because of the destruction of vital infrastructure and the damage to Japanese factories that

supply high-tech components. Because Japan is the world's third largest economy, the disaster will severely impact the rest of Asia and the global economy for years. The damage to housing and infrastructure is unprecedented. Japan will experience a huge surge in steel imports to build sturdier structures to replace all those that were damaged or destroyed.

Japan's Food Safety Commission has restricted shipments from Fukushima prefecture of vegetables that register higher than permissible levels of radioactive material. Also restricted are shipments of milk. Parents of babies <1 year old are advised not to use tap water for powdered milk or baby formula. As a result, people are buying up supplies of bottled water. The Japanese consume large quantities of seafood; they will need to find alternative food sources because of the damage in the areas where seafood is processed.

Japan's nuclear safety regulatory agency has taken a hard-headed approach to atomic power expansion. About 30% of the nation's electricity output comes from nuclear power. The government's goal was to increase that to 40% by 2020. Without more nuclear power, Japan will experience rampant blackouts in the future.

The Japanese people's comportment under such severe stress has been remarkable. No panic, no looting. A calm, disciplined, and stoic manner has prevailed, with people caring for one another. Few societies could maintain such order and solidarity during a catastrophe of this magnitude. Group interaction and cooperation are the foundation of Japanese society. The whole world has witnessed Japan's dignity and grace in the face of devastation. The capacity to endure the unendurable is the very essence of the Japanese character.

As of April 2, 2011, the number of deaths totaled 11,578, with 16,451 still missing. Since the March 11 earthquake, there have been 800 aftershocks, and these have registered up to >5.0 magnitude. Japanese scientists believe the last time the Sendai region of Japan was hit by an earthquake and tsunami with a magnitude as high as the March 11 event may have been AD 869. Some 18,000 Japanese troops and 7000 Americans have joined Japanese police, firefighters, and Coast Guard to search for bodies along hundreds of miles of the Japanese northeast coast, which was devastated by the tsunami (22). Sixty-five ships were involved in the effort.

How long can radioactivity hang around? Twenty-five years after the Chernobyl nuclear disaster in the Soviet Union, wild boars in Germany are still too radioactive to eat and the mushrooms the pigs dine on are not fit for consumption either (23). The German experience shows what could await Japan if the problems at the Fukushima Daiichi plant get any worse. The German boars roam in forests nearly 1000 miles from Chernobyl. Yet the amount of radioactive Cesium-137 within their tissue often registers dozens of times beyond the recommended limit for consumption and thousands of times above normal. Cesium's half-life is roughly 30 years. Cesium in high levels is thought to be a risk for various cancers. Nevertheless, an increase in cancers that might be linked to cesium has not occurred in Europe. Cesium also accumulates in the soil, which makes boars most susceptible. They snuffle through forest soil with their snouts and feed on the kinds of mushrooms that tend to store radioactive material. Japan's Fukushima plant so far has not leaked nearly as much radiation as Chernobyl, but authorities there have banned the sale of milk, spinach, cabbage, and other products from surrounding regions as a precaution.

NUCLEAR VS. COAL

According to Holman W. Jenkins Jr. (24), an UN-monitoring project has found no scientific evidence for an increase in overall cancer incidence or mortality rates among residents of the Chernobyl region in Russia, aside from a serious uptick in curable thyroid cancer among those exposed as children. But which is safer: nuclear or coal? Thousands more die in coal mine accidents each year (especially in China) than have been killed in all nuclear-related accidents since the beginning of nuclear power. Additionally, coal plants spew toxins like mercury and other metals—along with more radioactive thorium and uranium than a nuclear plant—which are no less amenable to elimination than from a nuclear plant. In 2004, the Environmental Protection Agency estimated that a new emission standard then being proposed would by itself save 17,000 lives a year. Jenkins has convinced me that if nuclear plants are placed in relatively safe areas, not on the Pacific Rim where earthquakes are common, they are safer over the long haul than is coal.

A METEOROLOGICAL AUTOPSY

A number of meteorologists have gathered to study the consequences of the monstrous tornados that struck some areas in the South in late April 2011 (25). They surveyed damage from the ground and air, asking questions about the buildings that were destroyed. Were they brick, wood, or a combination? Were they secured to a slab or set on concrete blocks? What type of roofs did they have? Answers to those questions will help explain how strong the twisters were. A mobile home, for example, will be demolished by winds of 110 to 136 mph. A well-built home can withstand much stronger winds. One meteorologist for the Weather Service's southern region headquarters in Fort Worth, Texas, likened a roof with a large overhang to a baseball cap with a brim; wind blowing in your face will press on the brim and lift the hat off, and the same can happen with a house. Assessing damage becomes more complicated as the meteorological investigators move along the track of a tornado. Once structures start to break apart, the wind collects debris and then they are moving grinders that impact all downstream structures. These investigators tried to determine if there was one tornado criss-crossing the entire state of Alabama or more than one. If it was a single twister, it would be one of the longest on record, rivaling a 1925 tornado that raged for nearly 220 miles. Thus, living in sturdy houses or buildings potentially saves lives and lowers medical costs.

In contrast to the civility of the Japanese toward one another after their recent earthquake and tsunami, the reaction of some citizens in the destroyed towns in the South after the recent tornado was striking. In Tuscaloosa, Alabama, and other cities, looters have been picking through the wreckage to steal the little the victims have left. One citizen remarked, "The first night they

took my jewelry, my watch, my guns. . . . They were out here again last night doing it again." Overwhelmed Tuscaloosa police imposed a curfew and got help from National Guard troops to try to stop the scavenging.

Along their flattened paths, the twisters blew down police and fire stations and other emergency buildings along with homes, businesses, churches, and power infrastructures. The number of buildings lost, damage estimates, and number of people left homeless were enormous. Tuscaloosa's emergency management center was destroyed. A fire station in nearby Alberta City, one of the city's worst-hit neighborhoods, was destroyed. The firefighters survived, but damage to their equipment forced them to begin rescue operations without a fire truck. A Salvation Army building was destroyed, costing Tuscaloosa much-needed shelter space. The Federal Emergency Management Agency, of course, has responded to all affected areas and has officials on the ground in Alabama, Mississippi, Kentucky, Georgia, and Tennessee. The death toll has reached well over 350, and almost 75% of the deaths occurred in Alabama.

MACONDO EXPLOSION A YEAR LATER

After BP's Macondo well in the Gulf of Mexico blew out in April 2010, many feared that the resulting oil spill would turn the Gulf into a dead sea, destroy its beaches, kill its vibrant seafood and tourism industries, and mortally wound the economies of states from Florida to Texas (26). It didn't happen. The spill's long-term effects on the environment are still a serious question, but the Gulf turned out to be surprisingly resilient, and so far the news has been unexpectedly good. Most of the oil is gone. Fishing has resumed, the beaches are clean (with a few exceptions), tourists' bookings are up, and Gulf seafood is safe to eat.

The most important change in the past year was the death of the illusion that the oil industry is infallible—a conviction built by 40 years without a major drilling-related accident in US waters. The Macondo accident, which killed 11 men and took 87 days to bring under control, will cost BP an estimated $40 billion. The accident resulted in shutting down temporarily most deep-water drilling operations in the Gulf, and only about half of them have been allowed to resume drilling. The new process for obtaining permits has been slowed enormously. Local economies that depend on Gulf drilling are suffering from this slow-motion recovery. If another such accident occurred, deep sea drilling would probably be finished. Someday, as an editorial in *USA Today* indicated, the roughly 250 million vehicles on US highways might be able to run on clean energy, but until then, drilling in deep water will be essential for a nation that now buys half its oil from the volatile world market. It is crucial that we drill safely, and it's also crucial that we drill.

Where did all the oil go? Government and university scientists are still trying to reach consensus on where all the oil went. Some of the oil was eaten by microbes, and some of it ended up or will become imbedded on the seafloor or on beaches or marshes. The heavier stuff will wash up on beaches 20 years from now, according to physical oceanographer Robert Weisberg of the University of South Florida. Even the amount of oil that was spilled remains a mystery. Federal officials estimated the amount at >200 million gallons of crude.

What are the health effects of the Deepwater Horizon oil spill? Immediate physical problems linked to the spill have not materialized. Lichtveld and colleagues (27) are especially concerned about the effect that eating potentially contaminated seafood might have on pregnant women and their babies.

METROPOLITAN AREA POPULATION GAINS

According to 2010 Census data released in April 2011, Dallas–Fort Worth–Arlington is the fourth largest metropolitan area in the USA, with nearly 6.4 million persons (28). During the decade of 2000 to 2010, its population increased 23.4%. During the last decade, Houston–Sugar Land–Baytown grew 26.1% (to nearly 6 million); San Antonio grew 25.2% (to 2.2 million); and Austin–Round Rock grew 27.3% (to 1.7 million). Ten of the 51 largest metropolitan areas grew faster than did the Dallas–Fort Worth–Arlington area in the last decade. Areas with the greatest increases in population were Las Vegas–Paradise and Raleigh–Cary, NC, which both increased 41.8%. In contrast, the New York–Northern New Jersey–Long Island population is nearly 19 million, and it grew only 3.1% during the last decade.

THE WORLD'S MEGA CITIES

There are 22 cities with ≥10 million people living in them (29): Paris, 10 million; Cairo, Istanbul, Lagos, Moscow, and Osaka, 11; Beijing, Manila, and Rio de Janeiro, 12; Buenos Aires, Karachi, and Los Angeles, 13; Dhaka and Kinshasa, 15; Kolkata, 16; Shanghai, 17; Mexico City, 19; New York City, 19.4; Mumbai, 20; San Paulo, 20.3; Delhi, 22; and Tokyo, 36.7. By 2025, the following cities (with present-day populations) also will be >10 million: Bogota, 9 million; Lima, 9; Lahore, 7; Jakarta, 9; Chongqing, 9.4; Shenzhen, 9; and Guangzhou, 9. It is these megacities where the growth is, and as they get bigger almost surely health will get worse. A population of 1 million used to be a large city.

FIGHTING AND DRINKING

I am not advocating alcohol, but as Bob Lynn, Alaska state representative and Vietnam veteran, advocates, "If you get shot at, you can have a shot" (30). His effort is to establish a drinking age of 18 for active-duty service members. It's an idea that has gotten consideration in other states, and it makes sense. Unfortunately, Mr. Lynn's proposal would violate the 1984 Federal Uniform Drinking Age Act. The "old enough to fight, old enough to drink" argument has force. In fact, 18-year-olds in the USA are old enough to do pretty much everything except drink alcohol. They can join the military, marry, sign contracts, and take student loans. Colleges encourage students to go into six-figure debt—which can't be discharged in bankruptcy—but forbid them to drink alcohol on campus because they are deemed insufficiently mature to appreciate the risk. To be fair, as Glenn Harland Reynolds writes, over 130 college presidents, as part of something called the Amethyst Initiative, have called for an end to the drinking age of 21.

The higher drinking age, of course, does not stop college students from drinking. It drives drinking out of bars and restaurants and into dorm rooms and fraternity houses, where there is less supervision from the nonintoxicated and less encouragement for moderation. Defenders of the status quo claim that highway deaths have fallen since the drinking age was raised to 21 from 18, but those claims obscure the fact that this decline merely continued a trend that was already present before the drinking age change—one that involved every age group, not just those 18 to 21.

What is really going on here is prohibition. A nation that cares about freedom—and that has already learned that prohibition was a failure—should know better. As *Atlantic Monthly* columnist Megan McArdle writes, "A drinking age of 21 is an embarrassment to a supposedly liberty-loving nation. If you are old enough to enlist, and old enough to vote, you are old enough to swill cheap beer in the company of your peers."

Alcohol is dangerous, as we all know, but so are governmental restrictions.

T. R. AND FOOTBALL

Head injuries are common, of course, in football. John Miller (31) reports that in the early 1900s, President Theodore Roosevelt inserted himself in the fight over violence in football and possibly saved the game, if not from extinction then at least from regulation to second-tier status in the world of athletics. Today, a major problem is concussions (32). One study sponsored by the National Football League found that professional football veterans >50 years of age are 5 times as likely as the general population to suffer from dementia.

These numbers are bad, but consider the situation in 1905 when 18 people died on the gridiron. Back then, critics likened the game to gladiator combat in Roman amphitheaters and launched a crusade to decrease its violence. Led by President Charles Eliot of Harvard and joined by the *Nation* magazine and muckraking journalists, progressive-era prohibitionists wanted to eliminate the increasingly popular sport. At one point, Harvard, Columbia, Northwestern, Stanford, the University of California, and several smaller colleges quit playing the game. Following the 1897 death of Richard Von Gammon, a fullback at the University of Georgia, the Georgia state legislature voted to ban football. The governor vetoed the bill after hearing from Gammon's mother, who urged him not to outlaw a sport that her son had loved. Written in a 1905 report, Harvard's President Eliot was adamant: "No honorable sport embraces the barbarous ethics of warfare." Roosevelt had little patience for such talk. "Harvard will be doing the baby act if she takes any such foolish course as President Eliot advises," he wrote. Roosevelt worried about producing "mollycoddles instead of vigorous men." T. R.'s interest dated back to 1876, when as an 18-year-old Harvard freshman he watched the second-ever game between his school and Yale. He never played football but became an enthusiastic fan. He thought football served a meaningful role in the socialization of boys, helping turn them into men.

Roosevelt, of course, became a noted outdoorsman and war hero in the 1880s and 1890s. He ranched in the Dakotas, hunted big game, and led the Rough Riders to victory in Cuba. In his memoir of the Spanish-American war, T. R. indicated that when he recruited his army unit he was looking for cowboys and football players. (He recruited his Rough Riders in San Antonio.)

In 1899, T. R. gave his famous speech on the cultivation of national virtues, "The Strenuous Life." When he revised those remarks for a children's magazine, he urged boys to play sports because they "had an excellent effect in increased manliness." He paid special attention to football: "In short, in life, as in a football game, the principle to follow is: Hit the line hard; don't foul and don't shirk, but hit the line hard!"

In 1905, Roosevelt took up brutality in football. He called a private meeting at the White House and invited Yale's Walter Camp—football's legendary founding father—and coaches from Harvard and Princeton. T. R. told them, "Football is on trial. Because I believe in the game I want to do all I can to save it." Without dictating a solution, Roosevelt urged the men to take a critical look at the sport. That winter with a little additional nudging from the president, they formed the National Collegiate Athletic Association. They also passed a series of rule changes: they increased the number of yards needed for a first down from 5 to 10, created a neutral zone at the line of scrimmage, and legalized the forward pass. It took a few years to perfect the new rules, but the forward pass changed the way the sport was played. Deaths and injuries subsided as football abandoned its rugby-like origins and became a distinctly American game.

MARATHON RUN

Kenyan Geoffrey Mutal recorded the fastest marathon time ever on April 18, 2011. He won the Boston Marathon in 2:03:02 hours, nearly 3 minutes faster than the previous Boston record and speedier than the 2008 world record of 2:03:59. Running those 26.2 miles in 123 minutes means an average of 4.69 miles/minute. When I was in high school, that time would win the 1-mile race!

WARREN BUFFET PRINCIPLES

The chief executive of a Berkshire Hathaway company told Al Lewis, columnist for Dow Jones Newswires in Denver, that Warren Buffet demanded three things of him: intelligence, energy, and integrity (33). "He said the third part was the most important because the last thing he wanted was a very bright, high-energy crook running one of his companies," Jerry Henry said in a 2003 interview. Mr. Henry was then CEO of Johns Manville, a building products company in Denver, a part of Berkshire Hathaway.

Al Lewis' column, of course, was prompted by Mr. Buffet's disclosure that one of his executives, David Sokol, had resigned after he had invested more than $10 million of his own money in Lubrizol and then recommended to Mr. Buffet that Berkshire Hathaway buy the company—netting a personal profit of $3 million. Mr. Buffet whitewashed Mr. Sokol's blazingly obvious ethical lapse in a written statement. Anyone who owns Berkshire Hathaway stock and receives Buffet's annual report will see how an episode such as the Sokol one could result in such a quick "retirement."

Berkshire Hathaway consists of 76 companies, and Mr. Buffet sends a memo to each of the company managers, whom he calls the "All Stars," every 2 years. Excerpts from his July 26, 2010, letter follow (34):

> As I've said in these memos for more than 25 years: "We can afford to lose money—even a lot of money. But we can't afford to lose reputation—even a shred of reputation." We must continue to measure every act against not only what is legal but also what we would be happy to have written about on the front page of a national newspaper in an article written by an unfriendly but intelligent reporter.

> Sometimes your associates will say "Everybody else is doing it." This rationale is almost always a bad one if it is the main justification for a business action. It is totally unacceptable when evaluating a moral decision. . . . If anyone gives this explanation, tell them to try using it with a reporter or a judge and see how far it gets them.

> If you see anything whose propriety or legality causes you to hesitate, be sure to give me a call. However, it's very likely that if a given course of action evokes such hesitation, it's too close to the line and should be abandoned. . . .

> Somebody is doing something today at Berkshire that you and I would be unhappy about if we knew of it. That's inevitable: We now employ more than 250,000 people and the chances of that number getting through the day without any bad behavior occurring is nil. But we can have a huge effect in minimizing such activities by jumping on anything immediately when there is the slightest odor of impropriety. Your attitude on such matters, expressed by behavior as well as words, will be the most important factor in how the culture of your business develops. Culture, more than rule books, determines how an organization behaves.

Pretty good principles.

CIVIL WAR'S 150TH ANNIVERSARY

April 2011 marked the 150th anniversary of the beginning of the Civil War. Over the next 4 years, battlefields and other historic sites across the country will host commemorations, celebrations, and reenactments. Elizabeth Samet, who teaches English at West Point, had a good piece on Ulysses S. Grant, who wrote his memoirs while dying of throat cancer (35). He composed much of it in a cottage at Mount McGregor, New York, now a state historic site on the grounds of a correctional facility. On display is the bed in which Grant died, as well as floral arrangements from his funeral, clothing, personal effects, and a bottle of the narcotics prescribed to dull his pain. Grant wanted to finish the book to save his family from bankruptcy and establish his written legacy. His extraordinary concentration allowed completion of the book, *Personal Memoirs of Ulysses S. Grant*, which was published about 6 months after Grant died on July 23, 1885.

Several years ago I visited the General Grant National Memorial, aka Grant's Tomb, which was dedicated in 1897. The mausoleum was once, as the historian Joan Waugh documents, "a sacred pilgrimage" for Civil War veterans and remained New York City's most popular attraction through the beginning of World War I. As late as 1929, tourists still visited in large numbers. Today, a visitor is alone there. When I visited with several of my offspring, we were the only ones in sight. The crypt by the sarcophagi containing Grant and his wife, Julia, is encircled by the bronze busts of five Union generals: Sherman, Sheridan, McPherson, Thomas, and Ord.

Grant wrote in his memoirs that after the first bloody day at Shiloh, he made his headquarters under a tree in a drenching rain. He moved for a time to a nearby cabin that had been turned into a field hospital: "All night wounded men were being brought in, their wounds dressed, a leg or an arm amputated as the case might require and everything being done to save life or alleviate suffering. The sight was more unendurable than encountering the enemy's fire, and I returned to my tree in the rain."

One of Grant's staff officers, Horace Porter, characterized the style of his commander's orders and dispatches as "vigorous and terse, with little of ornament; its most conspicuous characteristic was perspicuity." This, as Elizabeth Samet writes, is also an apt description of the *Memoirs*, which many writers from Matthew Arnold to Gertrude Stein have deeply admired.

Now, 126 years have passed since Grant's death and we are at war again: in Afghanistan and Iraq and Libya. Other fighting occurs in Egypt, Yemen, Syria, Tunisia, Bahrain, Iran, and the Ivory Coast, to name a few. General George Marshall observed: "If man does find the solution for world peace it will be the most revolutionary reversal of his record we have ever known."

WHY THE CIVIL WAR STILL MATTERS

James M. McPherson, the George Henry Davis Professor of History Emeritus at Princeton University and the winner of the 1989 Pulitzer Prize for *Battle Cry of Freedom: The Civil War Era,* had a piece in the spring 2011 issue of *American Heritage* entitled "Why the Civil War Still Matters." He asks, "Why do we care about a war that ended so long ago?" He writes (36):

Part of the answer lies in the continental scope of a conflict fought not on some foreign land but on battlefields ranging from Pennsylvania to New Mexico and from Florida to Kansas, hallowed ground that Americans can visit today. The near-mythical figures who have come to represent the war intrigue us still: Abraham Lincoln and Robert E. Lee, Ulysses S. Grant and Thomas J. "Stonewall" Jackson, William T. Sherman and Nathan Bedford Forrest, Clara Barton and Belle Boyd.

Most important, the sheer drama of the story, the momentous issues at stake, and the tragic, awe-inspiring human cost of the conflict still resonate. More than 620,000 Union and Confederate soldiers gave their last full measure of devotion in the war, nearly as many as the number of American soldiers killed in all the other wars this country has fought—combined.

Americans in both North and South were willing to fight on despite such horrific casualties because their respective nations and societies were at stake. Would America move toward a free-labor capitalist economy and a democratic polity in all regions, or would a slave-labor plantation economy and a hierarchical society persist in half of the country?

The war of 1861–1865 resolved two festering questions that the Revolution of 1776 and the Constitution of 1789 had left unresolved: whether this fragile republican experiment called the United States would survive as one nation, indivisible; and whether this nation born of a declaration that all men are created with an equal right to liberty would persist as the largest slave-holding country in the world. Many Americans, painfully aware of the unhappy fate of most republics through history, worried whether theirs would also be swept into the dustbin of history. Before the Civil War, some Americans had advocated the right of secession and periodically threatened to invoke it; eleven states did invoke it in 1860–61. But since 1865 no state or responsible political leader has seriously threatened secession. . . .

In 1854 Abraham Lincoln said that the "monstrous injustice of slavery . . . deprives our republican example of its just influence in the world—enables the enemies of free institutions, with plausibility, to taunt us as hypocrites." Since 1865 that particular "monstrous injustice" has existed no more.

MORE ON FEDERAL BORROWING

Thomas G. Donlan (37), writing in *Barron's,* points out the following: "All federal revenues—from income taxes, Social Security, and Medicare payroll taxes, corporate taxes, excise taxes, customs duties, estate and gift taxes and user fees—are consumed to pay Americans myriad federal benefits. These include Social Security, Medicare, Medicaid, veterans' benefits, food stamps, farm subsidies and the many other forms of social insurance and welfare, including economic stimulus and job-creation." In other words, the federal government borrows everything it needs to operate as a government, such as defense, highway construction, foreign aid, aid to states and localities, land management, pollution control, various regulations, scientific research, payment of federal employees' salaries, and payment of interest on the national debt. All of this is being borrowed! The US Treasury now owes 61% more than it did in March 2007, having issued $5.4 trillion in new debt during that period.

According to Donlan, the only thing that is saving us presently is the low interest rates that the federal government is paying to borrow all this money. When interest rates go up, they will be the fastest-growing budget item in the federal government. And they have no way to go but up.

OXYMORON

An oxymoron is usually defined as a phrase in which two words of opposite meaning are brought together. A friend recently sent me this list: clearly misunderstood; exact estimate; small crowd; act naturally; found missing; fully empty; pretty ugly; seriously funny; only choice; original copies; and happily married.

—William Clifford Roberts, MD
5 May 2011

1. Marsa L. The hot zone. *Discover,* December 2010, pp. 38–44.
2. Kim T, McCann I. Settling the water hog debate. *Dallas Morning News,* April 30, 2011.
3. Appleton R. High-tech study finds that Dallas has nearly five trees per person. *Dallas Morning News,* April 8, 2011.
4. Kivimäki M, Batty GD, Hamer M, Ferrie JE, Vahtera J, Virtanen M, Marmot MG, Singh-Manoux A, Shipley MJ. Using additional information on working hours to predict coronary heart disease: a cohort study. *Ann Intern Med* 2011;154(7):457–463.
5. Hsia J, Macfadyen JG, Monyak J, Ridker PM. Cardiovascular event reduction and adverse events among subjects attaining low-density lipoprotein cholesterol <50 mg/dl with rosuvastatin: the JUPITER trial (Justification for the Use of Statins in Prevention: an Intervention Trial Evaluating Rosuvastatin). *J Am Coll Cardiol* 2011;57(16):1666–1675.
6. Adams J. Double-down dieting with calorie labeling. *Wall Street Journal,* April 2–3, 2011.
7. Swallow your outrage. Let quality of Heart Attack Grill decide its fate. *Dallas Morning News,* April 2, 2011.
8. Ingraham AM, Cohen ME, Bilimoria KY, Ko CY, Hall BL, Russell TR, Nathens AB. Effect of delay to operation on outcomes in adults with acute appendicitis. *Arch Surg* 2010;145(9):886–892.
9. When painkillers kill 2 people every hour, it's time to act. *USA Today,* April 25, 2011.
10. McGuire C. No to prescription monitoring. *USA Today,* April 25, 2011.
11. Roberson J. C-sections may increase health costs. *Dallas Morning News,* April 30, 2011.
12. The march of health progress. *Wall Street Journal,* March 25, 2011.
13. Beck M. When a cuddly crib puts the baby in danger: new construction standards take effect in June, but rules don't cover risk of bedding, toys to infants under 1-year old. *Wall Street Journal,* April 19, 2011.
14. O'Donnell J. Deadly debate over crib bumpers. Industry report backs them, but advocates insist they're unsafe. *USA Today,* April 25, 2011.
15. Edwards JE. The congenital bicuspid aortic valve. *Circulation* 1961;23:485–488.
16. Szabo L. Puberty too soon: girls maturing faster than ever, and doctors aren't sure why. *USA Today,* April 11, 2011.
17. Shrank WH, Liberman JN, Fischer MA, Avorn J, Kilabuk E, Chang A, Kesselheim AS, Brennan TA, Choudhry NK. The consequences of requesting "dispense as written." *Am J Med* 2011;124(4):309–317.
18. Associated Press. Highway deaths fall to 60-year low. *Dallas Morning News,* April 2, 2011.
19. Copeland L. Nail-biters could kill a sports fan. *USA Today,* April 25, 2011.
20. Copeland L. Caution urged even as motorcycle deaths drop. *USA Today,* April 19, 2011.
21. Yew LK. Under extreme stress: Japan's dignity and grace. *Forbes,* May 9, 2011.
22. Associated Press. U.S. troops aid in massive hunt for bodies off coast. *Dallas Morning News,* April 2, 2011.
23. Associated Press. Boars show Chernobyl contamination. *Dallas Morning News,* April 2, 2011.
24. Jenkins HW Jr. Coal is more dangerous than nuclear. *Wall Street Journal,* April 13, 2011.
25. Rubinkam M, Eaton K. Scientists to retrace twisters' path. *Dallas Morning News,* April 30, 2011.
26. Vergano D, Jervis R, Weise E. True measure of damage is murky: despite saturation coverage of BP disaster, answers remain invisible. *USA Today,* April 18, 2011.
27. Goldstein BD, Osofsky HJ, Lichtveld MY. The Gulf oil spill. *N Engl J Med* 2011;364(14):1334–1348.
28. US Census Bureau. 2010 Census and Census 2000.
29. Laneri R. Slumdog millions. *Forbes,* May 9, 2011.
30. Reynolds GH. Old enough to fight, old enough to drink. *Wall Street Journal,* April 12, 2011.
31. Miller JJ. How Teddy Roosevelt saved football. *Wall Street Journal,* April 21, 2011.
32. Brady E, Falgoust JM. Concussions: new game plan. Head injuries now hot issue as leagues toughen policies. *USA Today,* April 13, 2011.
33. Lewis A. Rethinking the Oracle. *Post and Courier,* April 10, 2011.
34. Berkshire Hathaway Inc. *2010 Annual Report.* Available at http://www.berkshirehathaway.com/2010ar/2010ar.pdf; accessed May 5, 2011.
35. Samet E. From Shiloh to Kandahar. *Wall Street Journal,* April 22, 2011.
36. McPherson JM. Why the civil war still matters. *American Heritage,* Spring 2011.
37. Donlan TG. No accounting for benefits. *Barron's,* May 2, 2011.

Chapter 4

October 2011

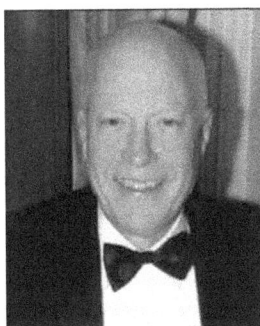

William C. Roberts, MD

DYSTHYMIA

The word was new to me, but according to Melinda Beck, who summarized several articles in medical journals for *The Wall Street Journal*, it is when someone has a dark mood on most days for at least 2 years (1–3). Persistent feelings of hopelessness, irritability, low self-esteem, and low energy are among its signs and symptoms. Even mild depression that is unrelenting can have severe consequences for work, family, and social life, as well as a high risk for suicide.

Researchers at the New York State Psychiatric Institute of Columbia University analyzed government surveys of 43,000 Americans and found that those with dysthymia were more likely to have physical and emotional problems and be on Medicaid or Social Security Disability than those with acute depression. They were also less likely to work full-time. Major depression shares some of the same symptoms, but it is 3 times as common and is more severe. It also tends to come in acute episodes, sometimes requiring hospitalization. Many people with dysthymia do not even realize they are depressed and never mention that feeling to their physicians. Some studies have found that nearly 80% of people with dysthymia also have episodes of major depression—sometimes known as "double depression." People with chronic depression are more likely to attempt suicide than those with more acute forms.

Officially, dysthymia affects only about 1.5% of the US population in any given year and 5% at some point during their lives. The current definition of dysthymia excludes anyone who had an episode of major depression during the past 2 years. Some experts have recommended combining dysthymia, double depression, and chronic major depression into a single category of chronic depression because symptoms often wax and wane over the years. In about half the cases the gloomy moods, chronic pessimism, and low self-esteem begin before age 18, and the disorder can look like shyness or irritability in young children. Dysthymia frequently runs in families, but it is unclear how much of that is due to nature or nurture. Children who suffer abuse or trauma have high rates of dysthymia, often

have trouble in school and in social relationships, and are less likely to get married than their peers.

Dysthymia that starts later in life is often triggered by a major life stress, such as the loss of a job, the death of a loved one, or the break-up of a marriage. It can also masquerade as chronic pain or other physical symptoms, further complicating diagnosis. Like other mood disorders, dysthymia is diagnosed about twice as often in women as in men, but men may simply be more stoic, be less willing to seek help, or attempt to self-medicate.

Dysthymia has not been studied as extensively as major depression, but treatment is generally the same. About one third of people with chronic depression respond briskly to antidepressants. Others try several medications or combinations of them to find relief. Talk therapy has been helpful also for chronic depression. Cognitive behavioral therapy is useful to teach patients to challenge negative thought patterns that bring them down. Treatment for chronic depression also generally takes longer than for the more acute forms. Relapse rates are high, and many people find they need to stay on medication long term. About 25% of people with dysthymia never find relief.

BRAIN SHRINKAGE

Robert Lee Hotz summarized a study in the *Proceedings of the National Academy of Sciences* that highlights what researchers call "the unique character of human aging" (4). The human brain can shrink up to 15% as it ages, a change linked to dementia, poor memory, and depression. Until now, researchers had assumed that this gradual brain loss in later years was universal among primates.

In the first direct comparison of humans to chimpanzees, a brain-scanning team led by anthropologist Chet Sherwood found that chimpanzees do not experience such brain loss. Using magnetic resonance imaging scans to measure changes in five key brain structures involved in memory, reasoning, and other mental processing, as well as overall brain volume, they compared measurements from 87 adult humans, aged 22 to 88 years, with the brain volumes of 99 adult chimps, aged 10 to 51 years. On average, human brains weigh about 3 pounds; chimp brains, about 1 pound. The researchers found that the human brain lost significant volume over time whereas the chimpanzee brain did not. Unlike chimpanzees and other primates, older humans are prey to a host of neurodegenerative diseases such as Alzheimer's disease. Stress, depression, and diet were also found to affect brain size.

Human brain shrinkage may simply be the price our species pays for living so much longer than other primates. Barring serious illness or injury, humans can expect to live about 80 years or more, almost twice the normal lifespan of a chimpanzee in the wild. During those extra decades of life, natural cell-repair mechanisms wear out and neural circuits wither. Natural grooves in the brain widen. Tangles of damaged neurons become dense thickets of dysfunctional synapses. So the chimpanzees have something on us humans.

ALZHEIMER RISK FACTORS

Barnes and Yaffe (5) from the University of California–San Francisco described seven conditions or behaviors that contribute to about 50% of Alzheimer's cases, which number 3 million in the USA and 34 million around the world. With no cure or treatment to reverse the mind-robbing disease, preventing new cases, of course, is crucial. They determined that physical inactivity had a 21% contribution to development of Alzheimer's; depression, 15%; smoking, 11%; hypertension, 8%; obesity, 7%; low education, 7%; and diabetes mellitus, 3%.

INSOMNIA

According to Petersen (6), about 30% of American adults have insomnia symptoms each year. About 10% of the population has chronic insomnia (difficulty sleeping at least 3 times a week for a month or more), leading to feeling tired, cranky, or foggy-headed during the daylight hours. Some people have a tough time falling asleep, others wake in the middle of the night and have trouble getting back to sleep, and still others rise for the day too early. Insomnia can increase the risk for other conditions, including heart disease, diabetes mellitus, and depression.

Americans spent about $2 billion on prescription sleep drugs in 2010. Although the number of prescriptions written rose 23% to about 60 million in 2010 from 49 million in 2006, total dollar sales decreased as generic versions of drugs like Ambien have entered the market. Sales of prescription sleeping pills in 2006 in the USA were $3.6 billion. This cost does not include self-treatment with alcohol or over-the-counter medications, such as Tylenol PM and Benadryl, which contain an antihistamine.

The most common sleep-aid drugs, called benzodiazepine receptor agonists, alter the activity of gamma-aminobutyric acid, a neurotransmitter thought to facilitate sleep. These sedatives slow the brain down and put it to sleep. These drugs have side effects, including daytime drowsiness (the "hangover effect"), memory problems, and balance problems. They can be dangerous when combined with other sedatives like alcohol, and there are some concerns that they can be addictive and abused.

The good news is that several pharmaceutical companies are working on newer approaches to treat insomnia. The compounds are meant to work differently than the current leading sleep-aids such as Ambien and Lunesta, which while generally safe can have troubling side effects. By contrast, many of the drugs being developed target particular systems responsible for sleep and wakefulness. The hope is that they will have fewer side effects and less potential for addiction and cognition problems the next day. Merck and Company is investigating a compound that inhibits the action of orexin receptors, which in turn interfere with the activity of orexin, a chemical in the brain that produces alertness. The company hopes to file for Food and Drug Administration approval by 2012. Other companies are working on similar products.

PREPARING FOR DEATH

George Burns stated something to the effect that we all die but he was looking for another way out. Saabira Chaudhuri (7) has provided a list of 25 documents we all need before we die, and their preparation could save our heirs great frustration and financial pain. These items are a marriage license; divorce papers; personal and family medical history; durable health care power of attorney; authorization to release health care information; living will; do not resuscitate order; housing, land, and cemetery deeds; escrow mortgage accounts; proof of loans made and debts owed; vehicle titles; stock certificates, savings bonds, and brokerage accounts; partnership and corporate operating agreements; tax returns; life insurance policies; individual retirement accounts (IRAs); 401(k) accounts; pension documents; annuity contracts; list of bank accounts; list of all user names and passwords; list of safe deposit boxes; will; letter of instruction; and trust documents.

An original will is the most important document to keep on file. It allows one to dictate who inherits what assets and the guardians for any underage children. Dying without a will means losing control of how one's assets are distributed. Instead, state law will determine what happens. Wills are subject to probate—legal proceedings that take inventory, make appraisals of property, settle outstanding debt, and distribute remaining assets. Not having an original document means this already onerous process could be much more of an ordeal, since family members can challenge a copy of a will in court.

A "letter of instruction" can be a useful supplement to a will, though it does not hold legal weight. It is a good way to make sure one's executor has the names and contact information of one's attorneys, accountants, and financial advisors. While the will should be stored with one's attorney or in a courthouse, the letter of instruction should be more readily accessible, particularly if it contains instructions on funeral arrangements. Heirs should also have access to a durable financial power of attorney form. Without it, no one can make financial decisions on one's behalf if one is incapacitated.

The most recent 3 years of tax returns should be available to one's heirs. These returns offer a snapshot of what assets the heirs should be looking for. These returns also help one's personal representative file a final income tax return and, if necessary, a revocable-trust return.

The most important health care document to fill out in advance is a durable health care power of attorney form. This allows one's designee to make health care decisions on one's behalf if one is incapacitated. The document should be compliant with federal health information privacy laws, so that physicians, hospitals, and insurance companies can speak with the designee. An authorization to release protected health care information is also useful to have.

The living will and the power of attorney constitute what are called "advance directives"; some states consolidate these into a single form. (AARP offers a state-by-state listing of advance directive forms on its website.) Terminally ill patients may wish to have their physicians make a do not resuscitate order.

Copies of life insurance policies are among the most important documents for one's family to have. Family members need to know the name of the carrier, the policy number, and the agent associated with the policy. Chaudhuri cautions that one should be especially careful with life insurance policies granted by an employer upon retirement since those are the kind that financial planners most often miss.

Estate planners also recommend drawing up a list of pensions, annuities, IRAs, and 401(k)s for one's spouse and children. An IRA is considered dormant or unclaimed if no withdrawal has been made by age 70½. According to the National Association of Unclaimed Property Administrators, tens of millions languish in unclaimed IRAs every year. One can track unclaimed pensions, 401(k)s, and IRAs at *Unclaimed.com*.

It is important for a spouse to know the location of the marriage license. For divorced people, it is important to leave behind the divorce judgment and decree or, if the case was settled without going to court, the stipulation agreement. These documents lay out child support, alimony, and property settlements and may also list the division of investment and retirement accounts.

URBAN VS. SUBURBAN VS. RURAL HEALTH

The County Health Rankings, a research project, recently issued its second annual report of state-by-state comparisons of health measures in every US county, and the findings were summarized by Melinda Beck in *The Wall Street Journal* (8). Many cities that were once notorious for pollution, crime, crowding, and infectious diseases have generally cleaned up, while rural problems have festered. Rural residents are now more likely than any other Americans to be obese, be sedentary, and smoke cigarettes. They also have higher rates of diabetes mellitus, stroke, heart disease, and high blood pressure. Although city dwellers have more air pollution, crime, sexually transmitted diseases, low-birthweight babies, and alcoholism, overall urbanites are healthier and are less likely to die prematurely than are rural Americans. In many measures, residents of suburban areas are the best off. They generally rate their own health the highest and have fewer premature deaths than either their urban or rural counterparts. Suburbanites also have the fewest low-birthweight babies, homicides, and sexually transmitted diseases.

Much of the health advantage in cities and suburbs may be a function of age, income, and education levels. The average annual household income in central cities is $53,000 according to the county ranking report, compared with $39,000 in rural areas and $60,000 in suburbs, and rural residents tend to be older and less educated than their urban counterparts. Rural residents also have less access to health care. About 25% of the US population lives in rural areas, but they are served by only 10% of the country's physicians. They are also less likely to have private health insurance, prescription drug coverage, or Medicaid coverage. Rural America is a place where those most in need of health care services often have the fewest options.

Unhealthy habits can start early. Rural children aged 2 to 5 are nearly twice as likely as urban kids to consume 24 ounces of sweetened beverages a day. From age 6 to 11, rural kids consume on average 80 g of fat a day, compared with 73 g for urban children. Patterns of TV watching and physical inactivity are roughly similar between the two groups. Obesity hits the rural areas the hardest. Overall, 19% of rural children aged 2 to 19 are obese, with a body mass index (BMI) >30 kg/m², and 36% of them are overweight, with a BMI of 26 to 30 kg/m². By comparison, 15% of urban kids the same age are obese and 30% are overweight.

Several factors make country living less healthy. Deaths from traffic accidents are more common in rural areas, not just because speed limits are higher, but also because the average emergency medical response to an accident is 18 minutes compared with 10 minutes in urban areas. Country living, of course, has some advantages. Children who grow up on farms tend to have less asthma and fewer allergies and autoimmune disorders than city kids. City dwellers have higher rates of mental health problems than rural residents. People who move from a city environment to the country or vice versa generally bring their health habits with them.

SUDDEN CARDIAC DEATH IN COLLEGE ATHLETES

The National Collegiate Athletic Association (NCAA) consists of a unique group of athletes. In any given year, there are approximately 400,000 student athletes aged 17 to 23 years who compete in 40 sports in three different NCAA divisions. Every institution uses a medical staff, which includes at least a certified athletic trainer, and each institution has a designated media staff. Although there is no mandatory reporting of deaths, NCAA athlete deaths are less likely to go unnoticed or unreported than deaths of other groups of athletes, and media searches may be more likely to identify deaths. In addition, the NCAA publishes records of the number of athletes participating each year in each sport as well as their sex and ethnic makeup.

Harmon and colleagues (9) from Seattle, Washington, and Indianapolis, Indiana, identified deaths among NCAA athletes between January 1, 2004, and December 31, 2008. During the 5-year period, there were a total of 1,969,663 athlete participant-years, with 843,106 female and 1,126,557 male athlete participant-years and 300,835 black and 1,583,635 white athlete participant-years. There were 273 deaths, and 187 (68%) were nonmedical and occurred off the playing field; these included accidents (51%), suicide (9%), homicide (6%), and drug overdose (2%). A cause of death could not be attributed in 6 (2%) of the 273 cases. Medical causes of death numbered 80 (29%), and the 45 with cardiac causes accounted for 56% of the medical deaths.

The risk of death varied by sport. Basketball was by far the highest-risk sport, with an overall annual death rate of 1:11,394. The risk of sudden cardiac death was 1:5743 in black basketball athletes and 1:21,824 in whites per year. There were 36 medical deaths that occurred with exertion. The others either occurred at rest or could not be classified. Of the exertional deaths, 27 of 36 (75%) were related to cardiac causes, with the remaining exertional deaths related to heat stroke. The sports with the next highest overall risk were swimming and lacrosse, followed by football and cross country.

INDOOR TRAMPOLINE PARKS

As of July 2011, about 50 indoor trampoline parks were operating in 12 states, with revenues approaching $100 million (10). The parks, which charge $8 to $14 an hour, feature wall-to-wall trampolines. They may be good exercise, but they are also a good source of broken ankles, arms, legs, and even necks. The American Academy of Orthopedic Surgeons does not recommend recreational use of trampolines. Be careful!

E. COLI, VEGETABLES, AND FRUITS

According to David Rising (11), as of early June 2011, >1800 people in Germany have been sickened by *E. coli* infection, mainly during the month of May. Of those sickened, 520 have had a life-threatening complication (like kidney failure) and 18 have died. The World Health Organization said that as of June 2011, 10 other European nations and the USA have reported 90 people sick with the same bacterium, and all but two of them had recently visited northern Germany. The source of the *E. coli* has been unclear, but raw tomatoes, cucumbers, and lettuce have been the main focus. To avoid food-borne illnesses, the World Health Organization recommends washing hands, keeping raw meat separate from other foods, thoroughly cooking the food, and washing fruits and vegetables, especially if eaten raw. Peeling raw fruits and vegetables is also recommended.

FEEDING A WARMING PLANET

The rapid growth in farm output that defined the late 20th century has slowed to the point that it is failing to keep up with the demand for food. Driven by population increases and rising affluence in once poor countries, consumption of the four staples that supply most human calories—wheat, rice, corn, and soybeans—has outstripped production for most of the past decade, drawing once large stockpiles down to low levels. The imbalance between supply and demand has resulted in two huge spikes in international grain prices since 2007, with some grains more than doubling in cost. Those price jumps, though felt only moderately in the West, have worsened hunger for tens of millions of poor people, destabilizing politics in scores of countries.

The previously discounted climate change is playing a role in the destabilizing of the food system. Many of the failed harvests of the past decade were a consequence of weather disasters, some of which were caused or worsened by human-induced global warming. Temperatures have risen rapidly during the growing season in some of the most important agricultural countries, and this increase has shaved several percentage points off of potential yields, adding to the price gyrations. Farmers everywhere, according to Justin Gillis writing for *The New York Times*, are facing water shortages and flash floods (12). Their crops are afflicted by emerging pests and diseases and by blasts of heat beyond anything that they remember.

The Green Revolution in agriculture several decades ago was led by Norman E. Borlaug, a young US agronomist who helped Mexico increase its wheat production sixfold. (Borlaug won the Nobel Prize in 1970 and is the only agronomist ever to win.) As the output rose, staple grains—which feed people directly or are used to produce meat, eggs, dairy products, and farmed fish—became cheaper and cheaper. Overall, the percentage of hungry people in the world shrank. By the 1980s, food production seemed under control. Governments and foundations began to cut back on agricultural research. During the past 20 years, Western aid for agricultural development in poor countries fell by almost half, with some of the world's most important research centers suffering mass layoffs. The consequence of this loss of focus began to show up in the world's food system toward the end of the last century. Output continued to rise, but fewer innovations were reaching farmers and the growth rate slowed.

That lull occurred just as food and feed demand was starting to take off, thanks in part to rising affluence in much of Asia. Erratic weather began eating into yields, such that the low grain supplies in 2007 and 2008 led to the doubling and in some cases tripling of prices. Whole countries began hoarding food, and panic buying ensued in some markets, notably for rice. Food riots broke out in >30 countries.

Farmers responded to the high prices by planting as much as possible, and healthy harvests in 2008 and 2009 helped rebuild stocks to a degree. That factor plus the global recession drove prices down in 2009. But by 2010, more weather-related harvest failures sent them soaring again. This year, rice supplies seem adequate but bad weather threatens the wheat and corn crops in some areas. Some experts fear that the era of inexpensive food is over. There would be no shortage if most of the grains did not go to feeding the nonhuman animals rather than directly to feeding people.

SHORTENING TIME TO MEDICAL SCHOOL

A program currently being developed will allow students throughout the University of Texas system to start college in 2013 and graduate from medical school in spring 2020, 1 year faster than earlier (13). Presently, medical education is the longest and most expensive of any profession. Students now spend 4 years in college, 4 years in medical school, and then 3 to 7 years more in training in their chosen specialty. For medical school alone, average student debt is $160,000.

The time and cost is considered a factor in the physician shortfall, expected to be 150,000 physicians in 15 years. Texas, the nation's second most populous state, already ranks last in the ratio of physicians to population. When I entered medical school in 1954, many medical schools accepted students who had finished only 3 years of college. The present "innovation" is simply a return to a previous program.

GRADUATE MEDICAL EDUCATION

On June 23, 2010, the Accreditation Council for Graduate Medical Education (ACGME) posted on its website new program requirements for residency training in the US, and these have been summarized by Dr. John W. Caruso of Jefferson Medical College (14). These guidelines contain the duty-hour regulations that will likely frame the work schedules of housestaff for the next decade. The guidelines were highly anticipated by the academic medical community and were heightened by the release in 2008 of the Institute of Medicine report: "Resident duty hours enhancing sleep, supervision and safety." This report raised concerns that the ACGME 2003 duty-hour regulations did not go far enough to ensure the safety of patients and residents. Specifically, the Institute of Medicine identified research models that found safety gains from more restrictive shift lengths and highlighted other industries that have aggressively regulated hours at work and at rest.

The new ACGME guidelines went into effect July 1, 2011. Specific changes to resident duty hours affect all years of postgraduate training. The 2003 requirements allowed for shifts of 24 hours plus an additional 6 hours for educational activities and patient sign-out. This effectively resulted in residents at all levels working for periods of up to 30 consecutive hours. The new guidelines are more restrictive and are differentiated for level of training. For PGY-I residents (interns), duty periods may no longer exceed 16 total hours. For PGY-II residents and above, the new limit is 24 total hours, and it was strongly suggested that this time period include an opportunity for "strategic napping" between the hours of 10:00 PM and 8:00 AM. These upper-level residents will now be allowed only an additional 4 hours for patient transition, instead of the 6 hours in the previous iteration of the duty-hour requirements.

Time off between duty periods is also stipulated by the ACGME requirements. Similar to the earlier regulations, residents must have at least 8 hours off between work periods and "should have 10 hours off." A new component stipulates that these work-free intervals must be >14 hours for upper-year residents following any 24-hour shift. The total limit of 80 hours per week is similar to the 2003 regulations. A new caveat requires all moonlighting activities of residents to be counted against this limit. This stipulation addressed a frequent concern that sleep deprivation of residents was also influenced by activities some individuals pursued outside of their appointed training programs. The requirements for call no more frequently than every third night and 1 day free from duty each week were not changed.

While the duty-hour requirements have generated the most attention, several other new stipulations intended to improve the safety of patient care in a training environment have been instituted. One initiative is outlined within the core competency category of "systems-based practice." Here it is stipulated that residents "must systematically analyze practice using quality improvement methods, and implement changes with the goal of practice improvement." This competency statement further

dictates that residents "work in interprofessional teams to enhance patient safety and improve patient care quality" and also that they "participate in identifying system errors and implementing potential system solutions." The program director must ensure that residents are "integrated and actively participate in interdisciplinary clinical quality improvement and patient-safety programs." Finally, the ACGME added that "residents and faculty members must demonstrate an understanding and acceptance of their personal role in the monitoring of their patient-care performance and improvement indicators."

These requirements will ensure that residency programs go further to involve residents and faculty in safety and quality efforts. The current ACGME requirements are easily satisfied with conferences; programs have most often used the "morbidity and mortality" format to do so. The new requirements will require training programs to make certain that residents are active participants in the process. Creating multidisciplinary efforts will be a new paradigm for many programs, and the monitoring and use of performance indicators for residents will likely be a challenge for some.

Another new focus has been placed on resident sign-outs or handovers ("transitions of care"). The new guidelines ask that programs create clinical schedules that minimize these transitions. It is specified that there be "structured handover processes to facilitate continuity and safety" and that programs ensure that "residents are competent in communicating with team members" in the handover process. These new features will require training programs to develop systems and solutions that are beyond the current norms.

Finally, the ACGME has formally outlined supervision models for residents. The new requirements define these levels as "direct," "indirect," and "oversight." They further outline that PGY-I residents be directly supervised or indirectly supervised, with the latter model allowable only if the supervisor is immediately available. While this intensified need for supervision will be a shift for some programs, it is likely the single most important safety measure to be adopted. It is no longer acceptable for the least experienced team member to make critical decisions without the input of senior residents and faculty. The goal here is to lessen the likelihood of a PGY-I learning of a flawed decision only during teaching rounds that occur hours after the clinical events that ensued.

In summary, the new ACGME requirements go beyond the well-publicized ones intended to ensure that residents are less fatigued. Quality and safety are further stressed in these requirements. Medical life, as in other areas, is getting more and more complicated.

US POPULATION GROWTH

The average number of children among women aged 40 to 44 in the USA among Asians is 1.8; blacks, 2.0; whites, 1.8; and Hispanics, 2.3 (15). The growth of Latinos in the USA, once driven by immigration, is now fueled by births, chiefly by Mexicans and Mexican-Americans, according to a new analysis of US Census Bureau data. The number of Hispanics in the USA has increased 43% since 2000 and more than doubled since

1990. With a population of 50.5 million in 2010, Hispanics now account for nearly 1 in 6 US residents and for 23% of people under the age of 18. The population of Latinos of Mexican origin, who represent nearly two thirds of US Hispanics, grew by 7.2 million between 2000 and 2010 as a result of births and only about 4.2 million due to immigrant arrivals.

In the previous 2 decades, the number of new Mexican immigrants in the US either matched or exceeded the number of births. The current surge in births follows the massive wave of Hispanic immigration to the US that began in the 1970s. The tilts suggest that descendants of immigrants could be the main engine of US population growth for decades to come. It is predicted that >80% of US population growth through 2050 will come mainly from Hispanic immigrants and their children. In 1970, <1 million Mexicans lived in the USA. By 2000, that number had jumped to nearly 10 million, and by 2007, it had reached 12.5 million. Since then, the Mexican population in the US has remained constant because the influx of immigrants has slowed dramatically—400,000 in 2010 compared with about 1 million in 2006. In the last decade, the Hispanic share of the population grew in every US state. Texas' Hispanic population increased 41%, accounting for two thirds of the state's growth.

DECREASING PERCENTAGE OF CHILDREN IN THE US POPULATION

The 2010 census data show that the percentage of children in the US is 24%, falling below the previous low of 26% in 1990 (16). The share is projected to slip to 23% by 2050, even as the percentage of people ≥65 is expected to increase from 13% today to 20% by 2050 because of the aging of baby boomers. In 1900, the share of children reached as high as 40%, compared with a 4% share for those ≥65 years. The percentage of children in subsequent decades was >30% until 1980, when it fell to 28% amid declining birth rates, mostly among whites. With the low percentage of children now, this generation will grow up to become a shrinking workforce that will have to support the nation's expanding elderly population—bad news for health care, pensions, and other programs.

The children of immigrants make up one in four people <18 years of age in the US and are the fastest growing segment of the nation's youth, an indication that both legal and illegal immigrants as well as minority births are lifting the nation's population. Nationwide, the number of children has grown by 1.9 million, or 2.6%, since 2000. That represents a drop-off from the previous decade, when even higher rates of immigration by Latinos, who are more likely than other ethnic groups to have large families, helped increase the number of children by 8.7 million, or nearly 14%.

Twenty-three states and the District of Columbia had declines in the number of children in the first 10 years of this century, with Michigan, Rhode Island, Vermont, and the District of Columbia seeing some of the biggest drops. In contrast, states with some of the biggest increases—Texas, Arizona, Florida, Georgia, Nevada, and North Carolina—also ranked in the bottom third of states in terms of child well-being (levels of poverty,

single-parent families, unemployment, high-school dropouts, and other factors).

The slowing population growth in the US mirrors to a lesser extent the situation in other developed nations, including Russia, Japan, and France, which are seeing reduced growth or population losses due to declining birth rates and limited immigration. Depending on future rates of immigration, the US population is estimated to continue growing through at least 2050. Currently, 54% of the nation's children are non-Hispanic white, while 23% are Hispanic, 14% black, and 4% Asian. Over the past decade, the number of non-Hispanic white children declined 10% to 40 million, while the number of minority children rose 22% to nearly 35 million.

EXTREME CHILDHOOD OBESITY

A piece in the July 13, 2011, *Journal of the American Medical Association* argues that parents of extremely obese children should lose custody for not controlling their kid's weight (17). The journal piece argues that putting children temporarily in foster care is in some cases more ethical than obesity surgery. University of Pennsylvania bioethicist Art Kaplan argues that the debate risks putting too much blame on parents. Obese children are victims, he opines, of advertising, marketing, peer pressure, and bullying—things that parents cannot control. Roughly 2 million US children are extremely obese. Their obesity-related conditions, such as type 2 diabetes mellitus, breathing difficulties, and liver problems, might kill them by age 30. It is these kids for whom state intervention, including education, parent training, and temporary protective custody in the most extreme cases, should be considered.

AGING AND GAINING WEIGHT

Because gaining weight is so common in our population, many believe it is a normal part of getting older. Mozaffarian and colleagues (18) studied the weight, eating, and living habits of nearly 121,000 men and women from the Nurses' Health Study and the Health Professionals Follow-Up Study. Participants were tracked every 4 years for 20 years. They gained an average of 3.35 pounds over the 4-year periods and almost 17 pounds over the 20-year period. People who made the most unhealthy dietary changes gained nearly 4 pounds more in 4 years than those who had the healthiest dietary changes. People who ate an extra serving of chips a day gained an average of 1.7 pounds more in 4 years than those who didn't eat that extra serving. People who drank one more sugar-sweetened beverage added an extra pound more in 4 years than those who didn't. Other factors also led to weight gain: decreased physical activity, increased alcohol intake, <6 or >8 hours of sleep a night, and increased television viewing. And it's more than just watching the fat intake. Some foods such as nuts that are high in fat helped prevent weight gain. Other foods that are generally low in fat, such as white bread and low-fiber cereal, contributed to weight gain. People who increased their physical activity gained less weight than those who didn't. There are clearly healthy foods, less healthy foods, and the least healthy foods, and all of us must make the choices.

MOSQUITOES DYING FROM BITING HUMANS

Ivermectin, an inexpensive deworming pill used in Africa for 25 years against river blindness, was recently shown by Kobylinski and associates (19) to have a power that scientists had long suspected but never before demonstrated: mosquitoes die when they bite people who have recently swallowed the drug. While the mosquito-poisoning tool is effective, it is not very practical: for it to work effectively, nearly everyone in a mosquito-infested area must take the pill simultaneously. And, getting thousands of villagers to do that is a logistical nightmare. The mosquito effect appears to fade out within a month, so it would need to be repeated monthly. The investigators vacuumed mosquitoes from the walls of huts in three villages whose inhabitants had recently been given ivermectin and in three villages whose inhabitants had not and tested to see how many mosquitoes had malaria parasites. The ivermectin villages had almost 80% fewer. Interestingly, only older mosquitoes transmit malaria since they must get it first from humans.

THE WAR ON DRUGS

The Global Commission on Drug Policy, a 19-member panel chaired by former Brazilian President Fernando Henrique Cardoso, has declared America's "war on drugs" a failure with "devastating consequences for individuals and societies around the world" (20). The commission's report was released in June 2011 and recommended "far reaching changes including . . . decriminalization and experiments in legal regulations."

In July 2011, Representatives Barney Frank and Ron Paul introduced a bill in Congress to remove marijuana from the list of federally controlled substances, leaving it up to the states to decide if they wanted to legalize it. As Joseph A. Califano Jr. and William J. Bennett argue in *The Wall Street Journal*, legalization will only make harmful substances cheaper, easier to obtain, and more socially acceptable to use (20). The US has some 60 million smokers, 20 million alcoholics and alcohol abusers, and 21 million illicit drug users (over 7 million of whom are addicts). If illegal drugs were easier to obtain, the latter figure would rise sharply. Moreover, these two authors argue that more readily available drugs would increase criminal activity. Most violent crimes, such as murder, assault, and rape, occur when the perpetrator is either on drugs or drunk, and a high percentage of property crime involves people seeking money to buy drugs and alcohol.

Approximately 30% of our federal and state health care spending is attributable to the use and abuse of addictive substances, including tobacco, alcohol, and illegal drugs. The National Center on Addiction and Substance Abuse at Columbia University (CASA) estimated the total financial cost to taxpayers to be $500 billion annually. The human misery is incalculable. Increased use of illegal drugs will increase these costs and this misery.

A Medicaid patient with drug and alcohol problems costs $5000 to $15,000 a year more in health care costs than one without such problems. Most Medicaid hospital patients readmitted within 30 days are those with drug and alcohol problems.

The notion that taxing sales of marijuana and drugs like cocaine and heroin will provide a windfall for our public coffers also is illusory. For every $1 of taxes collected from the sale of tobacco and alcohol, we incur $9 in state and federal health care, criminal justice, and social service costs. These costs will skyrocket if legalization becomes the norm, draining our public coffers at an even more alarming rate.

Legalization in other countries has had disastrous results. In the 1990s, Switzerland experimented with what became known as Needle Park, a section of Zurich where addicts could buy and inject heroin without police interference. Policymakers saw it as a way to restrict a few hundred legal heroin users to a small area. It soon morphed into a grotesque tourist attraction of 20,000 addicts that had to be closed before it infected the entire city. In the Netherlands, where marijuana can be bought in "coffee shops," adolescent use, citizen anger, and international irritation have soared. Responding to the outcry from its own citizens and from other countries, the Dutch government has reduced the number of marijuana shops, limited the amount that can be purchased, and raised the age of legal buyers to 18 from 16. In May 2011, the Dutch government also announced that it will prohibit tourists from purchasing marijuana at "coffee shops" by the end of 2011.

Facing an onslaught of angry citizens whose neighborhoods were overrun with marijuana users, the Los Angeles City Council in 2010 closed 437 of the 1000 or more "medical marijuana shops" that opened after California's medical marijuana law passed in 1996.

Sweden provides an example of a successful restrictive drug policy. Faced with rising drug use in the 1990s, the government tightened drug control, stepped up police action, mounted a national action plan, and created a national drug coordinator. The result: drug use is a third of the European average.

Califano and Bennett strongly support greater emphasis on prevention and public health initiatives to reduce drug use, especially among children and teens. They argue that legalization, a policy certain to increase illegal drug availability and use among the nation's children, hardly qualifies as sound prevention. The facts are indisputable: 20 years of CASA research shows that a child who reaches 21 without using illegal drugs is virtually certain never to do so. Unfortunately, the US has shown little capacity to keep our two legal drugs, tobacco and alcohol, out of the hands of children and teens. There is little reason to believe that we can legalize drugs like marijuana, cocaine, and heroin only for adults and keep them away from children and teenagers. Califano and Bennett conclude: "We must remember one thing: drugs are not dangerous because they are illegal; they are illegal because they are dangerous."

These two individuals should know what they are talking about. Mr. Califano is the founder and chairman of the National Center on Addiction and Substance Abuse, and Mr. Bennett was secretary of education during the Reagan administration and the first director of the Office of National Drug Control Policy during the George H. W. Bush administration.

SYNTHETIC PSYCHOACTIVE DRUGS

Packaged and sold as innocent products such as "herbal incense" and "bath salts," synthetic psychoactive drugs are touted by users as legal alternatives to marijuana, cocaine, and other controlled substances that can bring stiff penalties and jail time (21). The bath salts are psychoactive stimulants that mimic cocaine, amphetamines, and other drugs. The synthetic marijuana includes JWH-O18, sprayed on potpourri or herbs to mimic marijuana. Some research chemicals are psychedelics, including 2C-E and similar chemicals that mimic LSD and other drugs.

But, the consequences of using these alternative products are proving to be devastating. According to Pam Louwagie, poison control centers have received >6000 calls about designer synthetics in 2011, 10 times more than in the first half of 2010. Synthetic drugs have been linked to or suspected in 20 deaths nationally in the past year. Emergency rooms are treating more patients who have overdoses on sometimes tiny amounts. The severity of the cases is what makes it so bad. The symptoms are severe and people are a threat not only to themselves but to those around them.

The new drugs are easy to find. Merchants promote the drugs on the Internet, and some are available on the shelves of record stores and smoke shops. Authorities believe the drugs are often manufactured by rogue chemists in foreign countries. Federal officials say many of the new designer drugs are already illegal under existing laws. To strengthen the hands of police and prosecutors, lawmakers in Washington, DC, and in many state capitols are trying to combat the burgeoning crisis by banning specific substances in designer synthetics and their chemical cousins. Thus far, few prosecutors have brought charges under the laws, which have yet to be fully tested in court.

SIXTEEN POUNDER

Janet Johnson, a 39-year-old woman with diabetes mellitus, gave birth to a 16 pound, 1 ounce baby by cesarean section on July 8, 2011 (22). Guinness World Records says the heaviest newborn ever recorded weighed 23 pounds, 12 ounces, born to an Ohio woman in 1879. Johnson's baby was born almost 2 years to the day after the hospital delivered its smallest baby, which weighed 15 ounces.

MEDICARE'S 45TH ANNIVERSARY

Medicare went into effect in 1966 (23). Initially it covered senior citizens only (those ≥65 years). Former President Harry S Truman, then 81, received the first Medicare card. Now Medicare and Medicaid cover not only seniors but young disabled adults and low-income children. In 2010, Medicare covered 47.2 million people and cost $525.7 billion in the federal budget; Medicaid covered 53.9 million and cost $272.8 billion. Medicare primarily provides insurance for hospitalization, physician visits, and prescription drugs. Medicaid not only covers these expenses but also provides dental services, eyeglasses, home health services, nursing home care, and many services necessary for children. Unlike Medicare, Medicaid is run by the states. Although there are broad federal guidelines, states have a great deal of flexibility to set eligibility and benefits and to determine how much providers are paid. The federal government pays an average of 57% of Medicaid costs and states provide the rest. How ObamaCare is going to change these programs is unclear.

GOVERNMENT SPYING ON PHYSICIANS

Alarmed by a shortage of primary care physicians, the Obama administration is recruiting a team of "mystery shoppers" to pose as patients, calling doctors' offices and requesting appointments to see how difficult it is for people to get care when they need it (24). The administration says the survey will address a "critical public policy problem": the increasing shortage of primary care physicians, including specialists in internal medicine and family practice. It will also try to discover whether physicians are accepting patients with private insurance while turning away those in government health programs that pay lower reimbursement rates. Federal officials predict that >30 million Americans will gain coverage under the health care law passed in 2010, and these newly insured Americans will need to seek out new primary care physicians, further exacerbating the problem. The survey is planned to take place in Texas and in eight other states.

The so-called "mystery shoppers" will not identify themselves as working for the government. According to government documents, the mystery shoppers will call medical practices and ask if doctors are accepting new patients and, if so, how long the wait would be. The government wants to know if doctors give different answers to callers depending on whether they have public insurance, like Medicaid, or private insurance, like Blue Cross and Blue Shield. Most doctors accept Medicare patients. In many parts of the country, Medicaid, the program for low-income people, pays so little that many physicians refuse to accept them. This, of course, could become a more serious problem in 2014 when the new health care law will greatly expand eligibility for Medicaid.

The administration has signed a contract with the National Opinion Research Center at the University of Chicago to help conduct the survey. Access to care has been a concern in Massachusetts, which provides coverage under a state program many in Congress have cited as a model for President Obama's health care overhaul. In a recent study, the Massachusetts Medical Society found that 53% of family physicians and 51% of internal medicine physicians were not accepting new patients. When new patients could get appointments, they faced long waits, averaging 36 days to see family physicians and 48 days to see internists.

MAKING PREDICTIONS

Dan Gardner, a Canadian journalist, recently authored *Future Babble: Why Expert Predictions Are Next to Worthless, and You Can Do Better* (25). The book is ultimately a devastating case for the inability of our so-called seers to call it right, regardless of the field in question. He demonstrates that history is rife with failed predictions. In 1990, Japan was the odds-on favorite to dominate the 21st century, a role now filled by China. Might India be the next nominee for the world's winners circle? Gardner rebukes our modern pundits with a rigorous analysis of their lack of accountability and an explanation of why humans continue to seek them out, even as failed forecasts follow failed forecasts. Humans crave future knowledge and have an aversion to uncertainty. We dislike randomness and consequently see patterns where none exist.

Among those who receive well-deserved scorn is Paul Ehrlich. His 1968 book, *The Population Bomb,* sold millions of copies and confidently predicted that famines in the 1970s would kill hundreds of millions. It didn't happen. Nobel Prize–winning economist and columnist Paul Krugman foresaw a depression if currency controls weren't introduced during the 1997 Asian financial crisis. Controls mostly were not introduced, and Asia was booming again in relatively short order.

A good part of the book is spent describing less dramatic psychological research on human decision making. Such studies of negativity bias, confirmation bias, and the importance of social status, among others, provide useful explanations of why humans crave predictions.

One key value of the book is the author's coverage of a groundbreaking study by Philip Tetlock, now professor at the University of California at Berkeley. In a 1984 study with 284 experts, he collected 27,450 judgments about the future. Results showed that their predictions would beat a dart-throwing chimp by a whisker, making the forecasts no more accurate than random guesses. Tetlock later found that the more famous the expert, the worse the accuracy. The overall findings remained valid irrespective of whether the predictions were pessimistic or optimistic, and whether they came from the political left or right.

HUMAN SPACE TRAVEL

The space shuttle *Atlantis* landed back on Earth on July 21, 2011, bringing an era to an end (26, 27). For the first time in 30 years, NASA has no program for human space travel. Lawrence Krauss opined in a recent piece in the *Wall Street Journal* that the space-shuttle program failed to live up to its primary goal of providing relatively cheap and efficient human space travel (26). There were a total of 135 shuttle flights at a cost of approximately $1 billion per flight, or $55 billion in the last decade alone. The $100 billion space station orbiting no further from Earth than Washington is to New York City cost $100 billion. Either aboard the shuttle or the International Space Station, astronauts have explicitly demonstrated that what we learned from sending people into space is not much more than how to keep them alive up there. The lion's share of cost associated with sending humans into space was devoted, as it should have been, to making sure that they survived the voyage. No other significant science has emerged from a generation's worth of roundtrips in near-Earth orbit.

There were some highlights. The Hubble Space Telescope launch and repair missions were useful. Certainly the shuttle program cannot be justified on the grounds that it helped us build the International Space Station. The station, according to Krauss, is a largely useless international make-work project that was criticized by every major science organization in the USA. The station now houses a $2 billion particle-physics experiment, the results of which have been inconsequential. The best science done by NASA consisted of sending robots to places humans could never survive and peering into the far depths of the cosmos, back to the early moments of the Big Bang, with instruments far more capable than our human senses, all for a small fraction of what it cost to send a living person into Earth's orbit. The first rovers went to Mars for what it would cost to make a movie about sending Bruce Willis to Mars. Professor Krauss concludes: "If we are going to spend hundreds of billions of dollars on human space travel, we need to have a rational plan and one that can excite the imagination of the next generation of would-be scientists and explorers." The space shuttle did not provide such a plan or inspiration.

Giving up space ventures probably is a bad idea, according to Al Neuharth (27). After the Sputnik Satellite was launched by the USSR in 1957, President John F. Kennedy concluded that any nation wanting to be number one on Earth must also be number one in space. Ironically, as Al Neuharth writes, we are again at the mercy of the Russians. We are a distant second in space behind Russia and may soon be third behind China, which has announced that it will put a man on the moon after 2020, in hopes of later exploring Mars or Venus. The critics of the space program have long said that it cost too much, but it cost only an eighth of the cost of the wars in Iran and Afghanistan up to this point. Is nation-building in places like Afghanistan 8 times more important than exploring the universe? Probably by the time we start the US space program again, Russia, China, Japan, and India will be ahead of us.

BIN LADEN'S PORN

According to Asra Q. Nomani (The DailyBeast.com), pornography is the Muslim world's "dirty little secret" (28). US intelligence sources found a cache of video porn in Osama Bin Laden's hideout in Abbottabad. Called *fuhsha* in Arabic, pornography is strictly forbidden under Islamic law, though Muslim nations that repress and segregate women also have the highest rates of pornography use in the world. Porn invariably turns up in raids of al Qaida safe houses. The finding of the x-rated material in Bin Laden's home points to the tortured hypocrisy at the heart of militant Islam's restrictive culture. Although Islam "has very rich traditions of sacred sexuality and eroticism, extremists have turned that tradition rancid with their misogyny; by dehumanizing women and making sex dirty and forbidden, they actually encourage young men's porn fetishes." Bin Laden's stash apparently is inspiring mocking tabloid headlines throughout the world.

AUTO THEFT

Car theft is greater during the summer than at any other time of the year (29). According to comments from members of the Tarrant Regional Auto Crime Task Force, car theft is much less likely if things are hidden from view, the car is locked, and keys are removed from the car. Many thieves apparently see items in a car to steal and then discover keys once inside. Half of the stolen cars had been left unlocked, and nearly one third had the keys in the ignition. One member of the Reduce Auto Theft in Texas group indicates that crime groups are increasingly targeting trucks: the top three stolen vehicles in Texas are Ford, Chevrolet, and Dodge pickups. Lock the car. Put potentially valuable items in the trunk. Keep the keys in your pocket or purse.

THE KNOWN KNOWNS, THE UNKNOWN KNOWNS, AND THE UNKNOWN UNKNOWNS

These are phrases used by Donald Rumsfeld when he was secretary of defense. Thomas Sowell in a recent column gave examples of these phrases (30). Known knowns might be that we know how many aircraft carriers some other country has. An example of unknown knowns would be our knowing that another country has troops and tanks but not knowing how many of each. An example of the unknown unknown would be having no clue, for example, that on September 11, 2001, somebody was going to fly two commercial airplanes into the World Trade Center. We have many unknown knowns and unknown unknowns in medicine.

MANAGING FEDERAL MONEY

Al Neuharth, who founded *USA Today*, is now 87 years old and writes a weekly column in the newspaper he started. He rates the top five most important federal expense categories in this order: health, education, transportation, military, and exploration (31). The present Congress does put health as number one, and the Medicare and Medicaid bill for 2011 is expected to be nearly $850 billion. But the military (mislabeled Defense Department) is a close second at $712 billion. The nation-building misadventures in Afghanistan and Iraq account for $154 billion of the military budget. By comparison, our budget for public education is $77 billion, half of what we spend in Afghanistan and Iraq! Maybe that's why Japan, China, and India are putting too many of our young students to shame. Maybe Congress not only needs to raise the debt limit, but also put education ahead of the military.

TAXES

Tax the rich; down with the corporate jets—that's the present-day theme. But, some facts: 50% of Americans who file tax returns pay almost 100% of the income taxes; the top 25% of filers pay 86% of the taxes; the top 10% pay 67% of the taxes; and the top 1% pay 38% of the tax revenues (32). In 2008, that was $392 billion paid by that 1% out of a total take of $1003 billion. The rich are doing their share. It is not good to play one part of our population against another. What we need is more rich people, and then more taxes would be paid.

—WILLIAM CLIFFORD ROBERTS, MD
8 August 2011

1. Beck M. When gray days signal a problem. *Wall Street Journal*, July 26, 2011.
2. Fawcett J. *Report of the DSM-V Mood Disorder Work Group*. Arlington, VA: American Psychiatric Association, April 2009. Available at http://www.psych.org/MainMenu/Research/DSMIV/DSMV/DSMRevisionActivities/DSM-V-Work-Group-Reports/Mood-Disorders-Work-Group-Report.aspx; accessed July 28, 2011.
3. Hellerstein D. Medications, therapy, exercise in treating depression . . . all remodel the brain. *Psychology Today*, July 22, 2011.
4. Hotz RL. Brain shrinkage: it's only human. *Wall Street Journal*, July 26, 2011.
5. Barnes DE, Yaffe K. The projected effect of risk factor reduction on Alzheimer's disease prevalence. *Lancet Neurol* 2011 Jul 18 [Epub ahead of print].
6. Petersen A. Dawn of a new sleep drug? *Wall Street Journal*, July 19, 2011.
7. Chaudhuri S. The 25 documents you need before you die. *Wall Street Journal*, July 2–3, 2011.
8. Beck M. City vs. country: who is healthier? *Wall Street Journal*, July 12, 2011.
9. Harmon KG, Asif IM, Klossner D, Drezner JA. Incidence of sudden cardiac death in National Collegiate Athletic Association athletes. *Circulation* 2011;123(15):1594–1600.
10. Horovitz B. Trampoline parks growing by leaps and bounces. *USA Today*, July 14, 2011.
11. Rising D. *E. coli* illness spreading more slowly. Associated Press, June 4, 2011.
12. Gillis J (*New York Times*). Fighting to feed a warming planet. *Dallas Morning News*, June 26, 2011.
13. Ackerman T (*Houston Chronicle*). Plan reduces time to become doctor. *Dallas Morning News*, July 12, 2011.
14. Caruso JW. The 2011 ACGME program requirements: a new model for quality and safety. *Health Policy Newsletter of the Thomas Jefferson University* 2011;24:1–2.
15. Jordan M. Births fuel Hispanic gains. *Wall Street Journal*, July 15, 2011.
16. Yen H (Associated Press). Share of kids in U.S. hits new low. *Dallas Morning News*, July 13, 2011.
17. Murtagh L, Ludwig DS. State intervention in life-threatening childhood obesity. *JAMA* 2011;306(2):206–207.
18. Mozaffarian D, Hao T, Rimm EB, Willett WC, Hu FB. Changes in diet and lifestyle and long-term weight gain in women and men. *N Engl J Med* 2011;364(25):2392–2404.
19. Kobylinski KC, Sylla M, Chapman PL, Sarr MD, Foy BD. Ivermectin mass drug administration to humans disrupts malaria parasite transmission in Senegalese villages. *Am J Trop Med Hyg* 2011;85(1):3–5.
20. Califano JA Jr, Bennett WJ. Do we really want a "needle park" on American soil? *Wall Street Journal*, July 1, 2011.
21. Louwagie P. Synthetic drugs cause mayhem, baffle police. *Dallas Morning News*, July 31, 2011.
22. Associated Press. Bigger in Texas: baby checks in at 16 pounds. *Dallas Morning News*, July 12, 2011.
23. Neuharth A. Medicare anniversary 45 years with changes. *USA Today*, July 1, 2011.
24. Pear R. Survey targets doctor deficit. *Dallas Morning News*, June 27, 2011.
25. Gardner D. *Future Babble: Why Expert Predictions Are Next to Worthless, and You Can Do Better*. New York: Dutton, 2011 (320 pp.).
26. Krauss L. The shuttle was a dud but space is still our destiny. *Wall Street Journal*, July 22–24, 2011.
27. Neuharth A. Giving up space lead puts the same on us. *USA Today*, July 22, 2011.
28. Nomani AQ. Bin Laden's secret stash of porn. *The Week*, May 27, 2011.
29. Brown M. New campaign focuses on auto theft. *Dallas Morning News*, July 7, 2011.
30. Sowell T. Trapped by unknowns. *Dallas Morning News*, July 14, 2011.
31. Neuharth A. How should Congress manage your money? *USA Today*, July 29, 2011.
32. Donlan TG. A glimpse of economic health. *Barron's*, August 1, 2011.

Chapter 5

January 2012

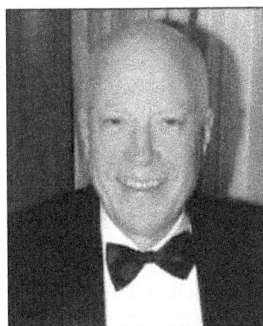

William C. Roberts, MD

KAIHOKEN

In Japanese, the word means "health insurance for all" (1). In 2011, Japan celebrated 50 years of universal health insurance, which started there in 1961, assuring access to a wide array of health services for the entire population. Since then, benefits have become more egalitarian while health expenditures have remained comparatively low: 8.5% of the gross domestic product (GDP) and 20th of countries in the Organization for Economic Co-operation and Development (as of 2008). This achievement is particularly remarkable because the percentage of the population aged 65 years and older has increased nearly fourfold (from 6% to 23%) during these past 50 years. Many factors contributed to this impressive performance, including public health policies, high literacy rates and educational levels, the traditional diet, exercise, economic growth, and a stable political environment.

As described by Reich and colleagues (2) from both Japan and the USA, with the inauguration of Emperor Meiji in 1868, the Japanese government embarked on rapid westernization throughout society. In health care, the government over time succeeded in changing the basis of medical practice from Chinese to Western medicine. Unlike other Asian countries, Japan did not allow independent schools in Chinese medicine to coexist with schools teaching Western medicine. Moreover, the transition was achieved with minimal cost and limited social disruption. For hospitals, however, Japan needed to adopt a new method of delivering care because virtually no public or religious institutions could serve this role. Japan developed hospitals for specific purposes: those for teaching and research, those for army and navy personnel, those for quarantining patients with communicable and venereal diseases (the public hospitals), and—the most numerous—private hospitals that expanded from clinics. In all four cases, the hospital was regarded as the doctor's workplace, and a doctor served as director with clinical and administrative responsibilities. The medical staff of these new hospitals was typically controlled by the professors of prestigious medical schools, notably the University of Tokyo. Physicians were rotated, at the decision of the professor, within the closed network of the university clinical department and its affiliated hospitals.

The most successful private hospitals continued to expand until they rivaled the large hospitals in the public sector. Thus, there was not much distinction between physicians' offices and hospitals. Large medical centers maintained outpatient departments, which patients could visit without referrals. There was also not much distinction between specialists and general practitioners. Those who went into private practice mostly provided primary care because they did not have access to hospital facilities. This basic structure continues today.

In 1945, at the end of World War II, Japan's major cities had been destroyed and an estimated 3.2 million people had died (3, 4). Deep poverty and malnutrition scarred the entire country. Japan's surrender was followed by 7 years of US occupation that sought to restructure the health care system as part of its goal of democratizing the society. The occupying forces strengthened community health institutions. Astounding gains in health status occurred. Between 1947 and 1955, average life expectancy in Japan increased by nearly 14 years. These achievements were attributed to public health policies that were started before the war and facilitated during the occupation, along with reconstruction efforts, and were expanded by the Japanese government after it regained sovereignty in 1952. These early postwar health gains included employee-based health insurance and community health insurance which covered over 70% of the population. Medical education continued during that early postwar period. The hierarchical structure with the University of Tokyo at the top remained intact. Japan now has the world's longest life expectancy.

Japan is currently undergoing several sociocultural changes that are challenging its society, including the rise of part-time and temporary employment for young workers, a growing number of young women who postpone marriage and childbearing, the ever-expanding number of older people, a widening inequality in income, and diversity in values. Japan's fertility rate has declined to 1.37 live births per woman—about the same rate as in Italy and Germany, slightly higher than the rate in Singapore and South Korea, and much less than the replacement rate (2.2 children per woman aged 15 to 45 years). These demographic changes have profound implications for Japan's health care system in the future.

ACUTE MYOCARDIAL INFARCTION WITH LOW-DENSITY LIPOPROTEIN CHOLESTEROL LEVELS <70 MG/DL

Lee and 19 other authors (5) from South Korea analyzed 1054 patients with acute myocardial infarction (AMI) who had baseline low-density lipoprotein (LDL) cholesterol levels <70 mg/dL and survived between November 2005 and December 2007. The patients were divided into two groups according to the prescribing of statins at discharge (statin group, N = 607; nonstatin group, N = 447). Statin therapy significantly reduced the risk of the composite endpoint (death, recurrent AMI, target coronary artery revascularization, and coronary artery bypass grafting) at 1 year. Statin therapy reduced the risk of cardiac death by 53% and the risk of coronary revascularization by 55%, but there was no difference in the risk of the composite of all-cause death, recurrent AMI, and repeated percutaneous coronary intervention rates. This study indicates that patients with LDL cholesterol levels <70 mg/dL who take statins have better outcomes than those who do not, despite the relatively low baseline LDL level. Another lesson is that an LDL of 70 mg/dL is not low enough and <50 mg/dL almost certainly would be better.

HOSPITALIZATION AND MORTALITY RATES IN HEART FAILURE PATIENTS ≥65 YEARS

Heart failure (HF) imposes one of the highest disease burdens of any medical condition in the US, with an estimated 5.8 million patients having HF in 2006. The risk of developing HF increases with advancing age, and as a result, HF ranks as the most frequent cause of hospitalization and rehospitalization in older Americans. Heart failure is also one of the most resource-intensive conditions, with direct and indirect costs in the US estimated at $39 billion in 2010.

As the US population grows older, the HF hospitalization rate would be expected to increase, but this may not be the case. Chen and associates (6) from several US medical centers examined changes in HF hospitalization rates and 1-year mortality rates in the US in the years 1998 to 2007. They included only Medicare beneficiaries hospitalized during that time where the principal discharge diagnosis was HF. The adjusted HF hospitalization rates declined from 2845 per 100,000 person-years in 1998 to 2007 per 100,000 person years in 2008, a relative decline of 30%. The overall 1-year mortality rate declined slightly over that decade but remained high. This finding, of course, is good news. As the Framingham study has taught, approximately 90% of patients who eventually develop HF have preexisting systemic hypertension. Thus, if patients with hypertension were treated (and adequately), the number who develop HF would almost certainly decline.

OBESITY AND DIABETES MELLITUS IN HIGH-POVERTY URBAN AREAS VERSUS LOW-POVERTY AREAS

Ludwig and colleagues (7) from several US centers assigned 4498 women with children living in public housing in high-poverty urban areas (in which ≥40% of residents had incomes below the poverty threshold) to one of three groups: 1788 were assigned to receive housing vouchers, which were redeemable only if they moved to a low-poverty center tract (where <10% of the residents were poor) and received counseling on moving; 1312 were assigned to receive unrestricted, traditional vouchers with no special counseling on moving; and 1398 were assigned to a control group that was offered neither of these opportunities. The prevalence of a body-mass index (BMI) ≥35 kg/m², a BMI ≥40, and a glycated hemoglobin level of ≥6.5% were lower in the group receiving the low-poverty vouchers than in the control group, but not significantly different between the group receiving traditional vouchers and the control group. This study indicates that the opportunity to move from a neighborhood with a high level of poverty to one with a lower level of poverty was associated with a reduction in the prevalence of extreme obesity and diabetes mellitus. Better income is associated with better health.

INFANT MORTALITY

According to the World Health Organization and other groups in 2009, 3.3 million babies died around the world before they were 1 month old (8). Many apparently could have been saved by such simple techniques as ensuring that the mothers gave birth on clean surfaces, breastfed their babies, and kept them warm by holding them close. Among the 193 countries examined, the highest newborn death rate in the world is in Afghanistan, where one of every 19 babies dies before the first-month birthday. By comparison, one of every 233 newborns dies in the USA, 1 in 909 in Japan, 1 in 455 in France, 1 in 385 in Lithuania, and 1 in 345 in Cuba. The US is #41 worldwide in newborn death rates.

Some factors considered in explaining our high newborn death rate include the mother's health before pregnancy. Maternal obesity, smoking, high blood pressure, and diabetes mellitus increase the chances that babies will not survive. African American babies have higher death rates than European American babies, no matter how rich or poor the mothers are. And the USA has an unusually high rate of premature births, which reduce a baby's chance of survival. Possibly fertility treatments, common in the USA, lead to premature births and therefore higher newborn death rates.

SUICIDAL BEHAVIOR IN THE USA

The Centers for Disease Control and Prevention (CDC) in October 2011 presented its results from a study of >90,000 adults in 2008 and 2009 (9). The participants did not include homeless people, those in the military, or those hospitalized with psychiatric problems. An estimated 1 million adults in the USA per year reported making a suicide attempt in 2008 and 2009; 36,035 committed suicide in 2008. Suicide is the tenth leading cause of death in the US. An estimated 666,000 people visited US hospital emergency rooms in 2008 for self-inflicted violence. More adults in the Midwest and West have suicidal thoughts than those in the rest of the country. In the US in 2008, 8.3 million people had suicidal thoughts (3.7% of the population), 2.2 million people made suicidal plans (1% of the population), and 1 million people attempted suicide (0.5% of the population). According to the CDC, 0.8% to 1.5% of adults in Texas in 2008 and 2009 attempted suicide. The state with the highest rate of suicidal thoughts was Utah (6.8%), and the state with the lowest was Georgia (2.1%). Actual suicide attempts were highest in Rhode Island (1.5%) and lowest in Delaware and Georgia (0.1%).

MULTIVITAMINS AND DIETARY SUPPLEMENTS

Two articles published in prominent medical journals in October 2011 suggest that multivitamins and many other dietary supplements often do not have health benefits and indeed in some cases may cause harm (10). Some nutrition researchers say taking vitamins is a waste of money for those without a specific nutrient deficiency or chronic illness. It appears from a number of studies that supplements do not make healthy people healthier. Vitamins B6 and B12, for example, are often touted as being good for the heart, but several studies have found that they do not lower the risk of cardiovascular disease. Vitamin C has not been shown in many studies to lower a person's risk of getting a cold. Calcium, while important to bone health, does not lower the risk of heart disease or cancer and may increase the risk of kidney stones. Researchers and nutritionists still recommend dietary supplements for the malnourished and people with certain nutrient deficiencies or medical conditions. Folic acid, the supplement of folate, reduces the likelihood of a common birth defect when taken by pregnant women. It appears that a "balanced diet" is the best way to get needed vitamins, particularly when the diet consists of plant-rich foods. Vitamin C is found in citrus such as oranges and limes; dairy products are heavy in calcium; almonds are heavy in vitamin E; leafy greens such as spinach are heavy in folate.

HIRING SMOKERS

I remember reading years ago a $1.00 biography of Ted Turner who founded CNN and was one of the great innovators of the 20th century. Early on at CNN, he interviewed all prospective employees and was said to ask each one, "Do you smoke cigarettes?" If the potential employee said "yes" he apparently would reply, "If you are so dumb as to smoke cigarettes, you are not smart enough to work here."

Baylor Health Care System announced that starting on January 1, 2012, it will no longer hire smokers in its North Texas facilities (11). Baylor Dallas has for some time aggressively pushed a "stop smoking" program for its current employees, and those who smoke face a surcharge in their health insurance cost. A ban on hiring smokers is controversial, but it is the right move. Baylor Dallas is not alone in the "no-smokers" hiring policy. Memorial Hermann Hospital in Houston, Texas, and the Cleveland Clinic in Cleveland, Ohio, already have done the same.

As we all know, tobacco use is the leading preventable cause of death in the USA. Dr. Donald Berwick, head of the Centers for Medicare and Medicaid Services, emphasized that persuading people to stop smoking is a top priority of a federal campaign to empower Americans to make lifestyle changes to prevent certain diseases.

ONE SPERM DONOR AND 150 CHILDREN

Jacqueline Mroz of *The New York Times* described a woman who used a sperm donor to conceive a baby 7 years earlier and hoped that one day her son would get to know some of his half-siblings (12). She searched a web-based registry for other children fathered by the same donor and helped to create an online group to track them. Over the years, she watched the number of children in her son's group grow and grow and grow. Today there are 150 children, all conceived from the same sperm donor, in this group of half-siblings, and more are on the way.

As more women choose to have babies on their own and as the number of children born through artificial insemination increases, large groups of donor siblings are starting to appear. Although so far 150 is the largest, many others now comprise 50 or more half-siblings cropping up on websites and in chat groups where sperm donors are tagged with unique identifying numbers.

Now there is growing concern among parents, donors, and medical experts about potential negative consequences of having so many children fathered by the same donor, including the possibility that genes for rare diseases could be spread more widely through the population. Of course, accidental incest between half-sisters and half-brothers, who often live close to one another, obviously could occur.

Fertility clinics and sperm banks apparently earn huge profits by allowing lots of children to be conceived with sperm from popular donors. Families want more information on the health of donors and the children conceived with their sperm. Critics are calling on legal limits on the number of children conceived using the same donor sperm and a reexamination of the anonymity that cloaks many donors.

Other countries, including Britain, France, and Sweden, limit how many children a sperm donor can father. There is no such limit in the USA. There are only guidelines issued by the American Society for Reproductive Medicine, a professional group that recommends restricting conception by individual donors to 25 births per population of 800,000.

No one really knows how many children are born in the USA each year using sperm donors. Some estimates put the number at 30,000 to 60,000. Mothers of donor children are asked to report a child's birth to the sperm bank voluntarily, but just 20% to 40% of them do so. Because of this dearth of records, many families turn to the registry's website, www.donorsiblingregistry.com, for information about a child's half-brothers or half-sisters. On the website, parents can register the birth of a child and find half-siblings by looking up a number assigned to a sperm donor. Many parents are shocked to learn just how many half-siblings a child has. It looks like there may be some legislation in this area in the near future.

ADOLPHE QUETELET AND BODY MASS INDEX

One of the first academics to seek correlations between measurement of body size (anthropometry) and social conditions was Belgian-born Lambert Adolphe Jacques Quetelet (1796–1874) (13) *(Figure)*. A prodigy in mathematics, he also studied sculpture and painting, published poetry, and coauthored

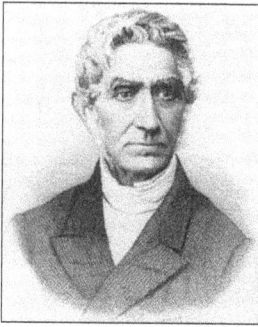

Figure. Adolphe Quetelet.

a libretto. Quetelet founded the first astronomical observatory in Belgium in 1826. But soon he turned his attention from the stars to the study of the human form. When recruited to design a national census of the Netherlands, Quetelet—influenced by seminal thinkers in probability theory, including Joseph Fourier and Siméon Poisson—established the principle that a random sample from a representative diversified group could be used to estimate the characteristics of a total population. Over the ensuing decades, Quetelet contended that "the study of man" could be aided by the study of averages of physical characteristics, as well as rates of birth, marriage, and growth. These data, over time, might provide insights into social differences between regions and countries. In 1831 and 1832, he conducted what is believed to be the first study of newborns and children based on their heights and weights and then extended his survey to adults.

Three years later, Quetelet published his seminal work, *A Treatise on Man and the Development of His Aptitudes.* Part of the book identified the growth spurts following birth and puberty. Quetelet's ultimate aim was to define the characteristics of the "average man," and he initially looked to the familiar bell-shaped curve that had been used by scientists to describe natural phenomena. But he had problems fitting people's heights and weights into such a normal distribution. Quetelet ultimately devised novel formulas to link height and weight and is credited with providing the calculations for what we currently term the *body mass index*, the ratio of weight in kilograms and height in meters squared (thus a measure of weight standardized by height), and key measures of growth and development.

With this metric in hand, Quetelet and other academics of his era gathered in Brussels in 1853 at the first International Statistical Congress. Among the many projects launched by the meeting was one to prepare a "uniform nomenclature of the causes of death applicable to all countries." These data could then be linked to body size and the risk of various diseases, as well as social variables like geography, migration, war, and famine. While keen to apply statistics to social science, Quetelet, who still performed exacting astronomical measurements, was alert to the dangers of overinterpreting numbers associated with factors that might contribute, like crime rates, suicide rates, and intellectual aptitude. Thus was born the BMI, which, in my view, should replace the respiratory rate as one of the "vital signs" of the physical examination.

EXTREME WEATHER IN 2011

From February's "snowmageddon" to spring's deadly tornadoes, from Hurricane Irene to Texas' raging wildfires, 2011 was an extraordinarily bad year for weather (14). The director of the National Oceanic and Atmospheric Administration's National Weather Service described 2011 as the first year since 1980 (when such measurements began) in which 10 separate weather events each caused more than $1 billion in damage. These figures are partly due to increased population density: the more people living in a particular area, the more property that can be damaged when a storm hits. Extreme conditions happen in places that usually do not experience them and are therefore less prepared. A hurricane on the Eastern seaboard can be expected to cause flooding in coastal North Carolina and New Jersey—but not in northern Vermont. The average global land temperature from January through July was among the warmest since recordkeeping began over 100 years ago. Warmer temperatures lead to more severe and frequent extreme weather events, like tornadoes, droughts, and floods.

CHILDHOOD ALTRUISM

A recent social science study, published in September 2011 in the online journal *PLoS One*, asked 136 children aged 3 and 4 years old to step one at a time into a playroom where each was handed six sets of colorful stickers (15). They were told that they could keep all of their stickers or give some or all to a child they didn't know. The social scientist was attempting to determine if children are altruistic. About two thirds of the children chose to give one or more sets of stickers to an unknown recipient who had none. There were no significant differences in generosity between boys and girls. Among those who declined to share, many had something in common: a variation in a gene known as *AVPR1A* that regulates a hormone in the brain associated with social behaviors. Researchers found that this genetic variant was associated with a significant decrease in willingness to share. Of the 136 children invited to share some of their sets of stickers, two participants gave away their entire supply. Asked in a videotaped interview why he gave away all his stickers, one child responded: "That's how you become happy."

Of the 136 children in the Israeli study, the largest group gave away one sticker; the second largest group gave away none. Twenty-two children gave away more than one sticker. Thus, altruism in young children, as in adults, exists in near equal parts with selfishness.

Another study, also published in *PLoS One* in October 2011, found a sense of fairness and altruism in 15-month-old babies, tested in part on their willingness to share a favorite toy (15).

While genetics may play a part in people's willingness to share, environmental influences from home, school, and the world at large may play a larger role, according to social scientists. Even children too young to talk seem able to absorb and imitate acts of empathy and generosity. Positive reinforcement can help cultivate generous behavior. Upon witnessing generosity in a child, parents are advised to resist any impulse to bestow a gift and instead offer praise of the child's character as well as his or her behavior. Generosity apparently can be habit-forming. Magnetic resonance imaging has shown that being generous and being described as generous can engage the so-called reward circuitry in the brain, prompting release of dopamine-like neurotransmitters that are associated with positive feelings.

According to Kevin Helliker, writing in *The Wall Street Journal*, most research to study the roots of generosity takes place in adults. Studies have found that about 70% of adults choose to share when cash is used in the same exercise as that performed with the Israeli children. It is a common exercise used by researchers known as "the dictator game," in which the participant, the dictator, has to decide how to split a thick sum of money between himself and a recipient who is unknown and therefore not likely to reciprocate.

Experiments with children typically are staged free of parents, siblings, and other acquaintances from whom the child might expect a reward of some kind. In a large study of British school children aged 4, 6, and 9, psychologist Joyce Benenson (16) found a strong correlation between socioeconomic status and willingness to give. Acts of generosity were less common among children in poverty, because as she says, "Poverty is linked with myriad differences in socialization practices, including less interaction with unfamiliar adults" and greater exposure to violence.

LEFT-HANDEDNESS

Only about 10% of Americans are left-handed, yet since the end of World War II, nearly half of American presidents have been lefties (Harry S Truman, George H. W. Bush, William J. Clinton, and Barack Obama). Is there something special about left-handed people? Rik Smits (17), a left-handed science writer, attempted to answer this and other questions in *The Puzzle of Left-Handedness*. He writes that lefties and righties don't differ in personality, ability, creativity, or any other measurable characteristic. Smits debunks a number of myths about "handedness," but what makes us righties or lefties has not been determined. *The Puzzle of Left-Handedness* offers some interesting comments on handedness, but Smits' speculations ultimately leave one scratching his or her head—with either hand.

PHARMA IN THE JUNGLE

Not long ago my ex-wife (Carey Cansler Roberts) sent me the book *State of Wonder* by Ann Patchett (18). (The book reminded her of our trip together to the Amazon, Menaus, and the Rio Negro many years earlier.) The book is about an American drug company based in Minnesota that wanted to develop a fertility drug to allow women to get pregnant at any age. The stockholders were overjoyed at the possibility. Deep in the Amazon rainforest along the banks of the Rio Negro, the Lakashi tribe had been living quietly, procreating without fanfare well into their eighth decade. An elusive but brilliant scientist, Dr. Annick Swenson, had discovered that these women gnawed on the bark of a rare tree deep in the jungle and that the bark imparted fertile longevity.

But Dr. Swenson took her own sweet time on the research, and the pharmaceutical company grew impatient—especially since she had eschewed all forms of contact. They did not even know exactly where she was. So the company sent a fellow scientist, Anders Eckman, to track her down and report on the state of drug development. Unfortunately, the Minnesotan did not do well in the Amazon, and within weeks Eckman was dead of a febrile illness.

Then, his lab partner, who became the heroine, was dispatched to the jungle. Marina Singh, a loner pharmacologist, had quit her obstetrics-gynecology residency after a horrendous medical error, oddly enough under the auspices of the department chair, none other than Dr. Annick Swenson. The senior physician, as a consequence, abandoned her junior physician at the time in the face of medicolegal calamity.

Marina suffered the various insults of the tropics during her hunt for the elusive Dr. Swenson: flotilla of insects, lost luggage, venomous snakes, psychogenic side-effects of antimalarial drugs, intermittent fevers, and generalized disorientation.

The pharmacological drama shows that the bark of the magical tree turned out to confer immunity to malaria, in addition to providing fertile longevity. The scientists realized that the drug company would quickly pull the financial plug if it became aware that the goal of the scientists was to help the world's poor fight mosquito-borne parasites, rather than to help wealthy Western women achieve pregnancy in their sixth and seventh decades. The industry wanted a blockbuster fertility drug, not a pennies-per-pill malarial agent. Hence, the secrecy of Dr. Swenson and her refusal to update the drug company and its anxious stockholders on her progress.

That the good Dr. Swenson had been nibbling the ambrosia bark herself and became pregnant and preeclamptic at the age of 72 years, and that her former underling, who quit midway through training, was the only available physician to perform the emergency C-section in the teeming Amazonian jungle, is not how most medical errors get worked out.

PREGNANT MARATHON

A few hours after completing the 26.2-mile Chicago marathon, Ms. Miller gave birth to a 7-pound, 13-ounce healthy baby. Ms. Miller is an experienced marathoner and was 38 weeks and 5 days pregnant during the marathon (19).

THE IRONMAN WORLD CHAMPIONSHIP

Thirty-eight-year-old Craig Alexander had won this event in 2008 and in 2009, and in 2011 he did it again (20). In 2011, he beat the previous record set in 1996 by approximately 1 minute. He completed the 2.4-mile ocean swim, the 112-mile bike ride, and the 26.2-mile marathon run in 8 hours, 3 minutes, 56 seconds. Britain's Chrissie Wellington, 34 years old, won her fourth world title, finishing at 8:55:08. It is amazing what the human body is capable of.

Jacque Steinberg has written *You Are an Ironman* (21). The ironman and ironwoman triathlon must be completed within 17 hours. The ironman originally started in Hawaii with a field of 15. It now is an event held throughout the USA in which more than 50,000 athletes cross the finish line.

Jacque Steinberg's book follows three men and three women, most in their 40s, who pay a nonrefundable $525 a year in advance to sign up for the 2009 Ironman Arizona. The reader follows the six as they put their normal routines on hold and adopt rigorous training regimens. One of the six was Leanne Johnson, who made a vow while cheering on her husband to his first ironman finish. Her husband, Scott, was born with cystic fibrosis and underwent a double-lung transplant before setting his sights on an ironman. It was now his wife's turn, and the

30-year-old nurse drew the same support from her husband that she gave to him. Another of the six was a nurse with two teenagers who got the idea after overhearing two triathletes swap stories. Another was a former social worker and mother of five who took up running as an adult. Another was an English teacher inspired by the broadcast of the original ironman in Hawaii he had seen as a child.

HAPPILY MARRIED

Some people have considered it the top oxymoron. Lindsey Townsend (22), writing in the *Dallas Morning News,* had an interesting piece on marriage, a subject of which I am far from an expert. She states that "most of us still expect to be rocked by passion while nestled in security." But she indicates that some of her friends who have been more or less happily married for years admit "after the second drink" that they resent the lack of passion in their lives. She calls that the "Raisin Bran syndrome": "Even if you really like Raisin Bran, do you want to eat it every morning for the rest of your life?" She suggests that the real trouble starts when boredom leads to bad manners. "We stop behaving ourselves and all too often our beloved ends up getting the worst part of us, while we save the good stuff for strangers and friends." She speaks of the pastor who was asked to give words of wisdom to a newlywed couple. He said, "After 50 years of counseling couples, it's a bit humbling to admit that the best advice I have to offer is to be kind to each other." She goes on to say, "I have realized that no matter what it looks like from the outside, no one ever really knows the story of a marriage except the two people who are living it." It reminds me of the song "Behind Closed Doors." I like her comments.

INSURANCE

*Consumer Report*s recently listed several kinds of insurance policies that most people do not need (23):

- *Mortgage life insurance:* It is less expensive to use term life to cover your mortgage debt, should you die.
- *Credit card loss prevention insurance:* It usually costs more than $100 per year, but by law losses due to card theft are capped at $50 per card.
- *Cancer insurance:* Regular health insurance plans often cover medical expenses related to cancer treatment.
- *Accidental death insurance:* Since one is extremely unlikely to die in an accident, term life insurance is a more logical investment.
- *Involuntary unemployment insurance:* It is better to maintain an emergency fund that can cover living expenses for 6 months or more.
- *Flight insurance:* Flight crashes are extremely rare. If one worries about premature death, term life insurance is a better way to go. Even life insurance can be unnecessary for some people—those single or childless, for example, and those who have no one depending on their income.

VIRTUES OF SOLITUDE

Diana Senechal's fourth book, *Republic of Noise: The Laws of Solitude in Schools and Culture,* will be published in January 2012 (24). She is a former teacher in the New York Public Schools. She takes schools to task for a tight focus on rapid activity and instant results. She argues that schools need to make room for the things of solitude, such as literature, science, art, friendship, and matters of conscience. I am reminded of Johann von Goethe's comment: "Talents are best nurtured in solitude; character is best formed in the stormy billows of the world." Carl Sandberg said, "One of the greatest necessities in America is to discover creative solitude." Henry-Marie Beyle stated, "One can acquire everything in solitude but character."

When I was at the National Institutes of Health for many years, I virtually always went into my office on Saturdays. The reason was peace and quiet. It was a time I could think out projects and manuscripts I was working on—how to package them, how to put a pink ribbon around them and get them through the editorial boards of various medical journals. Without that peaceful quiet think time, my publication list would be enormously shorter. Today, with e-mails, cell phones, car radios, and busy homes, it is more difficult for many to find sites where creativity comes alive.

THE 1% VERSUS THE 99%

Everyone likes a tax paid by someone else, so it is not surprising that 99% of us would rather the other 1% paid more taxes. As Scott Burns indicates, in 2009 the top 1% of all income tax returns in the USA with a positive-adjusted gross income pulled in a total of $1.3 trillion (25). Of that amount, 24% was paid in federal income taxes, or $318 billion. The top 1% received nearly 17% of all income and paid 37% of all federal income taxes. The bottom 75% of all taxpayers (annual income <$66,000) had a total of $2.75 trillion in income and paid $110 billion in income taxes, about 4.1% of income. The top 1% income people (those with adjusted gross incomes of $344,000 annually) paid 6 times as large a proportion of their income than the bottom 75%. The top 5% had household income of $155,000 or more; the top 10%, $112,000 or more; the top 25%, $66,000 or more; and the bottom 30%, <$32,000 annually. Those were figures for 2009.

Can people in the top 1% pay more? Of course, but how much of their $1.3 trillion can we take? Only $1 trillion is left because the top 1% already pay $318 billion in taxes. Since the official federal deficit is estimated at $1.3 trillion for the 2011 fiscal year, even if the top 1% paid 100% of their income in taxes, the federal budget would not be balanced. As Scott Burns indicates, "The 1% vs. the 99% is a powerful side byte for a political debate, but it is deeply trashy economics."

JOBS, HOPE, AND CASH

Peggy Noonan (26), writing in *The Wall Street Journal,* starts a recent column this way: "Ten years ago, Steve Jobs was alive, Bob Hope was alive, Johnny Cash was alive. Now we are out of jobs, out of hope and out of cash." She stated that she heard that from a Transportation Security Administration agent in New York. The agent's joke, she indicated, was a good summation of the current moment and the public mood.

SEVEN BILLION PEOPLE

The world's population hit 7 billion in October 2011 (27, 28). The world's population reached 1 billion in 1804; 2 billion in 1927; 3 billion in 1959; 4 billion in 1974; 5 billion in 1987; 6 billion in 1998; and now 7 billion in 2011. The United Nations projects that the world population will reach 8 billion by 2025 and 10 billion by 2083. The numbers, of course, could be much higher or lower depending on such factors as access to birth control, infant mortality rates, and average life expectancy, which has risen from 48 years in 1950 to 69 worldwide today.

China remains the most populous nation with 1.34 billion people. In the past decade, it added 74 million, more than the population of France and Thailand. Nonetheless, its growth has slowed dramatically, and the population is projected to start shrinking in 2027 and by 2050 to be smaller than it is today. Three decades of strict family planning rules that limit urban families to one child and rural families to two helped China achieve a rapid decline in fertility.

India, with 1.2 billion people, is the second most populous country and is expected to overtake China around 2030 when its population will reach an estimated 1.6 billion. Nevertheless, India's fertility rate, now 2.6 children per woman, should fall to 2.1 by 2025 and 1.8 by 2035. More than half of India's population is under 25.

Europe is having the opposite problem. Spain used to give parents $2500 Euros (more than $3000) for every newborn child to encourage families to reverse the country's low birth rate. But the checks stopped when Spain's austerity measures took hold. Who will pay the bills to support the older ones in the years ahead is a bothersome question. In many European countries, birth rates are shrinking and populations are aging. Women have chosen to have their first child at later ages, and the difficulties in finding jobs and affordable housing are discouraging some couples from having any children. In 2010, for the fourth consecutive year, more Italians died than were born. Italy's population, nonetheless, grew slightly to 60.6 million due to immigration, a highly charged issue across Europe now.

Unlike many countries in Europe, France's population is growing slightly but steadily every year. It has one of the highest birth rates in the European Union, with around 2 children per woman. One reason is immigration to France by Africans with large family traditions, but it's also due to family-friendly legislation. The government offers public preschools, subsidies to all families with >1 child, generous maternity leave, and tax exemptions for employers of nannies.

Like France, the USA has one of the highest population growth rates among industrialized nations. Our fertility rate is just below the replacement rate of 2.1 children per woman, but our population has been increasing by almost 1% annually due to immigration. With 312 million people, the US is the third most populous country after China and India.

Most of the population growth, of course, is coming from the developing nations, not from the developed nations. Since 1950, with projection to 2050, the developed nations are estimated to increase by 0.8 billion people and the undeveloped, by 1.3 billion. Thus, those with the least are having the most.

In response to the earth's reaching 7 billion people, a professor at Columbia University commented, "The consequences for humanity could be grim." A *New York Times* columnist declared that "the earth is full" and that "we are eating into our future." Another editorial mentioned "a human swarm that is over breeding." We are overbreeding in a way that "prosperous, well-educated families" from the developed world do not.

Certainly this population growth has disproved Paul Ehrlich's thesis in his 1968 *The Population Bomb,* which opened with this sentence: "The battle to feed all humanity is over. In the 1970s the world will undergo famines—hundreds of millions of people are going to starve to death in spite of any crash programs embarked upon now." The book was wildly popular, but the mass starvation he predicted never materialized, and the people in India whom he thought could never feed themselves are now eating better than ever despite a population more than twice the size it was when *The Population Bomb* appeared.

Thomas Robert Malthus' ominous warnings about a growing population's outstripping the food supply were not borne out in his day (the late 1700s and early 1800s) or since. The predictions of Malthus proved to be wrong. The premise of his work, however—that there must be some limit to population growth—is hard to argue with. As William McGurn writes in *The Wall Street Journal,* "The main flaw in Malthus is . . . his premise. Malthusian fears about population follow from the Malthusian view that human beings are primarily mouths to be fed rather than minds to be unlocked. In this reasoning, when a pig is born in China, the national wealth is thought to go up, but when a Chinese baby is born the national wealth goes down" (28).

Matt Ridley, author of *The Rational Optimist,* suggests that human progress is driven when people connect with one another and exchange ideas as well as goods. In our own day, he believes, this interaction has been accelerated by the revolution in technology that has made distance largely irrelevant. That is one reason he takes a generally benevolent view of population growth. Matt Ridley goes on to say: "The mixing of ideas made possible by the Internet makes the drying up of innovations almost impossible to achieve, even if we wanted to, and the improvement in living standards almost inevitable" (28).

Maybe William McGurn is right: "Instead of looking for ways to reduce the number of people at the banquet of life, we would do better to look for ways to lay a better and more bounteous table" (28).

CHINA VS. USA

According to the World Bank, the size of China's economy is $10.1 trillion and that of the USA, $14.6 trillion, both based on purchasing power parity (29). But China is narrowing the gap quickly. Over the past 10 years, the annual real growth of China's GDP averaged 10.5% compared with 1.7% in the USA. The Chinese economy increased at an annual rate of 9.6% in the first half of 2011 versus a rate of <1% in the USA. Thomas Friedman, in a recent *New York Times* column, states: "We are the United States of Deferred Maintenance. China is the People's Republic of Deferred Gratification. They save, invest, and build. We spend, borrow, and patch" (30).

The US's reign as the largest world economic power began a little before 1890, when it supplanted the previous global giant, namely China, which had boasted the largest economy in the world from 1500 until nearly 1890. Yet during those 5 centuries when its economy was the world's largest, China was never even close to being the world's wealthiest country. Italy was almost twice as rich in 1500, the Netherlands almost 3 times as rich in 1700, and the UK 6 times as rich in 1870. Today, though the GDPs of the US and China are roughly equal, the average person in China lives on an income that can buy only 16% of the goods and services that the average person in the USA can buy, and it will take decades for that gap to close.

As Charles Kenny argues in *Bloomberg Businessweek*, second place is not all bad (29). In that position, the US probably would not have to be the world's police. US military spending now accounts for more than two fifths of the world's total, and it sucks up a larger percentage of GDP than the military spending of any other member of the Organization for Economic Co-operation and Development, which numbers 20 nations. And if the US is #2, it would probably be more popular around the world than it is presently. Our image abroad has improved enormously since 2007 and that of China has fallen. Nevertheless, the US still outperforms China on almost every conceivable quality-of-life indicator, including happiness polls, where China is in 70th place. The average American lives 5 years longer than the average Chinese, and our mortality rates for children <5 are less than half the Chinese levels. We have a democracy and elect the president. The same cannot be said of the leadership of the Communist Party of China. And certainly there are advantages to life, liberty, and the pursuit of happiness that we have in greater abundance.

IRAQ AND AFGHANISTAN

The Iraq War started in 2003 and ended in December 2011 (31, 32). It was not a victory and not a defeat; it was just over. A total of nearly 4500 troops died in the war. They come home to no parades or pleasant memorials. Whether Iraq will prove to be a democratic ally in the Middle East or retreat into sectarian violence, encouraged by neighboring Iran, remains to be seen.

An important lesson from the war is not about how it ended but about how it began—with the disastrously mistaken belief that the US could advance its interests by intervening militarily in the Middle East. Instead, the hubris bred hostility among Muslims and appears likely to make Iran the big winner in Iraq.

Although we are leaving Iraq, we are still trying nation-building in Afghanistan (33, 34). Three countries have tried before: the British tried it three times, from 1839 to 1842, from 1878 to 1880, and in 1919. They failed each time and lost 28,000 troops. Russia (then USSR) tried it for 10 years (1979–1989) and failed, losing 14,000 troops. Our 10-year misadventure in Afghanistan has taken the lives of over 1800 military men and women. As Al Neuharth writes, "The National Guard, which was formed to protect our nation at home, sacrificed 172 of those lives. If the National Guard were used to protect our airports, seaports and borders, we'd be far safer at far less cost in lives and dollars rather

than invading Afghanistan in 9/11/2011 to try to get Osama bin Laden and his small gang of perpetrators" (34).

STEVE JOBS (1955–2011)

There is no question that Steve Jobs shook the world (35–44). He first redefined the personal computer, accelerating the decline of many of the first-generation computer companies that had focused on centralized mainframes. His 1984 advertisement for the first Macintosh (introduced that year) made other personal computers look Orwellian. With the Internet he became a broader disruptive force, first radically changing the music industry. His iPod (introduced in November 2001) let listeners buy one song at a time instead of the CDs planned by music publishers. And then there was the iPhone, which upended the mobile industry, and the iPad (introduced in April 2010), which defined the tablet.

But it was not always a straightforward line for Steve Jobs. He was the product of Joanne Schieble, a graduate student in speech therapy at the University of Wisconsin (now known as Joanne Simpson). His father was Syrian-born Abdulfattah Jandali, who was also at the University of Wisconsin working on his PhD in political science. (He was awarded his doctorate in 1956.) While a student in Madison, Wisconsin, he became romantically involved with Joanne, who became pregnant in 1954, but her father didn't approve of the relationship with Mr. Jandali. Ms. Simpson went to San Francisco for a few months to get away while she was pregnant. She eventually put her son, Steve Jobs, up for adoption. Ms. Simpson returned to Madison and soon afterwards her father died, enabling her and Mr. Jandali to marry. After he graduated, they moved to Syria, he planning to become a diplomat, but a transitional government prevented that. Ms. Simpson was also unhappy in Syria, and they moved back to Green Bay, where she gave birth to their second child, Mona, who in 1993 published the novel *The Lost Father*. A few years later, Mr. Jandali and Ms. Simpson divorced, and she later remarried. Mr. Jandali was never involved in Mona's life as she was growing up.

In 1955, Steve Jobs, as he stated in his commencement address at Stanford University in 2005, was adopted by Paul Jobs, a high school dropout who became a machinist, and Clara Jobs, who never graduated from college. He grew up in San Francisco. Jobs later had a relationship with his birth mother and sister but he never, despite opportunities, wanted to meet his biological father.

In 2006, widowed Mr. Jandali remarried, and he now lives in a gated Reno, Nevada, suburb. He apparently constantly reads books, usually on his iPad, and he has outlined several fiction and nonfiction books that he hopes to finish writing when he retires. He now manages a Reno casino in Boomtown.

Steve Jobs finished only one semester in college. After dropping out of Reed College in Portland, Oregon, Jobs traveled to India, shaved his head, wore local clothing, and became a Buddhist. The lessons of that philosophy stayed with him for the rest of his life.

In 1976, Jobs (age 21) and Stephen Wozniak founded Apple. Wozniak was a self-made engineer of brilliance. (In 1981, Wooz crashed his Beachcraft Bonanza and spent months recuperating; he returned to Apple only nominally thereafter. From then on, Jobs was "the man.") No one quite knew what Jobs was. He was not an engineer or technologist, and he was no conventional businessman. He made himself up as he went along.

In 1979, Jobs led a group from Apple to visit Xerox. They emerged with the ideas that transformed the industry. At Xerox in the 1970s, a group of brilliant researchers invented the personal computer—they called it the *Alto*—complete with onscreen windows, menus, icons, graphics, and the mouse, all more or less what we know today. Allan Kay was foremost among these genius innovators. Kay built, in turn, on the 1960s inventions of Douglas Engelhart, who was the first to develop the mouse, the onscreen window, and the whole idea of computers that did more things than compute. Corporate Xerox was unimpressed with the Alto. It was expensive, and who needed a personal computer anyway? Xerox ushered in a group from Apple into their top-secret research arena in Palo Alto and allowed them to look and ask questions. Jobs led the Apple group and understood right away that the Xerox researchers had done something tremendous. They had made an easy-to-use computer that spoke pictures instead of numbers. Jobs saw that a cheap version of this elegant computer might be gigantically popular and hugely important. And he ran the project that rolled out the Apple Macintosh in 1984. That Mac was a milestone of modern history. The 1984 Mac had only 128,000 bytes of memory and a tiny 9-inch screen. It looked like an upright shoebox plus keyboard and mouse. But that was the beginning.

Two years later, in 1986, Jobs was fired from Apple, the company he started. Rather than become bitter or seek vengeance, Jobs came to recognize his firing as the best thing that ever happened to him. He maintained a cordial and respectful relationship with his former company. In the interim, he formed NeXT and Pixar. In 1997, Apple bought NeXT, and soon Jobs was CEO of Apple again.

Business historian John Steele Gordon described Jobs' iPhone. In addition to its being a phone, "it's an address book, a date book, a camera (both still and moving), a notebook, a clock that tells the time in any city in the world, a compass, a metric converter and a calculator. It takes dictation. You can send and receive written messages with it. It will tell you where you are and help you get where you need to go. It will keep track of your investments and tell you your net worth as of that second. You can deposit a check into your bank account with it while lying in bed. It will give you the latest news, via every major news organization. It's a dictionary, an encyclopedia and a field guide to birds. It gives you the weather, both where you are and in any city in the world. It will tell you the phase of the moon, send you a bulletin when a new exoplanet has been discovered, tell you the sunrise and sunset times for any place on Earth, show you the cloud cover around the globe and tell you what that bright star in the sky is named" (44). It can do more than 350 things other than being a phone.

The iPhone and its larger brother, the iPad, are remaking the world before our eyes. Already, communications, journalism, publishing, the music business, and the movies will never be the same. "The iPhone and iPad are but the latest in a long series of innovations by Jobs that have fundamentally shaped the technical revolution made possible by the microprocessor, . . . a cheaply manufactured computer on a chip, . . . the most consequential invention since the steam engine about 250 years ago—and probably since agriculture, the invention that started humankind down the road to civilization itself some 10,000 years ago" (44).

As John Steel Gordon indicates, Jobs was not a magician; he is the Henry Ford of our time. Ford didn't invent anything. Instead, he took something that had largely been invented by others and turned it into a world-transforming technology by making it accessible to the common man. Jobs didn't invent the microprocessor any more than Ford invented the automobile. Indeed, he and his companies did not invent much of the technology that makes the iPhone and such so extraordinary. They put together the pieces invented elsewhere to produce something profoundly new that the public loved and could also afford.

Jobs along the way made Apple the second most valuable company in the world. Jobs owned 5.4 million shares of Apple and, according to the *Forbes 400*, was worth $7 billion, making him the 39th richest person in the world. (His fierce rival—Bill Gates—is #1, worth $59 billion.)

—WILLIAM CLIFFORD ROBERTS, MD
2 November 2011

1. Japan: universal health care at 50 years. *Lancet* 2011;378(9796):1049.
2. Reich MR, Ikegami N, Shibuya K, Takemi K. 50 years of pursuing a healthy society in Japan. *Lancet* 2011;378(9796):1051–1053.
3. Summerskill W. Museum: hope after Hiroshima. *Lancet* 2011; 378(9796):1063.
4. Kirby T. Kenji Shibuya: promoting global health in Japan. *Lancet* 2011;378(9796):1064.
5. Lee KH, Jeong MH, Kim HM, Ahn Y, Kim JH, Chae SC, Kim YJ, Hur SH, Seong IW, Hong TJ, Choi DH, Cho MC, Kim CJ, Seung KB, Chung WS, Jang YS, Rha SW, Bae JH, Cho JG, Park SJ; KAMIR (Korea Acute Myocardial Infarction Registry) Investigators. Benefit of early statin therapy in patients with acute myocardial infarction who have extremely low low-density lipoprotein cholesterol. *J Am Coll Cardiol* 2011;58(16):1664–1671.
6. Chen J, Normand SL, Wang Y, Krumholz HM. National and regional trends in heart failure hospitalization and mortality rates for Medicare beneficiaries, 1998–2008. *JAMA* 2011;306(15):1669–1678.
7. Ludwig J, Sanbonmatsu L, Gennetian L, Adam E, Duncan GJ, Katz LF, Kessler RC, Kling JR, Lindau ST, Whitaker RC, McDade TW. Neighborhoods, obesity, and diabetes—a randomized social experiment. *N Engl J Med* 2011;365(16):1509–1519.
8. In ranking of newborn deaths, 'we're No. 41' is USA's shame. *USA Today*, October 4, 2011.
9. Stobbe M. Death wishes vary widely. *Dallas Morning News*, October 22, 2011.
10. Wang SS. Is this the end of popping vitamins? *Wall Street Journal*, October 25, 2011.

11. Baylor's preventive measure. *Dallas Morning News*, September 28, 2011.
12. Mroz J. From one sperm donor, 150 children. *Dallas Morning News*, October 2, 2011.
13. Floud R, Fogel RW, Harris B, Hong SC. *The Changing Body: Health, Nutrition, and Human Development in the Western World Since 1700*. Cambridge: Cambridge University Press, 2011 (431 pp.).
14. Price C. Extreme weather: the 2011 edition. *Parade Magazine*, October 2, 2011.
15. Helliker K. "It's mine!" The selfish gene. *Wall Street Journal*, October 11, 2011.
16. Benenson JF, Pascoe J, Radmore N. Children's altruistic behavior in the dictator game. *Evol Hum Behav* 2007;28(3):168–175.
17. Smits R. *The Puzzle of Left-Handedness*. London: Reaktion, 2011 (384 pp.).
18. Patchett A. *State of Wonder*. New York: Harper, 2011 (368 pp.).
19. Wire reports. Woman gives birth after marathon. *USA Today*, October 11, 2011.
20. Associated Press. Aussie wins third Ironman title. *Dallas Morning News*, October 9, 2011.
21. Steinberg J. *You Are an Ironman: How Six Weekend Warriors Chased Their Dream of Finishing the World's Toughest Triathlon*. New York: Viking, 2011 (304 pp.).
22. Townsend L. Is 'happily married' a myth? *Dallas Morning News*, October 15, 2011.
23. Best to skip some insurance. *Dallas Morning News*, October 25, 2011.
24. Senechal D. *Republic of Noise: The Loss of Solitude in Schools and Culture*. Lanham, MD: Rowman & Littlefield, 2012.
25. Burns S. Doing the math shows tax debate in a new light. *Dallas Morning News*, October 23, 2011.
26. Noonan P. This is no time for moderation. *Wall Street Journal*, October 15–16, 2011.
27. Crary D. 7 billion and no end to fears. *Dallas Morning News*, October 25, 2011.
28. McGurn W. And baby makes seven billion. *Wall Street Journal*, October 25, 2011.
29. Kenny C. The case for second place. *Bloomberg Businessweek*, October 17–23, 2011.
30. Friedman TL. A word from the wise. *New York Times,* March 2, 1010.
31. The end in Iraq. *Dallas Morning News*, October 25, 2011.
32. After nine years in Iraq, time for troops to come home. *USA Today*, October 24, 2011.
33. Associated Press. U.S. in Afghanistan: 10 years later. Longest war marked by progress, despair. *Dallas Morning News*, October 7, 2011.
34. Neuharth A. Dollars and sense of 10 Afghan years. *USA Today*, October 14, 2011.
35. Isaacson W. *Steve Jobs*. New York: Simon & Schuster, 2011 (627 pp.).
36. Gelernter D. Steve Jobs and the coolest show on Earth. *Wall Street Journal*, October 7, 2011.
37. Jobs and Jobs. *Wall Street Journal*, October 7, 2011.
38. Crouch A. The secular prophet. *Wall Street Journal*, October 8–9, 2011.
39. Benzon A. For Job's biological father, the reunion never came. *Wall Street Journal*, October 10, 2011.
40. Steve Jobs 1955–2011. *Bloomberg Businessweek*, October 10–15, 2011.
41. Grossman L, McCracken H. The inventor of the future. *Time*, October 17, 2011.
42. Razzaque R. Steve Jobs put life and death in their place. *USA Today*, October 19, 2011.
43. Swartz J, Martin S. Jobs lived intriguing, yet inscrutable life. *USA Today*, October 26, 2011.
44. Gordon JS. Shaping the future, Henry Ford style. *Dallas Morning News*, September 11, 2011.

Chapter 6

April 2012

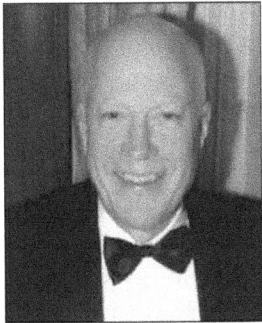

William C. Roberts, MD.

WATER SCARCITY

Benjamin Franklin stated in his *Poor Richard's Almanac*, "When the well is dry we learn the worth of water" (1). Steven Solomon, in his book entitled *Water: The Epic Struggle for Wealth, Power and Civilization,* stated that "water is overtaking oil as the world's scarcest critical natural resource" (2). He indicated that oil is substitutable, albeit painfully, by other fuel sources, or in extremis can be done without, but water's uses are pervasive, irreplaceable by any other substance, and indispensable. In his 2010 book he provides numerous observations, some of which are the following.

There is hardly an accessible freshwater source or a strategically placed waterway in an economically advanced part of the planet that has not been radically engineered by man. As the world population moves toward 9 million and with so many third world inhabitants moving toward consumption and waste-generation levels of the one fifth living in industrialized nations, demand for more fresh water is soaring. Yet no new breakthrough capable of expanding the usable water supply is anywhere evident.

Water scarcity is cleaving an explosive fault line between fresh water-haves and have-nots: among relatively well-watered industrial world citizens and those of water-famished developing countries; among those upriver who control river flows and their neighbors downstream whose survival depends upon receiving a sufficient amount; and among those nations with enough agricultural water to be self-sufficient in food and those dependent upon foreign imports to feed their populations. The new fresh water fault line is fomenting a more divisive competition among interest groups and regions for a greater allocation of limited domestic water resources: between heavily subsidized farmers on the one side and nonsubsidized industrial and urban users on the other; between the well-healed situated within close proximity to fresh water sources and the rural and urban poor remote from water sources; between those able to pay the top price for abundant, wholesome drinking water and the water destitute who glean the dredges; between those who dwell in locations with effective pollution regulations, modern wastewater treatment, and sanitation facilities, and those whose daily lives are contaminated by exposure to impure, disease-plagued water; between the privileged minority living in the planet's relatively well-watered and forested temporal zones and the largest part of the human race living on water-fragile dry lands, oversaturated tropics, or more exposed to the costly unpredictability of extreme precipitation that causes floods, mudslides, and droughts.

Every day across the planet, armies of the water poor, mainly women and children compelled by thirst to forego school and productive work, march barefoot 2 or 3 hours per day transporting water in heavy plastic containers from the nearest clear source for their barest household survivor needs—some 200 pounds per day for a four-person household. This portion of humanity includes over 1.1 billion people, almost one fifth of all humanity, who lack access to at least a gallon per day of safe water to drink. Some 2.6 billion, 2 out of 5 people on earth, are sanitary have-nots lacking the additional 5 gallons needed daily for rudimentary sanitation and hygiene. Far fewer still achieve the minimum threshold of 13 gallons per day for both basic domestic health and well-being, including water for bathing and cooking. The lives of the most abject of water have-nots are chronically afflicted and shortened by diarrhea, dysentery, malaria, dengue fever, schistosomiasis, cholera, and the other conditions that make waterborne diseases human beings' most prevalent scourge. Half the people in the developing world of Africa, Asia, Latin America, and the Caribbean suffer from diseases associated with inadequate fresh water and sanitation. This side of the humanitarian divide includes the 2 billion human beings whose lives are uprooted catastrophically every decade from inadequate public infrastructure protection from water shocks. By contrast, on the water-have side of the humanitarian divide, industrialized-world citizens use 10 to 30 times more water than their poorest, developing nation counterparts. In the water-wealthy USA, each person uses an average of 150 gallons of water per day for domestic and municipal purposes, including such extravagances as multiple toilet flushes and lawn watering.

Water rationing is increasingly commonplace in water have-not societies. So too are internecine conflicts and violent protests over scare supplies and high prices. Inadequate water supply commonly manifests itself in the form of insufficient food output, stunted industrial development, and a shortage of energy, which requires copious volumes of water for cooling and power generation. Chronic water scarcity undercuts the political legitimacy of governments, fomenting social instability and failed states. Water rights, bombings, deaths, and other violent warning signs occurred from 1999 to 2005 in conflicts over water in Karachi, Pakistan, in Gujarat, India, in provinces of arid North China, in Cochabamba, Bolivia, between Kenyan tribes, among Somalian villages, and in Darfur, Sudan. The wars in the last century were often about oil; in this century, water.

Up to half the world's wetlands disappeared or were severely damaged in the 20th century's drive to obtain more arable land and fresh water for agriculture. Worldwide expansion of irrigable farmland is now peaking for the first time in history. Mankind's withdrawal of useable, renewable fresh water from the surface of the planet is expected to rise about 60% by 2025!

In the first decade of the 21st century, an increasing number of nations were so critically water stressed that they could no longer grow all the crops they needed to feed and clothe their populations. Growing crops is a water-intensive enterprise: about three quarters of mankind's water is used for farm irrigation. Food itself is mainly water. To produce a single pound of wheat requires half a ton or nearly 250 gallons of water; a pound of rice needs between 250 and 650 gallons. Livestock for meat and milk multiplies the water requirements since the animals have to be nourished with huge quantities of grain; up to 800 gallons or over 3 tons of water is needed to produce a single hamburger and some 200 gallons for a glass of cow's milk. A well-nourished person consumes about 900 gallons of water each day in the food he or she eats. Production of an ordinary cotton t-shirt requires about 700 gallons of water.

As water-poor countries fall short of self-sufficiency, they are growing increasingly dependent upon importing grain and other foods from water-wealthier farming nations. By 2025, up to 3.6 billion people in some of the driest, most densely populated and poorer parts of the Middle East, Africa, and Asia will live in countries that cannot feed themselves. The growing bifurcation between water-poor food importers and water-rich exporters is further exacerbated by manmade ruination of crop land from soil erosion and polluting runoff. The upward spiraling international food prices as the era of cheap water and cheap food comes to an end is already causing grave consequences. What is needed is a new Green Revolution, perhaps including the development of genetically modified plant hybrids that grow with less water.

Man's access to this renewable fresh water supply is limited to a maximum of one third, since about two thirds quickly disappears in floods and into the ground, ultimately returning to the sea. Even so, that one third totals enough available renewable water to more than suffice for the planet's 7 billion people if it were distributed evenly. But it is not. A large share runs off unused in lightly inhabited jungle rivers like the Amazon, the Congo, and the Orinoco, and across Russia's Siberian expanses toward the Arctic, in the giant Yenisei and Lena Rivers. Thus, the amount of readily available fresh water per person is less

than the threshold annual 2000 cubic meter measure of water sufficiency. And it is declining sharply as the world population increases. Hot climates suffer much higher losses from evaporation than cool, temperate ones. In Africa, only one fifth of all rainfall transforms into potentially utilized runoff.

Thus, each region's actual water challenge varies enormously by environment, availability, and the population it has to support. Australia, by far the driest continent, has only 5% of the world's runoff, but it supports the smallest human population—a mere 20 million, or less than one half of 1% of the world's population. Asia, the largest continent, receives the most renewable water, about one third of the total. Nonetheless, it is the most water-stressed continent because it has to meet the needs of three fifths of humanity, contains some of the world's arid expanses, and receives over three quarters of its precipitation in the form of hard-to-capture seasonal monsoons. The water-richest continent is South America, with 28% of the world's renewable water and only 6% of its population. On a per-person basis, it receives 10 times as much fresh water each year as Asia and 5 times as much as Africa. Yet most of it flows away unused through jungle watersheds, while some high desert regions remain bone dry. North America is water wealthy, with 18% of the world's runoff and 8% of its population. Europe has only 7% of the world's water for its 12% share of population, but it is comparatively advantaged in its wet, northern, and central half because much of its water falls year round, evaporates slowly, and runs off in easily accessible navigable small rivers.

The planet's dry lands, encompassing one third of humanity, or over 2 billion people, have only 8% of the world's renewable supply of water in their surface streams and fast-recharging ground water tables. More than 90% of the dry-land inhabitants live in developing nations, making water famine one of the key vexing challenges of international economic development. It is hardly surprising that the vast dry land belt stretching from North Africa and the Middle East to the Indus Valley is also one of the world's politically volatile regions. At the other end of the spectrum are super water-have countries such as Brazil, Russia, Canada, Panama, and Nicaragua, with far more water than their populations can ever use. The USA and China have large hydrological imbalances: the modestly populated American far west feels constraints on its rapid growth, and the fertile northern plain of China is one of the most severely water-scarce, environmentally challenged regions on earth. India's huge population is outstripping the highly inefficient management of its fresh water resources, forcing farmers, industry, and households to pump ground water faster and deeper than prudent. Western European nations have managed successfully because they use their limited water resources more productively, using a higher proportion for industry and cities and less for agriculture.

Because water is so heavy and needed in such vast quantities, chronic shortages cannot be permanently relieved by transporting it over long distances. One reliable indicator of water wealth is the amount of water storage capacity each nation has installed per person to buffer it against natural shocks. The storage leaders are the world's wealthiest nations, while the poorest remain most exposed to the natural caprices of water.

Despite its growing scarcity and preciousness to life, water is also man's most misgoverned, inefficiently allocated, and profligately wasted natural resource in both democracies and authoritarian states. Modern governments routinely maintain monopolistic control over their nation's supply, pricing, and allocation; commonly, water is distributed as a social good, a political largesse to favored interest groups and to public projects. Governments treat water as if it were a limitless gift of nature to be freely dispensed by any authority with the power to exploit it. In contrast to oil, and nearly every other natural commodity, water is largely exempted from market discipline. Rarely is any inherent value ascribed to the water itself. Only the cost of capturing and distributing it is routinely accounted. Nor is any cost ascribed to the degradation of the water ecosystem from whence it comes and to which, often in a polluted condition, it ultimately returns. By belonging to everyone and being the responsibility of no one, water for most of history has been consumed greedily and polluted recklessly.

The result, compounded over time, is a colossal underpricing of water's full economic and environmental worth. This fact sends an insidious, illusionary economic signal that water supply is endlessly plentiful, promoting wasteful use. Man's most egregious waste of water came from the distortions caused by the chronic underpricing of water for irrigation. Irrigation farmers in Mexico, Indonesia, and Pakistan paid little more than 10% of the full cost of their water. Because Islamic tradition held that water should be free, many Muslim countries charge little or nothing for it. American government dam water subsidies were grandfathered upon a small number of farmers who cultivated a quarter of the irrigated crop land in the arid lands of the west. Inefficient flood irrigation is still subsidized in many water-poor regions. Underpriced water is also a disincentive to urban conservation. Through leaky infrastructure, thirsty Mexico City loses enough water every day—some two fifths of its total supply—to meet the needs of a city as large as Rome. The world faces a trillion-dollar-plus water infrastructure deficit in the years immediately ahead just to patch the leaks!

Water's peculiar treatment economically was contemplated in the 18th century by Adam Smith. In his *Wealth of Nations*, he pondered, "Nothing is more useful than water; but it will purchase scarce anything; scarce anything can be had in exchange for it." Why was water, despite being invaluable to life, so cheap, while diamonds, though relatively useless, so expensive? Smith's answer was that water is ubiquity and the relatively easy labor required to obtain it accounted for its low price. His theory was superseded within mainstream economics in the late 19th century by a more refined explanation. Water's price was determined by a sliding scale based on its availability for its least valued uses: watering lawns, filling swimming pools, quenching the thirst of wildlife. Its premium rose as it became scarce for its most precious uses, reaching its zenith as priceless drinking water. The worth of water is now rising and to reflect Smith's original observation, nothing is more useful.

Bottled water is the world's fastest growing beverage, with annual global sales of over $100 billion, increasing at 10% per year and reaching handsome profits for several corporate giants

(Nestle, Coca-Cola, and Pepsi-Cola). The markup is 1700 times over the cost of public tap water. Privatized management of water utilities is another huge global sector, as is wastewater services, dominated by corporate multinationals. In total, water is a fast-growing, highly fragmented, competitive $400 billion per year industry. Subjecting water to market forces has enormous capacity to stimulate badly needed efficiency gains and innovations. But water is too precious to human life and too politically explosive to be left to the merciless logic of market forces alone.

Water scarcity requires nothing less than a comprehensive re-evaluation of water's vital importance as the new oil—a precious resource that has to be consciously conserved, efficiently used, and properly accounted for on the balance sheet: from public health, food production, and energy production to national security and the sustainability of the human civilization.

Turn off the faucet!

ENERGY DRINKS

A June 2011 article in *Pediatrics* warned that "stimulant-containing energy drinks have no place in the diets of children or adolescents" (3). In October 2011, the National Federation of State High School Associations cautioned that caffeinated energy drinks—often confused with such products as Gatorade, a fluid replacement drink—should not be consumed before, during, or after physical activity because they could raise the risk of dehydration and increase the chance of potentially fatal heart illnesses. The organization also warned of possible interactions with prescription medications, including stimulants used to treat attention-deficit hyperactivity disorder.

The energy drink business is now a $7.7 billion industry. Most best-selling energy drinks (Monster, Red Bull, and Rockstar) contain about 80 mg of caffeine per 8 oz, though they are often sold in containers as large as 20 to 24 oz *(Table 1)*. Other more extreme products abound, some of them in mix-your-own powders or concentrates, in strengths researchers say range from about 50 to 500 mg per serving. At their maximum strength, energy drinks contain about 300 mg more than the 2-oz shots of 5-Hour Energy frequently seen near checkout counters. A 16-oz can of the top-selling energy drinks contain about 160 mg of caffeine. A 16-oz cup of Starbucks' robust Pike Place Roast contains 330 mg. Some researchers have complained that identifying caffeine content and other ingredients is difficult for consumers because US Food and Drug Administration (FDA) regulations do not require products marketed as dietary supplements—as many energy drinks are—to adhere to the same labeling requirements as food and beverages. Canada, in November 2011, moved to limit caffeine in energy drinks to no more than 180 mg in containers up to 20 ounces. In the USA, cola-type drinks are limited by the FDA to 71 mg of caffeine per 12-oz serving. But no such limit applies to energy drinks marketed as dietary supplements, and manufacturers are not required to list the caffeine content or all ingredients on the label, sometimes opting for the term "energy blend" or "proprietary blend."

Additives, including the herbal supplements guarana, green tea, and yerba mate, can boost the effective level of caffeine.

Table 1. Approximate caffeine content in selected drinks*

Beverage	Serving size (oz)	Caffeine (mg)
Soft drinks		
Coca-Cola	12	34
Diet Coke	12	46
Pepsi	12	38
Sprite	12	0
Coffee		
McDonald's brewed	16	100
Starbucks Caffe latte	16	150
Starbucks Pike Place Roast	16	330
Energy drink		
Amp	16	160
Full Throttle	16	197
Monster	16	160[†]
NOS	16	260
Red Bull	16	154
Rockstar	16	160
Spike Shooter	8.4	300
Wired X 344	16	344
Energy shots		
5-Hour Energy	2	207

*Reprinted with permission from Norwood, 2011 (3). Sources: Product labels, MayoClinic.com, company reports.

[†]Monster energy drinks do not include caffeine content on the label, but company and independent reports put it at about 160 mg per 16-oz serving.

Table 2. Estimated new cancer cases and deaths in the USA, 2012*

Site	New cases	Deaths
All	1,638,910	577,190
Oral cavity and pharynx	40,250	7,850
Digestive system	284,680	142,510
Respiratory system	244,180	164,770
Bones and joints	2,890	1,410
Soft tissues (including heart)	11,280	3,900
Skin[†]	81,240	12,190
Breast	229,060	39,920
Genital system	340,650	58,360
Urinary system	141,140	29,330
Eye and orbit	2,610	270
Brain and nervous system	22,910	13,700
Endocrine system	58,980	2,700
Lymphoma	79,190	20,130
Myeloma	21,700	10,710
Leukemia	47,150	23,540
Other or unspecified	31,000[‡]	45,900

*Adapted from Siegel et al., 2012 (8) with permission.

[†]Excludes basal and squamous.

[‡]Underestimated.

Less common additives such as yohimbine and bitter orange can increase heart rate, cause changes in blood pressure, and interact with certain antidepressive medications, according to the National Institutes of Health. Monster, the US leader in sales, does not list the amount of caffeine on its can, although independent sources place it at about 80 mg per 8-oz container, or 240 in Monster's 24-oz can. So far the FDA has not acted on petitions by academics and other experts to limit caffeine or change labeling requirements for energy drinks.

Emergency room visits associated with energy drink use increased more than 10-fold, from 1128 in 2005 to 13,114 in 2009, according to a report released in November 2011 by the federal government's Substance Abuse and Mental Health Services Administration; in 44% of visits, patients combined energy drinks with other substances such as alcohol, pharmaceuticals, or illicit drugs. Most adverse reactions were in those who consumed two to eight energy drinks or >200 mg of caffeine. A report from the Mayo Clinic by Higgins and colleagues (4) listed the side effects of these energy drinks as insomnia, nervousness, nausea, rapid heartbeat, and in rare cases seizures, cardiac arrhythmias, and cardiac arrest.

CANCER ESTIMATES FOR 2012

Each year the American Cancer Society estimates the numbers of new cancer cases and deaths expected in the USA in the current year and compiles the most recent data on cancer incidence, mortality, and survival based on data from the National Cancer Institute, the Centers for Disease Control and Prevention (CDC), the North American Association of Central Cancer Registries, and the National Center for Health Statistics (5). A total of 1,638,910 new cancer cases and 577,190 deaths from cancer are projected to occur in the USA in 2012 (Table 2).

During the most recent 5 years for which there is data (2004–2008), overall cancer *incident rates* declined slightly in men (by 0.6% per year) and were stable in women, while cancer *death rates* decreased by 1.8% per year in men and by 1.6% per year in women. Over the past 10 years (1999–2008), cancer death rates have declined by >1% per year in men and women of every racial/ethnic group with the exception of American Indians/Alaskan Natives, among whom rates have remained stable. The most rapid declines in death rates occurred among African American and Hispanic men (2.4% and 2.3% per year, respectively). Death rates continue to decline for all four major cancer sites (lung, colorectal, breast, and prostate gland), with lung cancer accounting for almost 40% of the total decline in men and breast cancer accounting for 34% of the total decline in women. The reduction in overall cancer death rates since 1990 in men and since 1991 in women translates to the avoidance of about 1,024,400 deaths from cancer.

Nevertheless, cancer is still the second leading cause of death in the USA behind heart disease. About 1 in 2 men and 1 in 3 women develop cancer during their lifetimes. The reduction in breast cancer deaths has been attributed to the decreased use of hormone replacement therapy, to earlier detection, and to better treatments. Both colonoscopy screening and mammography screening rates are higher than they were a year ago. Although the frequency of cancer in general is decreasing, seven cancers are increasing: mouth and throat cancers caused by human papillomavirus, the same virus that causes cervical cancer; esophageal adenocarcinoma, which is linked to chronic acid reflux, obesity, and smoking; melanoma, caused by exposure to ultraviolet radiation from the sun and tanning beds; liver cancer, which may be related in part to increases in hepatitis B and C infections; thyroid cancer, for unknown reasons, but maybe because of better detection; kidney cancer, which may be related to rising obesity; and pancreatic cancer, which is linked to smoking, obesity, and family history. Thus, preventing obesity will decrease the frequency of cancers of the esophagus, liver, kidney, and pancreas. Another reason to lose weight.

BINGE DRINKING

According to a January 2012 report from the CDC, 1 in 6 adults in the USA is a binge drinker, consuming an average of eight drinks per occasion and doing so four times a month (6). The risky behavior exists in all states, causing more than half of the 80,000 deaths and three quarters of the $23 billion in economic cost. Most alcohol-impaired drivers binge drink. Binge drinking means men drinking ≥5 drinks within a short period of time and women drinking ≥4 drinks. The authors analyzed self-reported data collected during 2010 of US adults aged ≥18 in 48 states and in the District of Columbia. The prevalence was twice as likely in men (23%) than women (11%). The highest prevalence of binge drinking was among those aged 18 to 34 years. The highest frequency was among the 65+ group. Those with an income of >$75,000 annually were more likely to binge drink. Those with an income of <$25,000 annually did it most often and drank the most per binge. Most people, however, who binge drink are not alcoholics.

STRESS

A survey by the American Psychological Association (APA) indicates that the average stress level in the USA in 2011 was 5.2 on a 10-point scale, down from 6.2 in 2007 (7). Among those surveyed, 39% indicated that their stress rose in 2011, 17% said it dropped, and 44% said it stayed the same. According to the APA, until 2011, stress has been rising each year since 2007. The newest survey involved 1226 adults aged 18 and older. Those reporting extreme stress, grade 8, 9, or 10, dropped from 32% to 22%, and 27% of adults said their stress had decreased in the past 5 years. Better economic conditions may be the explanation, because the 10 top causes of stress are money, work, the economy, relationships, family responsibilities, family health, personal health, job stability, housing costs (mortgage or rent), and personal safety. The APA also has recommendations to handle stress: *take a break, exercise, laugh, get support,* and *meditate.* Of these, the most successfully used stress management tool is exercise. The APA survey found that adults aged 18 to 32 (the so-called "Millennials") are less likely than older adults to feel stressed by the economy. Unlike older adults who have watched their nest eggs disappear, younger people have been most affected by the downturn's impact on jobs.

COMPASSION FATIGUE

Compassion fatigue is a combination of burnout and secondary traumatic stress from witnessing the suffering of others. The group that is affected the most is nurses, and compassion fatigue can lead to a feeling of sadness and despair that affects their health and well-being (8) *(Table 3)*. A number of hospitals are tackling the problem in the midst of a worsening shortage of nurses. Compassion fatigue has been linked to decreased productivity, lessened empathy, more sick days, and higher turnover, particularly among cancer-care providers.

A study led by the University of Nevada's nursing school in Reno found that about 12% of US registered nurses were not working. Of those, more than 25% cited burnout or stressful work environments. The high turnover increases the workload on remaining nurses, and that can result in higher death rates and lessened patient safety. Compassion fatigue was identified as a special problem for nurses in the early 1990s. The New York State Nurses Association conducted its first compassion-fatigue workshop at a hospital last year and is urging hospitals and nursing schools to offer such programs.

AIRPLANE GERMS

It's a common complaint: fly on a crowded airplane and come home with a cold. Air travelers suffer higher rates of infection than do non–air travelers. A reported number is 20% (9). Air that is recirculated through the cabin is most often blamed. But studies have shown that high-efficiency particulate air filters on most jets today

Table 3. Symptoms of compassion fatigue*

Work-related	Physical	Emotional
• Avoidance or dread of working with certain patients • Reduced ability to feel empathy towards patients or families • Frequent use of sick days • Lack of joyfulness	• Headaches • Digestive problems: diarrhea, constipation, upset stomach • Muscle tension • Sleep disturbances: inability to sleep, insomnia, too much sleep • Fatigue • Cardiac symptoms: chest pain/pressure, palpitations, tachycardia	• Mood swings • Restlessness • Irritability • Oversensitivity • Anxiety • Excessive use of substances: nicotine, alcohol, illicit drugs • Depression • Anger and resentment • Loss of objectivity • Memory issues • Poor concentration, focus, and judgment

*From Landro, 2012 (8).

capture 99.97% of bacterial and virus-carrying particles. When air circulation, however, is shut down, which sometimes happens during long waits on the ground or for short periods when passengers are boarding or exiting, infections can spread rapidly. A study in 1979 found that when a plane sat 3 hours with its engines off and no air circulating, 72% of the 54 passengers on board got sick within 2 days. The flu strain they had was traced to one passenger. For that reason, the Federal Aviation Administration issued an advisory to airlines in 2003 saying that passengers should be removed from planes within 30 minutes if there is no air circulating, but compliance is not mandatory. Much of the danger comes from the mouths, noses, and hands of passengers sitting nearby. The "hot zone" for exposure is generally two seats beside, in front of, and behind, according to a study in the July 2011 issue of *Emerging Infectious Diseases,* published by the CDC.

A number of factors increase the odds of bringing home a cold from an airplane. The environment at 30,000 feet enables easier spread of disease. Air in airplanes is extremely dry, and viruses tend to thrive in low-humidity conditions. When mucus membranes dry up, they are far less effective at blocking infection. High altitudes also tire the body, and fatigue plays a role in making people more susceptible to catching colds. Also, viruses and bacteria can live for hours on some surfaces; some viral particles have been found to be active up to a day in certain places. Tray tables can be contaminated, and seatback pockets, which get stuffed with used tissues, soiled napkins, and trash, can be particularly dangerous. It is also difficult to know what germs are lurking on airline pillows and blankets.

There are some basic precautions passengers can take to keep coughs away. 1) *Hydrate:* drinking water and keeping nasal passages moist can reduce the risk of infection. 2) *Keep hands clean:* frequently use an alcohol-based hand sanitizer. We often infect ourselves, touching mouth, nose, or eyes with our own hands that have picked up something. 3) *Use disinfectant wipes to clean off tray tables before using.* 4) *Avoid seatback pockets.* 5) *Open the air vent and aim it so it passes just in front of your face.* Filtered airplane air can help direct airborne contagions away from you. 6) *Change seats if you end up near a cougher, sneezer, or someone who looks feverish.* 7) *Inform the crew if air circulation is shut off for an extended period.* 8) *Avoid airline pillows and blankets.*

Fortunately, most people sitting near someone who is ill do not get sick.

TRUCK DRIVING AND BODY WEIGHT

According to a 2007 study in the *Journal of the American Diabetic Association,* 86% of the estimated 3.2 million truck drivers in the USA are overweight, and most are obese (10). The US Transportation Department requires truck drivers to pass a certifying medical exam every 2 years. Drivers are checked for severe heart conditions, high blood pressure, and respiratory maladies, including sleep disorders. The results are bleak. Driving is a sedentary activity. Most truckers are paid by the mile, so they tend to squeeze every minute out of the 11 hours they are allowed on the road in a 24-hour period. Recently, transportation carriers, industry organizations, and even truck

stops are unrolling initiatives to help truckers slim down, shape up, and improve their health. Employers are holding health seminars, building on-site gyms, bringing in nutritionists and fitness trainers, and offering financial incentives to employees who stop smoking or lose weight. Some drivers are cooking in their rigs, walking or biking around truck stops, and blogging about their experiences at sites like truckingsolutionsgroup.org and safetythruwellness.com.

SLEEP DISORDERS IN POLICE OFFICERS

Rajaratnam and colleagues (11) from Boston screened 4957 North American police officers who participated in either an online or an onsite screening and monthly follow-up surveys between July 2005 and December 2007, and 40% screened positive for at least one sleep disorder: 1666 (34%) for obstructive sleep apnea, 281 (6%) for moderate to severe insomnia, and 269 (5%) for shift work disorder. Respondents who screened positive for any sleep disorder had an increased prevalence of physical and mental health conditions, including diabetes mellitus, depression, and cardiovascular disease. Police officers need to be awake.

OBESITY AND MEDICARE

The US Medicare system recently announced that it will cover intensive behavioral counseling for willing participants with a body mass index of ≥30 kg/m². The plan, expected to cover more than 30% of the Medicare population, will mean 6 months of in-person therapy, extending to 12 months if the beneficiary has successfully lost 3 kg.

TREATING LOW BACK PAIN

Sherman and associates (12) from Seattle, Washington, and Portland, Oregon, designed a trial to determine whether yoga is more effective than conventional stretching exercises or a self-care book for patients with chronic low back pain. A total of 228 adults with chronic low back pain were randomized to 12 weekly classes of yoga, conventional stretching exercises, or a self-care book. Back-related functional status and bothersomeness of pain at 12 weeks were the primary outcomes. At both 12 weeks and 26 weeks, the outcomes for the yoga group were superior to those of the self-care group but not superior to conventional stretching exercises at any time point. Keep stretching and moving.

COST OF ASSISTED LIVING

As the baby boomer generation grows older, the average life expectancy also increases. In the USA, life expectancy in 2008, the last year available, was 78.1 years. The number of people living in nursing homes nationwide has dropped in the last decade as other services—such as home health care and assisted living—have become more readily available (13). In 2000, 1.72 million lived in nursing homes in the US, and that had dropped to 1.5 million by 2010. Daily rates for rooms in private nursing homes vary across the continental US from <$200 to >$350 per day. The average in Texas is $188 per day and in Alaska, $655 per day. The hourly cost of hiring a home health aide across the

US varies from $15 to $30 daily. In Texas, the average is $18. Adult day care centers in the US range from $40 to >$100 per day; in Texas the average is $40 per day.

Who should consider a long-term care insurance policy? Not the wealthy. Not those of modest means who qualify for Medicare. It is those in between, where paying long-term care expenses would impoverish the spouse. Many people believe Medicare covers long-term care, but generally it does not. One must meet certain conditions for Medicare to pay for these types of care. People are staying in assisted living facilities for a lot longer than in the past. They are a lot less institutional than nursing homes: their appearance is better, they smell nicer, and they offer nice activities, such as live bands every week.

CANINE POSTTRAUMATIC STRESS DISORDER

By some estimates, more than 5% of the approximately 6050 military dogs deployed by US combat forces are coming down with canine posttraumatic stress disorder (PTSD) (14). Of those, about half are likely to be retired from service. Although veterinarians have long diagnosed behavioral problems in nonhuman animals, the concept of canine PTSD is only about 18 months old, having come into vogue among military veterinarians who have been seeing patterns of troubling behavior among dogs exposed to explosions, gunfire, and other combat-related violence in Iraq and Afghanistan. Like humans with the analogous disorder, different dogs show different symptoms. Some become hypervigilant, others avoid buildings or work areas that they had previously been comfortable in, and some undergo sharp changes in temperament, becoming unusually aggressive with their handlers or clingy and timid. Many stop doing the task they were trained to perform. Treatment can be tricky since the patient (dog) cannot explain what is wrong; veterinarians and handlers must make educated guesses about the traumatizing events. Care can be as simple as taking a dog off patrol and giving it lots of exercise, play, and gentle obedience training. More serious cases receive what is called "desensitization counter conditioning," which entails exposing the dog at a safe distance to a site or sound that might trigger a reaction—a gunshot, a loud bang, or a vehicle, for instance. If the dog does not react, it is rewarded, and the trigger is moved progressively closer until the dog is comfortable with it.

DIABETES MELLITUS AND AMPUTATION

About 1 in 10 US adults has diabetes mellitus; it is the seventh leading cause of death in the USA, according to the CDC. A recent study (15) disclosed that the number of diabetic patients aged ≥40 years who had lost a toe, foot, or leg fell from 1988 through 2008 from >11 to 4 per 1000 people. Among nondiabetics during the same period, the frequency of amputation had not changed. Even though the frequency of type 2 diabetes mellitus is continuing to increase in the USA because of the great increase in body weight, some of the other dreaded complications of diabetes including blindness and kidney failure have also decreased during this 20-year period. The exact reason for the decrease in amputations is unclear,

but CDC officials believe that improved patient education, earlier diagnosis, better blood sugar monitoring, protective shoes and other medical devices, and better care of feet are paying dividends.

PEOPLE HURTING PEOPLE

Matthew White, a self-described atrocitologist, necromatrician, and quantifier of hemoclysms, has compiled the most comprehensive, disinterested, and statistically nuanced estimates available of the death tolls of history's major catastrophes in a book entitled *The Great Big Book of Horrible Things* (16). His scorn is directed at the stupidity and callousness of history's great leaders and at the indifference of traditional history to the magnitude of human suffering behind momentous events. The largest numbers of victims in the top 25 events are listed in *Table 4*. The Second World War heads the list with 60 million fatalities. The American Civil War (1861–1865) resulted in 620,000 soldier fatalities and 75,000 civilian fatalities, and it is listed at number 75 in the all-time list. The Korean War, which resulted in 3 million soldier and civilian fatalities, is number 30. Our enemies in World War II, namely Germany and Japan, now are our best friends internationally.

Table 4. The 25 deadliest multicides*

No	Event	Deaths (millions)
1	Second World War (1939–1945)	66
2	Chinggis Khan (1206–1227)	40
3	Hao Zedong (1949–1976)	40
4	Famines in British India (18th–20th centuries)	27
5	Fall of the Ming Dynasty (1635–1662)	25
6	Taiping Rebellion (1850–1864)	20
7	Joseph Stalin (1928–1953)	20
8	Midwest slave trade (7th–19th centuries)	18.5
9	Timur (1370–1405)	17
10	Atlantic slave trade (1452–1807)	16
11	Conquest of the Americas (after 1492)	15
12	First World War (1914–1918)	15
13	An Lushan Rebellion (755–763)	13
14	Xin Dynasty (9–24)	10
15	Congo Free State (1885–1908)	10
16	Russian Civil War (1918–1920)	9
17	Thirty-Year War (1618–1648)	7.5
18	Fall of the Yuan Dynasty (ca. 1340–1370)	7.5
19	Fall of the Western Roman Empire (395–455)	7
20	Chinese Civil War (1927–1937, 1945–1949)	7
21	Mahdi Revolt (1881–1898)	5.5
22	The Time of Troubles (1598–1613)	5
23	Aurangzeb (1658–1707)	4.6
24	Vietnam War (1959–1975)	4.2
25	The Three Kingdoms of China (189–280)	4.1

*From White, *The Great Big Book of Horrible Things*, 2012 (16).

PROFESSIONAL BASEBALL AND BODY WEIGHT

As Matthew Futterman described in a January 27, 2012, piece in *The Wall Street Journal,* in signing *C. C. Sabathia, Albert Pujols,* and *Prince Fielder* (son of big leaguer Cecil Fielder), the New York Yankees, Los Angeles Angels, and Detroit Tigers have committed $590 million to 825 pounds of baseball player (17). The Detroit Tigers reached a reported 9-year, $214 million deal with 71-inch, 275-pound 27-year-old Fielder. Albert Pujols (Prince Albert) is 75 inches tall and weighs 230 pounds at age 31. He signed a 10-year $254 million contract with the Los Angeles Angels. Sabathia at age 31 is 79 inches in height and weighs 290 pounds. He signed a contract extension last year to pitch for the Yankees for 5 more years for $122 million (plus a $25 million option for 2017). All three of these players need a nutritionist. Their late-night meals and free (to them) room service in hotels is too tempting for them.

TOMATOES

Thomas Jefferson thought they were poisonous, and although he grew many in his yard in Monticello they were for decoration only. Now, 90% of backyard gardens include tomato plants, and in 2009 Americans bought $5 billion worth of commercially grown fresh tomatoes. Barry Estabrook has recently written a book entitled *Tomatoland . . .* and he asks the question: "What has happened to the good flavor that used to be in tomatoes?" (18). He found that the lack of flavor in today's crop of tomatoes is the result of science and business working together to create fruits that have a long shelf life and are nearly impervious to bruising or harsh handling. Most tomatoes Americans eat whole (as opposed to in a sauce or ketchup form) are grown in Florida. The Sunshine State's sandy soil lacks the basic nutrients needed to produce good-tasting fruit, so farmers rely heavily on chemical fertilizers, pesticides, and herbicides to give the plants a boost. The high environmental and human cost of this chemical is a fruit devoid of tomato flavor and one that contains less vitamin C, thiamine, niacin, and calcium and 14 times as much sodium as a tomato grown in the 1960s. The best tomato is the one grown in one's backyard. If you can't grow your own, shop at the local farmer's market or find locally grown in-season tomatoes in the supermarket. Whole Foods sells only "organic" tomatoes that have not been sprayed with chemicals.

ERRORS IN NEWSPAPERS

Newspapers often focus on reporting errors produced by members of our society, particularly those in prominent positions. The *Washington Post* publishes its own errors, a total of 875 corrections in its print edition in 2011, a 17% decrease from 1054 in 2010 (19). The 875 number is the lowest for any year since the *Post* began counting in 2005, when it had >1300 corrections. Good for the *Post!*

EUROZONE GOVERNMENT DEBT

European leaders are trying to stop a debt crisis that is threatening to shadow their 12-year-old experiment: a common Euro currency (20). The monetary union has existed since the Euro was created in 1999, but the European Union, which includes the 17 Euro nations and 10 others that use their own currencies, has no central authority over taxing and spending. Government debt as a percentage of gross domestic product in 2010 among the European countries ranges from 7% in Estonia to 143% in Greece, and not one of the 17 countries is in the black. The unemployment rate in the 17 nations ranges from 5% (Cyprus) to 20% (Spain). The US cannot provide leadership because we also are broke. Individuals have a hard time saving money without frugality; nations must learn that virtue.

FINANCIAL WORTH OF LAWMAKERS ON CAPITOL HILL

In the 1970s, the members of Congress included a barber, a pipefitter, and a housepainter, and they organized into what was called the "blue collar caucus" (21). The financial gap between Americans and their representatives in Congress has widened considerably since then, according to an analysis of financial disclosures by *The Washington Post.* Between 1984 and 2009, the median net worth of a member of the House of Representatives more than doubled, from $280,000 to $725,000 in inflation-adjusted 2009 dollars, excluding home equity. Over the same period, the wealth of an American family declined slightly, with the comparable median figure sliding from $20,500 to $20,000 according to the Panel Study of Income Dynamics from The University of Michigan. The growing disparity between Representatives and the represented means that there is greater distance between the economic experience of Americans and those of lawmakers.

The growing financial comfort of members of Congress relative to most Americans is consistent with the general trend in the USA toward inequality of wealth. Members of Congress have long been wealthier than average Americans, and in recent decades the wealth of the wealthiest Americans has outpaced that of the average. In 1984, the earliest year for which consistent wealth statistics are available for members of Congress, the 90th percentile of US families had holdings worth 6 times those of the median families; by 2009, the 90th percentile had holdings worth 12 times those of the median families. These figures include home equity. Not only has the median wealth of members of Congress increased, but the proportion of Representatives who have little besides a home has shrunk. In 1984, 1 in 5 House members had 0 or negative net worth, excluding home equity; by 2009 that number had dropped to 1 in 12.

Another possible reason for the growing wealth of Congress is that running a campaign has become much more expensive, making it more likely that wealthy people, who can donate substantially to their own campaigns, gain office. Since 1976, the average amount spent by winning House candidates quadrupled in inflation-adjusted dollars, to $1.4 million. The congressional pay is not one of the reasons for the growing disparity between Representatives and their constituents. In inflation-adjusted dollars, a member of Congress in 1977 earned $215,000; today, a member of Congress earns $174,000. The growth of income inequality has tracked closely with measures of political polarization, which has been gauged using the average difference between the liberal/conservative scores for Republican and Democratic members of the House.

A person's financial circumstances affect a person's political outlook. People identified as lower or middle class have been more likely to see income inequality as a problem and to favor redistribution of income. A Representative's occupation before being elected influences how liberal or conservative he or she is in voting, according to a study from Duke University. In order from most conservative to most liberal: farm owners; business people such as bankers or insurance executives; private-sector professionals such as physicians, engineers, and architects; lawyers; service-based professionals, such as teachers and social workers; politicians; and blue-collar workers. Although party affiliation is the strongest determiner of voting records, the differences between legislators of different occupational backgrounds are striking. This information was gathered by Peter Whoriskey of *The Washington Post*.

SNOWFLAKES

Kenneth Libbrecht, a Cal-Tech physics professor, has been studying snowflakes under the microscope for nearly 2 decades (22). His photos of the frozen crystals of water grace more than 3 billion US postage stamps. He also has authored numerous articles on the molecular dynamics that dictate how ice crystals grow. The shape that snow takes depends on the temperature. From about freezing to 25°F, snow forms as flakes; when the temperature hits about 23°, the snow forms into needles; and at about 22°, into hollow columns. When the temperature drops to 10°, flakes start forming again, but when it gets to –8° or so, it once again turns to columns, and at –30°, snow stops forming altogether. A copy of one of his stellar dendrites is shown in the *Figure*.

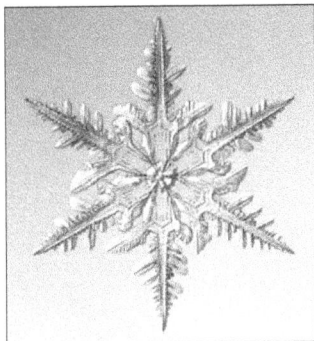

Figure. Snowflake.

PUBLIC-SECTOR PENSIONS

An Associated Press survey in 2011 found that the 50 states in the USA have a combined $690 billion in unfunded pension liabilities and just under $420 billion in retiree health care obligations (23). In California it was recently pointed out that a public education teacher there for 40 years can retire at age 59 with a pension of $174,000 a year for the rest of his or her life. Many cities, counties, and states in the US are struggling to pay pension bills, but changes are afoot. In November 2011, San Francisco voters supported a local ballot initiative to raise minimum retirement ages for some city workers. Laws increasing retirement ages for government workers have been signed in Rhode Island and Massachusetts in efforts to address underfunded pension systems. In New Jersey the retirement age was raised from 62 to 65. Most private-sector workers no longer receive defined benefit pensions that will pay them for life. Most must wait until age 65 or 67 to collect their full Social Security benefits or draw from 401k (closed) accounts that are invested in the stock market.

MATRIMONY

In 1960, 72% of adults 18 and older were married. That fell to 57% in 2000 and to 51% in 2011, according to Pew Researcher D'Vera Cohn (24). The share of marrieds could dip below 50% in a few years as single-person households, single parents, and couples living together outside of legal marriage multiply. The number of new marriages in the USA fell 5% from 2009 to 2010, a fall that may or may not be related to the bad economy. The decline is spread among age groups but is most dramatic among those under 30. Nearly 3 of every 5 adults aged 18 to 29 were married in 1960; but in 2011, it was only 1 in 5.

DISPOSING OF ELECTRONICS

Electronics contain lead, mercury, cadmium, and other potentially harmful chemicals, but only 25% of discarded devices (by weight) were recycled in 2009, the most recent year for which the Environmental Protection Agency has data (25). Seventeen states have banned electronic waste from landfills, requiring it to be recycled so its toxic materials do not leach into ground water. If we all recycled computers, computer displays, hard-copy devices, keyboards, mice, television sets, and mobile devices, we would all be better off.

FIRECRACKER INJURIES

Many Filipinos, largely influenced by Chinese tradition, believe that noisy New Year's celebrations drive away evil and misfortune. But many in the Philippines have carried that superstition to extreme, exploding huge firecrackers and firing guns to welcome the new year despite threats of arrest. Firecrackers in Manila on New Year's Eve 2011 injured 454, and 18 others were injured by stray bullets (26). The injured revelers included many children and filled hospital emergency rooms in Manila shortly after midnight. About a dozen plane flights, including two from the USA, were diverted or cancelled early New Year's Day after dark smog caused by a night of firecracker explosions obscured visibility at Manila's airports. Additionally, firecrackers ignited at least three fires that destroyed several houses in the capital area. Be careful with firecrackers.

US DEBT

The US debt is now about $16 trillion! The US population now is about 313 million people, and thus the debt for every adult and child amounts to $52,500. Countries in debt appear to be at the mercy of countries not in debt.

—WILLIAM CLIFFORD ROBERTS, MD
6 February 2012

1. Franklin B. *Poor Richard's Almanack*. New York: Peter Pauper Press (77 pp.).

2. Solomon S. *Water: The Epic Struggle for Wealth, Power and Civilization*. New York: HarperCollins, 2010 (596 pp.).

3. Norwood R. Young athletes, energy drinks: A bad mix? *USA Today*, December 2–4, 2011.

4. Higgins JP, Tuttle TD, Higgins CL. Energy beverages: content and safety. *Mayo Clin Proc* 2010;85(11):1033–1041.

5. Siegel R, Naishadham D, Jernal A. Cancer statistics, 2012. *CA Cancer J Clin* 2012;62(1):10–29.

6. Lloyd J. "Dramatic" findings on binge drinking. *USA Today*, January 11, 2012.

7. Jones S. Yeah, we're STRESSED but dealing with it. *USA Today*, January 11, 2012.

8. Landro L. When nurses catch compassion fatigue, patients suffer. *Wall Street Journal*, January 3, 2012.

9. McCartney S. Where germs lurk on planes. A survival guide. *Wall Street Journal*, December 20, 2011.

10. Ellin A (New York Times). Truckers driven to shape up. *Dallas Morning News*, November 27, 2011.

11. Rajaratnam SM, Barger LK, Lockley SW, Shea SA, Wang W, Landrigan CP, O'Brien CS, Qadri S, Sullivan JP, Cade BE, Epstein LJ, White DP, Czeisler CA; Harvard Work Hours, Health and Safety Group. Sleep disorders, health, and safety in police officers. *JAMA* 2011;306(23):2567–2578.

12. Sherman KJ, Cherkin DC, Wellman RD, Cook AJ, Hawkes RJ, Delaney K, Deyo RA. A randomized trial comparing yoga, stretching, and a self-care book for chronic low back pain. *Arch Intern Med* 2011;171(22):2019–2026.

13. Yip P, Alcott K. The cost of growing old. *Dallas Morning News*, December 19, 2011.

14. Dao J. Our furriest solders get PTSD, too. *Dallas Morning News*, December 5, 2011.

15. Li Y, Burrows NR, Gregg EW, Albright A, Geiss LS. Declining rates of hospitalization for nontraumatic lower-extremity amputation in the diabetic population aged 40 years or older: U.S., 1988–2008. *Diabetes Care* 2012;35(2):273–277.

16. White M. *The Great Big Book of Horrible Things*. New York: WW Norton, 2012 (669 pp.).

17. Futterman M. Will cholesterol kill baseball? *Wall Street Journal*, January 27, 2012.

18. Harris M. What happened to tomatoes? *Erickson Living*, January 2012.

19. Pexton PB. The year in corrections. *Washington Post*, January 1, 2012.

20. Act or face collapse, eurozone is warned. *Dallas Morning News*, November 29, 2011.

21. Whoriskey P. Congress looks less like rest of America. *Washington Post*, December 27, 2011.

22. Weise E. Wondering about snowflakes. *USA Today*, December 19, 2011.

23. Pear R. Hefty price tag thwarts payroll tax deal, others. *Dallas Morning News*, December 5, 2011.

24. Associated Press. Fewer Americans wedded to the idea of matrimony. *Dallas Morning News*, December 21, 2011.

25. Koch W. More states ban disposal of electronics in landfills. *USA Today*, December 19, 2011.

26. Gomez J. Philippines New Year firecrackers injure nearly 500. *Huffington Post*, January 1, 2012.

Chapter 7

July 2012

MAJOR PERSONALITY TYPES

In the late 1970s, while I was a visiting professor of cardiology at Duke University, I learned of the book titled *The Achievers: Six Styles of Personality and Leadership* by Gerald D. Bell (1), a professor in the School of Business at the University of North Carolina, Chapel Hill. The book had a major impact on me. I found its insights to be useful in my dealings with other people and as a consequence bought many copies for family, colleagues, and friends. While attending the American Osler Society meeting in Chapel Hill in April 2012, nearly 40 years after first learning about Bell's book, I was fortunate to meet the author, who was having a leadership conference also at the Carolina Inn. Professor Bell signed one of his books for me, and I enjoyed immensely speaking with him for a few minutes.

In his book, Bell described six personality styles: *the Commander, the Attacker, the Avoider, the Pleaser, the Performer, and the Achiever*, and he also described how to deal with each. He emphasized that we all have parts of these personalities within us but usually one of them dominates. The *Figure* summarizes in part the characteristic features of each of these personalities.

The Commander: This person demands an orderly environment. He or she is domineering, uses categorical thinking, sees only one aspect of communication, is close-minded, is self-disciplined, has a routine sexual style, performs well in orderly situations, sets high goals but takes below-average risks, and has moderate psychological health.

The Attacker: One of the six or seven publishers I have dealt with during my 30 years as editor of *The American Journal of Cardiology* was an attacker. I learned (from Bell) how to deal with an attacker. Bell's advice was to attack back. I did so and we became friends. The attacker, according to Bell, is shaped by a domineering, inconsistent, and harsh environment. The attacker is defiant, hostile, rejects responsibilities, acts uncommitted, gives variable commitment, disrupts, imputes evil to others, makes everything an emergency, forms an attack squadron, seldom admits being wrong, is cold personally, has an aggressive

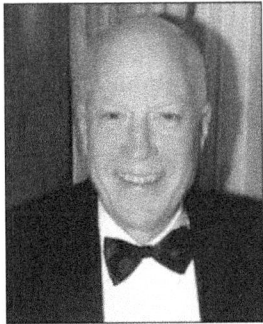

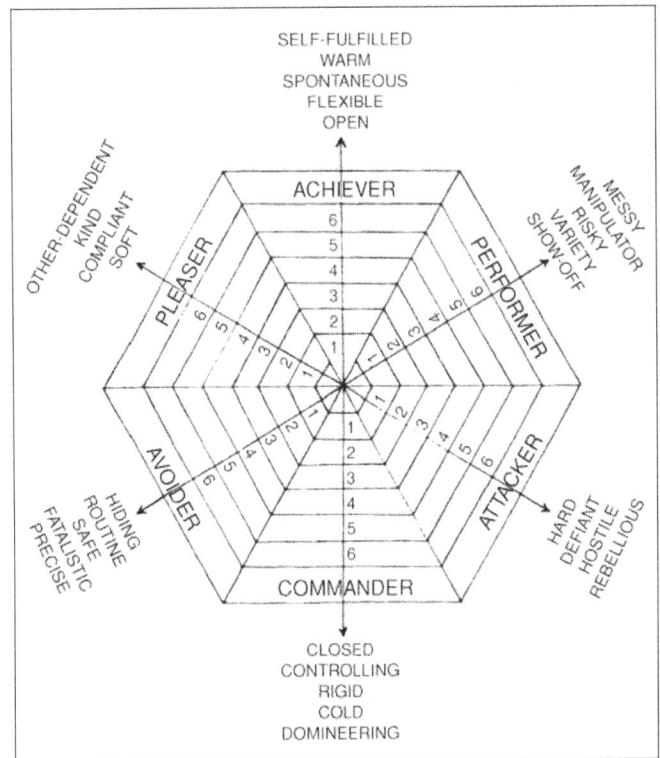

William C. Roberts, MD.

Figure. The six-M personality diamond.

sexual style, performs well in independent jobs, and has poor psychological health.

The Avoider: One of my bosses at the National Institutes of Health was an avoider. He told me one time to never make a decision until I was pressed against the wall and had to. Bell taught how to deal with that personality: Simply do not take issues to him on which he has to make decisions. I did that, and my boss and I became good friends. According to Bell, the avoider was raised in a fearful and overprotected environment, has low self-confidence, takes few risks, procrastinates, is dependent, is a nonexplorer, is unable to totally give of himself or herself in a relationship or freezes at the thought of intimacy, does not like feedback, performs well in easy jobs, and has poor psychological health.

The Pleaser: I also dealt with a pleaser for many decades and learned from Bell's book how to deal with one: let them please you. The pleaser's training environment is overcaring.

He or she needs to be accepted, is "other-directed," is highly persuadable, tends to be passive in lovemaking, has a reservoir of people-pleasing talents (releases tension with good humor, is sensitive and kind, is the "good guy"), performs well in social tasks, and has average psychological health.

The Performer: This is the dominant personality style in the US, making up just over 40% of the administrators and managers in the country. The performer's training environment stresses being successful and proper. The performer is an explorer, is skillful at manipulation, uses pseudoparticipation, is a deal-king, engages in joint-image management, takes credit for successes, parcels out compliments, uses anticipatory socialization (develops skills in learning the norms of the status group above him and then acts as they do to be accepted more quickly by them), uses proper timing, is an inside dopester, is counter-clever and is a good one-upsman, is hard to pin down—a fence-sitter, masters sensation transference (the process of transferring first impressions about an object into feelings about its contents), controls information, is purposefully courteous, dresses properly (perfectly groomed, fashionably dressed), selects proper friends, acquires proper knowledge (reads the latest books, sees the current "in" movie, knows the most popular music, uses proper habits, disguises his efforts), does not appear to be straining to look good—not too eager, and uses protective devices (shifts from one group to another, never gets close to others because it is exhausting to be on guard at all times around close associates). He uses two aspects of communication (what he says, the verbal part, and what he does, the nonverbal part). There is a lack of consistency between what he or she says and does; his sexual style is fleeting and distant and without intimacy; he bends the truth (uses false flattery, uses false modesty, lies to himself); he does well in prestigious jobs (when a first impression is important, when a flashy, polished image gets the job done, and when the positions are challenging and prestigious), and he has average psychological health.

The Achiever: I think the word used to describe this person is not quite accurate, but this is the ideal personality type. The achiever's environment warmly encourages independence. He or she has high self-confidence (is self-directed and nondefensive, has an acute awareness of inner feelings), is spontaneous and natural, is self-reliant (self-contained), is goal-oriented, is problem-centered instead of self-centered, is creative (an explorer), has deep genuine human relationships (feels without fear, is content, has compassion, is ethical, has fun), performs meaningful and challenging jobs well (is realistic), develops intelligence, and is 100% psychologically healthy. Bell opines that the only really successful marriages are between two achievers.

COMMONALITY IN GREAT LEADERS

Jack Welch, one of the great chief executive officers of the last century, and his wife, Suzy, ask "What do great leaders have in common?" (2). Their answer: *authenticity.* That makes people like you, trust you, and follow you. (He actually describes Bell's achiever.) They speak of "guarded behavior" as something that may minimize the ire of your enemies, but

it doesn't energize anyone either. They stress that leaders let go of the fear of offending people and embrace the authentic side. They offer a short list of "stuff authentic people say." First, Jack and Suzy quote Popeye, who stated that authentic people give you some version of "I yam what I yam and that's all that I yam." Authentic people are deeply comfortable with themselves; they acknowledge without phoniness where they have come from and who they have become, both the good and the not-so-good, through life's accidents and their own hard work and ambition. Second, authentic people say "I love" a lot. You name it, they are emoting about it. By the same token, authentic people also tend to throw around "I hate" quite a bit. They are overtly passionate. Maybe being candid gives you self-confidence—you are not hiding anything—and that self-confidence allows you to be exuberant about your beliefs, values, and opinions. Third, authentic people are not afraid to say "I screwed up, and I've been down, and it was awful." Authentic people seem to relish describing their mistakes in detail.

INTRIGUING HEALTH QUESTIONS

Catherine Price asked a number of medical experts some intriguing questions and recorded their answers (3). Here are some selections:

1) *Why do I get goosebumps during scary movies?* Goosebumps are produced by piloerection, a reflex that contracts the muscles around the base of each hair follicle, causing the hair to stand up and small bumps to emerge. Back when humans were hairier, piloerection had two benefits: it helped in keeping people warm by trapping heated air close to the skin, and in scary situations, it made them look bigger and more threatening. Watching a horror flick in an air-conditioned theater provides the perfect setup for piloerection. One is not only frightened but also probably cold.

2) *Why does it seem as if mosquitoes bite me preferentially?* The bloodsuckers are drawn to a tasty dinner by a variety of signals, including heat, carbon dioxide, movement, and the smell of skin secretions, like lactic acid. One study found that mosquitoes prefer people who have recently drank a beer. No one knows what precise combination mosquitoes find the most irresistible.

3) *Why do men get more hair in some places and less in others as they get older?* The "George Costanza effect" is a common sign of aging. It's caused by dihydrotestosterone, a sex hormone to which some men are genetically predisposed to become sensitive. When that sensitivity develops, the hormone often causes the hair follicles on the head to shrink and follicles elsewhere, like on the back or in the ears or nasal passages, to become stimulated.

4) *What are hiccups, and how can one stop them?* A hiccup is an involuntary contraction of the diaphragm and the muscles between our ribs. A bout of hiccupping is usually the result of overeating or drinking carbonated beverages. (Other causes include sudden excitement, stress, or too much alcohol.) Traditional remedies for bouts include holding our breath, sipping cold water, gurgling, swallowing a teaspoon

of dry sugar, gently pressing on our eyeballs, or leaning forward to compress our chest. Those with hiccups lasting >48 hours should see a physician. (I remember as a medical student seeing a hospitalized patient who had had hiccups constantly for 3 weeks. She was about the most exhausted human being I had ever seen.)

5) *Why does my nose run when it's cold outside?* Our nose helps perform a kind of climate control by heating and humidifying the air that we inhale so that it better matches the moist, warm conditions inside our lungs. Glands in our noses produce secretions that add moisture, and blood vessels in our nose dilate to warm the incoming air, acting like miniature radiators. When we breathe super-frigid air, those phenomena are amplified. Cold air tends to be drier, causing the glands in our nose to produce more secretions, and when we exhale warm, moist air out into the cold wind, some of the moisture condenses into droplets of water, which collect at the tip of the nose.

6) *Why do I huff and puff climbing stairs when I can easily run a mile on a treadmill?* As anyone who has used a rolling suitcase knows, it's a lot easier to pull a heavy object along a flat surface than it is to pick one up. When running on a treadmill, we barely lift any of our body weight up and down. Walking up a typical 45-degree staircase, on the other hand, requires moving 70% of our body weight against gravity.

ANTIBIOTICS IN FARMS

In March 2012, a federal court judge in Washington, DC, ordered the Food and Drug Administration (FDA) to take action on its own 35-year-old rule that would stop farmers from mixing antibiotics into animal feed, a practice that has led to a surge in drug-resistant bacteria (4). In 1977, the FDA concluded that the overuse of antibiotics in livestock, poultry, and other animals weakened the treatment's effectiveness in humans. The agency at that time issued an order that would have banned nonmedical use of penicillin and tetracycline in farm animals unless drug makers could show that the drugs were safe. But the rule was not enforced after vigorous opposition from Congress and lobbyists for the agriculture and drug industries. Judge Theodore Katz said the FDA must now begin steps to withdraw approval of antibiotics for routine use in animals, siding with four consumer-safety groups that brought a lawsuit against the agency. The court ruling, unfortunately, will not immediately halt the use of antibiotics in farms. The FDA must first give drug companies a chance to respond and schedule a public hearing.

Nearly 80% of all antibiotics sold in the USA are given to farm animals used in food production! Farmers mostly use the drugs in healthy animals to spur growth and to keep them from getting sick in crowded, unsanitary feedlots. Nevertheless, after constant use, some animals develop organisms that are immune to antibiotics. These germs, often called "superbugs," can then pass to farmworkers and their families or blow into neighboring communities in dust clouds or runoff into lakes and rivers during heavy rains or sometimes contaminate steaks and chops we eat. So, 35 years later, some effort is under way.

HOSPITALS CLOSING

According to the book *The New Health Age: The Future of Health Care in America* by David Houle and Jonathan Fleece, of the approximately 5764 registered hospitals in the USA in 2011 (housing 942,000 hospital beds along with 36,915,331 admissions), about one third will be closed or reorganized into entirely different types of health care service providers by 2020 (5). Hospitals make substantial imprints in the US; many are one of their community's largest employers and economic drivers. Of the total annual American health care dollars spent, hospitals account for more than $750 billion.

Several factors drive this "inevitable and historical shift." First, the US must bring down its health care costs. The average American worker costs his or her employer $12,000 annually for health care benefits, and this figure is increasing more than 10% every year. US businesses cannot compete in a globally competitive marketplace at this level of spending. Additionally, federal and state budgets are getting crushed by the cost of health care entitlement programs, such as Medicare and Medicaid. Hospitals, as a consequence, are vulnerable since they make up the highest percentage of health care costs in the USA. These authors suggest that health care reform will make connectivity, electronic medical records, and transparency commonplace in health care. This may mean that any American in the near future considering a hospital stay will go online to compare hospitals' relative infection rates, degrees of surgical success, and many other metrics. They suggest that the hospital market will become more open and competitive.

FIVE THINGS PHYSICIANS AND PATIENTS QUESTION IN CARDIOLOGY

The American College of Cardiology provided a list of five things for physicians not to do (6). 1) Don't perform stress cardiac imaging or advanced noninvasive imaging to evaluate patients without cardiac symptoms unless they have very high-risk markers. 2) Don't perform annual stress cardiac imaging or advanced noninvasive imaging for routine follow-up of asymptomatic patients. 3) Don't perform stress cardiac imaging or advanced noninvasive imaging for operative assessment in patients scheduled to undergo low-risk noncardiac operations. 4) Don't perform echocardiography as routine follow-up for mild, asymptomatic valvular disease in adults with no change in signs or symptoms. 5) Don't perform stenting of nonculprit lesions during percutaneous coronary intervention for uncomplicated hemodynamically stable ST-segment elevation myocardial infarction.

DEMENTIA IN PRISONS

Dementia in prisons is a fast-growing phenomenon, one that many prisons are unprepared to handle (7). It is a consequence of long sentences that have created a large population of aging prisoners. According to Pam Belluck of *The New York Times,* about 10% of the 1.6 million inmates in US prisons are serving life sentences, and an additional 11% are serving >20 years. And, many older people are being sent to prison. In 2010, a total of 9560 people aged ≥55 were sentenced, more than twice as many as in 1995. Also in 2010, the number of inmates ≥55 years almost quadrupled to nearly 125,000. Thus, the dementia population in prisons is obviously growing.

Many prisons would like to transfer inmates with dementia to nursing homes, but these individuals are often violent criminals, making states reluctant to parole them and nursing homes reluctant to take them. New York has established a separate unit for cognitively impaired inmates and uses professional caregivers at a cost of about $93,000 per bed annually compared with $41,000 in the general prison population. Other states, notably Louisiana and California, train prisoners to handle many of the impaired inmates' daily needs. These caregiving prisoners also protect inmates with dementia from prisoners who may try assaulting, abusing, or robbing them. Problems, problems.

MEDICAL TATTOOS

Some medical tattoos are taking the place of bracelets that list a person's allergies, chronic diseases, or even end-of-life wishes (8). Recently, a photograph was published of a physician who had "No CPR" tattooed over his sternum. Another had "type I diabetic" tattooed on her left forearm. But, medical tattoos do not appear to carry much legal weight. The National Tattoo Association, a nonprofit group that raises awareness about tattooing, does not track the number or styles of tattoos. A spokesman for the association, however, said he does about one medical tattoo a year at his shop in Orlando. Nine out of 10 medical tattoos relate to an allergy—usually, to penicillin or peanuts.

TEEN BIRTHRATES

US birthrates for teens aged 15 to 19 years in all racial and ethnic groups are the lowest since 1946 (9). In 2010, there were 34 births per 1000 teens, down from 62 births per 1000 teens in 1991. The all-time high was 96 during the Baby Boom year of 1957. The birthrate for Asian teens was 11; for whites, 23; for blacks, 51; and for Hispanics, 56. The report showed no change in the percentage of sexually active teen girls but significant increases in the use of contraception. The report also noted a decline in the percentage of teenage girls "who said they wanted to get pregnant." Good news.

VOLUNTEER DOCTORS AT ATHLETIC EVENTS

At running races and triathlons, volunteer doctors are getting fewer, and the reason appears to be an inability to get 1-day malpractice insurance to serve participants at these events (10). In 2011, 13 Americans died during running races and another eight died while competing in triathlons. About 13 million Americans enter running races each year, and 2.3 million compete in triathlons. The rising number of participants highlights the need for quality medical care at these events, and that usually comes from volunteer physicians. In the April 16, 2012, Boston Marathon, 27,000 started the race. About 70 physicians and 1300 first-aid volunteers, including nurses, medical students, and physical therapists, were on hand. About 1500 runners required some level of medical attention during or immediately following the race. Despite the worry about malpractice insurance, no American physician has been named in an event-related lawsuit, apparently because plaintiffs typically go after race organizers, who have deeper pockets. The Good Samaritan laws cover physicians only if they are bystanding fans and not official event volunteers.

Because of the shortage of physicians at these events, the World Road Race Medical Society and the medical director for the Chicago Marathon teamed with USA Track and Field and Sports Insurance Company to create policies specifically for volunteer medical teams. Beginning in 2009, all five major US marathons—Chicago, New York, Twin Cities, Boston, and Houston—bought the plan at a cost of $50 to $60 per physician. The US Triathlon began offering the program in 2011. But even at the $60 per-physician cost, not all event-marketing companies have jumped on board to cover their physicians. Some large adventure races hire paramedic services to be on standby. Still, smaller events use uninsured volunteers. There seems to be very few things where lawyers are not involved.

SOME AMAZING ATHLETES OVER 40 YEARS OF AGE

A recent article (11) highlighted numerous athletes over the age of 40. Here are some of the better-known examples:
- *George Foreman:* He earned the heavyweight crown at age 25 and successfully defended it twice before losing to Muhammad Ali in 1974. At age 45 (1994), he regained the title.
- *Nolan Ryan:* At age 44 he threw his seventh no-hitter.
- *Jack Nicklaus:* The "Golden Bear" at age 46 won his sixth Master's golf tournament and 20th major.
- *Dara Torres:* At age 41, she became the oldest swimmer ever to qualify for the Olympics and won three silver medals.
- *Martina Navratilova:* At age 49 and 11 months, she won her 49th Grand Slam title by winning the US Open mixed doubles tournament.
- *Kareem Abdul-Jabbar:* The 19-time NBA All Star led the Los Angeles Lakers to back-to-back titles after turning 40.

ELDERLY DRIVERS

They are safer than the younger ones. A recent 3-year study by the Insurance Institute for Highway Safety involving 1437 drivers aged ≥75 years found a decline of 45% in fatal accidents per 100 million miles traveled—a greater reduction than that in any other age group (12). Drivers ≥85 years still have a higher rate of deadly crashes than any other age group except teenagers. That is partly because seniors tend to avoid highway driving, where crash rates per mile are lower. Also, the older drivers are more likely than the younger ones to die in crash accidents because they tend to be more frail. Safe driving courses for older drivers are available through AARP and AAA. Many states require them, and most mandate insurance-premium discounts for seniors who take them. A free car assessment program, called "CarFit," cosponsored by AAA, AARP, and the American Occupational Therapy Association, is available in most states to help seniors adjust or modify their vehicles to be safer. Seniors, don't let anyone take those car keys away.

VACATION ACCIDENTS

I have become more conscious in recent times of accidents occurring during vacations. On a recent trip to Europe, while taking a picture, I twisted my knee and when visiting a museum I tripped and fell on the same knee. My walking has not been the same since. Vacations can be dangerous. A recent piece on deadly avalanches caught my attention. An avalanche in Washington State killed three skiers, and a fourth was saved by a safety device, a special backpack airbag system (13). The handle on the shoulder strap was pulled and a high-pressure cylinder filled with compressed air inflated the airbag. The airbag made the skier lighter and the skier floated to the surface of the avalanche and survived. It is called an avalanche airbag backpack. The airbag keeps the skier closer to the top of the avalanche. So far in 2012, 17 people, all in the western US mountains, have been killed by avalanches. In the past 10 years, an average of 25 people die per year in avalanches in the USA. Nearly all are exclusively winter sport enthusiasts exploring the back country—deep snow outside the boundaries of ski resorts. They include snowmobilers, climbers, snowboarders, snowshoe skiers, and hikers. These avalanche airbag backpacks cost from $600 to $1000. Sounds like good insurance to me.

WEATHER AND CLIMATE DISASTERS IN 2011

Tornadoes, droughts and fires, storms and flooding, and hurricanes contributed to a record 14 weather and climate disasters in the USA in 2011 that caused $1 billion or more in damage (14). Previously, the largest number of disasters was nine in 2008 and eight in 1998. The total cost for US natural disasters in 2011 was $55 billion, nowhere near the $160 billion price tag in 2005 ($144 billion of which was contributed by Hurricane Katrina). Although the cost was relatively low, 669 people died in these 2011 weather disasters. Half of these billion-dollar events were tornadoes, causing 551 fatalities. The Joplin, Missouri, tornado alone killed 161 people, the deadliest single tornado strike in the US since modern recordkeeping began. From spring to fall, heat and a lack of precipitation caused droughts and wildfires in the South. By the end of July, 84% of the southern plains had moderate to exceptional drought. In Texas, over 3 million acres were burned. Persistent rainfall, nearly 300% of normal precipitation amounts in the Ohio Valley, paired with melting snow caused historic flooding along the Mississippi, Missouri, and Souris Rivers. Seven states saw a record year. It was rain, not wind speed, that caused damage in 2011 from Hurricane Irene and Tropical Storm Lee. The Northeast saw extensive flood damage. Let's hope 2012 is better.

DRIEST YEAR IN TEXAS HISTORY

The driest year in Texas history (2011) caused a record $7.62 billion in agriculture losses, billions more than previously estimated (15). Texas is the nation's number three producer of agricultural products, behind California and Iowa, so when crops and cattle fail in the Lone Star State, prices rise nationally. The drought has cost Texas more than $14 billion in agricultural losses since 1998. Many ranchers sold off or slaughtered cattle

after ranch lands dried up and the price of hay skyrocketed. The state now has its smallest herd since the 1950s after losing about 660,000 cows during the drought. Cattle account for about half of Texas' agricultural production, which makes up 9% of its economy. Cotton losses are estimated at $2.2 billion and corn losses at $736 million. The remaining losses were largely in hay, wheat, and sorghum production. Let it rain.

THE JAPANESE DISASTER—A YEAR LATER

The massive earthquake and tsunami that struck Japan on March 11, 2011, killed >19,000 people and unleashed the world's worst nuclear crisis in >25 years (since Chernobyl) (16). The quake, a 9.0 on the Richter scale, was the strongest recorded in Japan's history. It set off a tsunami that inundated >50 square miles of land along 500 miles of the eastern coastline and damaged 29 railroads, 45 dikes, 78 bridges, nearly 4000 roads, and over 1,100,000 properties, 36,000 of which were inundated. Still today, some 325,000 people left homeless remain in temporary housing. While much of the debris has been gathered into massive piles, very little rebuilding has begun.

The Japanese government says that the damaged Fukushima Daiichi nuclear plant, where three reactor cores melted down after the tsunami knocked out their vital cooling systems, is stable and that radiation coming from the plant has subsided significantly. The plant remains, however, in a fragile state. Only two of Japan's 54 reactors are now running, while those shut down for regular inspection undergo special tests to check their ability to withstand similar disasters. They all could go offline by May 1, 2012, if none are restarted before then. The Japanese government has pledged to reduce reliance on nuclear power, which supplied almost 30% of the nation's energy needs before the disaster. The magnitude of that disaster is difficult to comprehend.

WASTED FOOD

CleanMetrics Corp, a software firm that analyzes the environmental impact of products and businesses, has found that vegetables are the most commonly wasted food in US homes, making up 25% of avoidable waste (17). Most grocery shoppers create food waste by overbuying. People tend to overestimate what they need at the store when they are well stocked at home and to underestimate what they need when they don't have enough. The average US family of four spends $500 to $2000 on food each year that ends up in the garbage. Of trash in a home, fruit and juices make up 16%; milk and yogurt, 13%; vegetables, 25%; and grains, 14%. Just over half of avoidable food and drink waste comes about because products were not used in time. About 40% of this waste is made up of leftovers, characterized as "cooked, prepared, or served too much." In the US, fears about foodborne illness and confusion about product "sell-by" dates are to blame for some food waste. In the UK, food waste is a public concern and a rallying point for politicians and corporations, similar to the issue of childhood obesity in the US. In recent years, UK grocery stores have tested ways to discourage overbuying, including "buy one, get one later" promotions at various chains. Today, spending on restaurant and take-out meals makes up about half of food expenditures in the USA. That probably decreases the scraps.

NOW IT'S THE PACIFIC OCEAN

Ben Lecomte in 1998 became the first person to swim across the Atlantic Ocean (18). A native of France, but now a US citizen, Lecomte undertook the 73-day, 3700-mile journey to raise money for cancer research in memory of his father, who died of colon cancer in 1991. He moved from France to Texas when he was 23 years old. Now, Lecomte, age 44, an alumnus of the University of Texas at Arlington, is training for his next adventure—a swim across the Pacific Ocean. His planned route is 5400 miles long. He hopes to start in May 2012 and finish in <6 months. His plan is the following: He will average about 40 miles a day, swimming 8 hours in two 4-hour segments. He will have a GPS device, which will help him when he takes breaks in the boat that will trail him; he will be able to start again exactly where he stopped. Aside from meals, he will have energy bars and fresh water. As with his first transoceanic swim, he will dedicate the adventure again to his father, who taught him how to swim. He will take on the Pacific, with the sharks and jellyfish and 30-foot swells.

DANIELLE STEEL

She has sold more than 800 million copies of her 100-plus books worldwide, 600 million in the US alone! Her novels have been on *The New York Times* bestseller list for 400 consecutive weeks, and 22 have been adapted for television (19). She often is writing, editing, or researching five books at a time, and she publishes three a year. She is a mother to nine children! Also, she is an avid art collector. She writes every day. She indicates that she had a horrible childhood, so as a little girl reading was her escape. When she turned 19 she started writing more books than she was reading. Now at the age of 70, writing is still an escape, she indicates, and she says that she is never lonely.

LATE DIVORCES

Although overall national divorce rates have declined since spiking in the 1980s, "gray divorce" has risen to its highest level on record (20). In 1990, only 1 in 10 people who got divorced were aged ≥50 years; by 2009, the number was 1 in 4. More than 600,000 people aged ≥50 years got divorced in 2009. A 2004 national survey found that women are the ones initiating most of these breakups: among divorces by people aged 40 to 69, women reported seeking the split 66% of the time. Cheating does not appear to be the driving force in "gray divorce." In the same 2004 survey, infidelity was cited by 27% as one of the three top reasons for seeking a divorce, a figure not out of line with estimated infidelity as a factor in divorce in the general population. The reason for these late divorces is unclear, but it springs at least in part from boomers' status as the first generation to enter into marriage with goals largely focused on self-fulfillment. Some marriages that in previous generations would have ended in death now end in divorce. In the past many people did not live long enough to reach the 40-year itch.

According to Susan Brown and I-fen Lin of Bowling Green State University, among people aged ≥50 years, the divorce rate has doubled over the past 2 decades. Professor Brown describes three phases of American views of marriage in the past century. First was the *institutional* phase, in the decades before World War II, when marriage was seen largely as an economic union. In the 1950s and 1960s, the *companionate* phase appeared, in which a successful marriage was defined by the degree to which each spouse could fulfill his or her role. Husbands were measured by their prowess as providers and wives by their skills in homemaking and motherhood. In the 1970s, the boomers initiated the *individualized* phase, with an emphasis on the satisfaction of personal needs—a more egocentric focus.

For many boomers, a late divorce is not their first marital split. Of the people >50 now getting divorced, 53% have done so at least once before. Having been married previously doubles the risk of divorce for those aged 50 to 64, and, for those aged ≥65, the risk factor quadruples. For boomers who have had trouble maintaining commitments in the past, hitting the empty-nest phase seems to trigger thoughts of mortality and of vanishing possibilities for self-fulfillment. Professor Brown predicts that the number of over-50 divorces by 2030, based on current trends, could top 800,000 per year.

NET WORTH OF US PRESIDENTS

In today's dollars, the following is the net worth (in millions) of some US presidents (21): George Washington (1789–1797), $525; Andrew Jackson (1829–1837), $119; John F. Kennedy (1961–1963), $1000; Lyndon B. Johnson (1963–1969), $98; Herbert Hoover (1929–1933), $75; Franklin D. Roosevelt (1933–1945), $60; William J. Clinton (1993–2001), $38; and George W. Bush (2001–2008), $20. The financially deprived: Ulysses S. Grant (1869–1877), Thomas Jefferson (1801–1809), Abraham Lincoln (1861–1865), and Harry S Truman (1945–1953). Mitt Romney's net worth is estimated at $250, and Barack Obama's, $5.

BILLIONAIRES IN THE USA

California has 94 billionaires; New York, 70; Texas, 48; Florida, 29; Illinois, 18; Michigan, 12; Connecticut, 11; Wisconsin, 10; Maryland, 9; and Washington, 8 (22). There are no physicians on the list, although Carl Icahn was a medical school dropout. The richest family in the USA is the Waltons, of Wal-Mart fame, divided among Christy, Jim, Alice, and Robson Walton. The wealthiest single individual in the USA is Bill Gates, with $61 billion from Microsoft, and next, Warren Buffet, with $44 billion from Berkshire Hathaway. The richest in the world is Carlos Slim Helu and family in Mexico, worth $69 billion.

ATTRACTIVE CITIES

The "hot-spots" survey, sponsored by CitiGroup, attempts to measure how attractive a city is to talent, capital, tourists, and businesses (23). The top 25 attractive cities are listed in the *Table*. Dallas tied for 25th with Vienna. New York was number

Rank/city		Score†
1.	New York	71.4
2.	London	70.4
3.	Singapore	70.0
T4.	Hong Kong	69.3
T4.	Paris	69.3
6.	Tokyo	68.0
7.	Zurich	66.8
8.	Washington	66.1
9.	Chicago	65.9
10.	Boston	64.5
11.	Frankfurt	64.1
12.	Toronto	63.9
T13.	Geneva	63.3
T13.	San Francisco	63.3
15.	Sydney	63.1
16.	Melbourne	62.7
17.	Amsterdam	62.4
18.	Vancouver	61.8
19.	Los Angeles	61.5
T20.	Seoul	60.5
T20.	Stockholm	60.5
22.	Montreal	60.3
T23.	Copenhagen	59.9
T23.	Houston	59.9
T25.	Dallas	59.8
T25.	Vienna	59.8

*Adapted from Economist Intelligence Unit. *Hot Spots: Benchmarking Global City Effectiveness.* London: Author, 2012:6. Available at http://www.citigroup.com/citi/citiforcities/pdfs/hotspots.pdf.

†Out of 100.

1, and London was number 2. Houston, Copenhagen, and Denmark tied for 23rd.

VACATIONING AT THE BEST HOTELS IN THE USA

According to a piece by Betsa Marsh (24), here are the top US hotels: The Greenbrier, White Sulfur Springs, West Virginia; The Grand Hotel, Mackinac Island, Michigan; West Baden Springs, French Lick, Indiana; Casa Monica, Saint Augustine, Florida; US Grant Hotel, San Diego, California; and Mohawk Mountain House, New Paltz, New York.

NEW LONDON, TEXAS, 75 YEARS AGO

In the 1930s, the Great Depression was in full swing, but the New London School District in New London, Texas, was one of the richest in the USA. A 1930 oil find in Rusk County had boosted the local economy, and educational spending grew with it. The New London School, a large structure of steel, was constructed in 1932 at a cost of $1 million (about $17 million in 2012 dollars). Its football stadium was the first in Texas to have electric lights. The school was built on sloping ground, and

a large dead-air space was contained beneath the structure. The school board had overridden the original architect's plans for a boiler and steam distribution system, instead opting to install 72 gas heaters throughout the building.

Late in 1936, the superintendent, with quiet approval from four board members, disconnected the school from commercial natural gas and tapped into a free unregulated and widely available byproduct of gasoline refining: waste natural gas. The switch would save the school district, perhaps the richest school district in the USA in 1937, $250 per month. Refineries pumped the waste gas back to oil rigs, where rig operators were required to dispose of it. Most released it into the air through tall pipes and burned it, lighting the night sky with orange flames. One of these waste gas lines passed 200 feet from New London School. The connection to the waste gas line was performed in early January 1937 by a school janitor, two bus drivers, and a welder that the school had hired.

On March 18, 1937, students prepared for the next day's interscholastic meet. At the gymnasium, the PTA met. At 3:17 PM, an instructor of manual training turned on a sanding machine in an area which, unknown to him, was filled with a mixture of gas and air. The switch ignited the mixture and carried the flame into a nearly closed space beneath the building, 253 feet long and 56 feet wide. Immediately, the building seemed to lift in the air and then smashed to the ground. Walls collapsed. The roof fell in and buried the victims in a mass of brick, steel, and concrete debris. The explosion was heard 4 miles away, and it hurled a 2-ton concrete slab 200 feet away.

Fifteen minutes later, the news of the explosion had been relayed over telephone and Western Union lines. Physicians and medical supplies came from Baylor Hospital in Dallas and from surrounding towns. Workers began digging through the rubble looking for victims. Flood lights were set up. The rescue operation continued through the night. Within 17 hours, all victims and debris had been taken away. Of the 500 students and 40 teachers in the building, 298 died. Only 130 students escaped serious injury. It was the worst school disaster in American history. The news spread around the world. Even Adolph Hitler sent condolences.

Today, fewer than 1000 live in New London. It contains a few buildings and houses; a convenience store that sells gas, microwave pizzas, sandwiches, lotto tickets, and a few groceries; a small bank branch office; a donut shop; and two churches. On a small island in the middle of State Highway 42, there is a pink granite cenotaph complete with classical figures carved into the apex. It is an imposing monument, particularly for a tiny town, flanked on one side by the school and on the other by a combination of café, soda fountain, and museum.

Two books on this disaster appeared in 2012 (25, 26). Saving money sometimes costs a lot of money and even lives.

RMS *TITANIC*: 100 YEARS LATER

On April 12, 1912, the RMS *Titanic* embarked on its maiden voyage, sailing from South Hampton, England, to New York City (27). It was the largest and most luxurious passenger liner ever built, and it was also considered "unsinkable." On April

14, however, the ship struck an iceberg, and 2.5 hours later it sank. Of the approximately 3000 people on board, about 1500 perished. Because of the tragedy, the *Titanic* became perhaps the best known ship in the world, capturing the public's imagination and inspiring books and movies. After the 1985 discovery of its wreckage, interest in the famed liner further increased.

The vessel was 883 feet long (three football fields), 92.5 feet wide, and 104 feet from keel to bridge. She had eight steel decks and a circular double bottom 5.25 feet through (the inner and outer "skins"). The ship was divided into 16 compartments by 15 transverse "water-tight" bulkheads, well above the water line. Communication from the engine rooms and boiler rooms was through water-tight doors that could be closed instantly from the captain's bridge. The crew numbered nearly 900, with 320 engineers and 65 navigators. The machinery and equipment of the *Titanic* were the finest attainable and represented the last word in marine construction. Her structure was of steel, of a weight, size, and thickness greater than that of any other ship. The cruising speed was 21 knots (24 miles per hour) with a maximum of 24 knots (28 miles per hour).

The *Titanic* was equipped with three engines—two reciprocating four-cylinder, triple-expansion steam engines and one centrally placed Parson's turbine—each driving a propeller. The two reciprocating engines had a combined output of 30,000 horsepower and the turbine, 16,000 horsepower. The two reciprocating engines were each 63 feet long and weighed 720 tons. They were powered by steam produced in 29 boilers and 159 furnaces. The boilers were nearly 16 feet in diameter and 20 feet long, and each weighed 91.5 tons and held 48.5 tons of water. They were heated by coal, 7703 tons of which could be carried on board. The furnaces required over 6 tons of coal a day to be shoveled into them by hand, requiring the services of 176 firemen working around the clock. One hundred tons of ash a day had to be disposed of by ejecting it into the sea. The work was relentless, dirty, and dangerous, and the firemen had a high suicide rate. *Titanic*'s rudder was nearly 79 feet tall and 15 feet long, and it weighed >100 tons. It required steering engines to move it. The ship had its own waterworks capable of heating and pumping water to all parts of the vessel via a complex network of pipes and valves. The main water supply was taken aboard while *Titanic* was in port, but in an emergency she could also distill fresh water from the sea.

Titanic was equipped with two 1.5 kW spark-gap wireless telegraphs located in the radio room on the Bridge Deck. One set was used for transmitting messages, and the other, located in a soundproof booth, for receiving them. The system, one of the most powerful in the world, had a range of 1000 miles.

The passenger facilities met the highest standards of luxury. The ship could accommodate 739 first-class passengers, 674 second-class, and 1026 third-class, plus 900 crew members. In all, she could carry 3339 people. Passengers could use an onboard telephone system, a lending library, and a large barbershop. The first-class section had a swimming pool, a gymnasium, a squash court, a Turkish bath, an electric bath, and a veranda café.

Although the *Titanic* was primarily a passenger ship, she also carried a substantial amount of cargo. Under contract with both Royal Mail and the US Postal Department, she had 26,800 cubic feet of space in her hull allocated for storage of letters, parcels, and specie (bullion, coins, and other valuables). The ship's passengers brought with them a huge amount of luggage; another 19,500 cubic feet was taken up by first- and second-class baggage. In addition, there was considerable cargo: furniture, food, and motor cars. *Titanic* was equipped with eight electric cranes, four electric wenches, and three steam wenches to lift cargo and baggage in and out of the hull. It was estimated that the ship used 415 tons of coal in South Hampton, simply generating steam to operate the cargo wenches, heat, and light.

Titanic carried 20 lifeboats: 14 standard wooden lifeboats with a capacity of 65 people each and four collapsible lifeboats with a capacity of 47 people each. All lifeboats were stored securely on the Boat Deck connected to davits by ropes. Additionally, two emergency cutters with a capacity of 40 people each were available. Each boat carried food, water, blankets, and a spare lifebelt. *Titanic* had the ability to carry up to 64 wooden lifeboats, which would have been enough for 4000 people. The White Star Line, however, decided that only 16 wooden lifeboats and four collapsible lifeboats would be carried, which could accommodate 1178 people, only one third of *Titanic*'s total capacity. The Board of Trade's regulations at the time required British vessels >10,000 tons to carry only 16 lifeboats with a capacity of 990 occupants, so *Titanic* actually provided more lifeboat accommodation than was legally required.

For the maiden voyage, 885 crew members were recruited. She did not have permanent crew and, like most vessels at the time, employed mostly casual workers who came aboard the ship only a few hours before she sailed from South Hampton. *Titanic*'s passengers numbered 1317: first class, 324; second class, 284; and third class, 709. The ship was considerably under capacity on her maiden voyage, as she could accommodate 2439 passengers. Some of the most prominent people of the day booked a passage aboard the *Titanic*. The exact number of people aboard is not known, as not all of those who had booked tickets made it to the ship; about 50 cancelled for various reasons, and not all of those who boarded stayed aboard for the entire journey.

On her third day out, Saturday, April 13, *Titanic* crossed a cold weather front with strong winds and waves up to 8 feet. These died down as the day progressed but by the evening of Sunday, April 14, it became clear, calm, and very cold. *Titanic* received warnings from other ships of drifting ice in the area of the Grand Banks of Newfoundland; nonetheless, the ship continued to steam at full speed, standard practice at the time. It was generally believed that ice posed little danger to large vessels. At 11:40 PM, one of the lookouts spotted an iceberg immediately ahead of *Titanic* and alerted the bridge. The first officer ordered the ship to be steered around the obstacle and the engines to be put in reverse, but it was too late. The starboard side of *Titanic* struck the iceberg, creating a series of holes below the waterline. Five of the ship's watertight compartments were breached. The ship was doomed as she could not survive >4 of its 16 compartments being flooded.

Titanic began sinking bow first with water spilling from compartment to compartment as her angle in the water became steeper. Those aboard *Titanic* were ill-prepared for such an emergency. The crew had not been trained adequately in carrying out an evacuation. The officers did not know how many they could safely put aboard the lifeboats and launched many of them barely half full. Most third-class passengers were trapped below decks as the ship filled with water. A "women and children first" protocol was generally followed for loading the boats, and most of the male passengers and crew were left aboard. Two hours and 40 minutes after *Titanic* struck the iceberg, her forward deck dipped under water and the sea poured in through open hatches and grates. As her unsupported stern rose out of the water, exposing the propellers, the ship split apart. The stern remained afloat for a few minutes longer. At 2:20 AM it sank, breaking loose from the bow section. The remaining passengers and crew were plunged into lethally cold water with a temperature of 28°F (–2°C). Almost all of those in the water died of hypothermia or cardiac arrest within minutes or drowned. Only 13 were helped into lifeboats, though these had room for almost 500 more occupants.

Earlier, distress signals had been sent by wireless devices, rockets, and lamps, but no ships responded or were near enough to reach her before she sank, except the *Californian*, which saw her flares but failed to assist. At about 4:00 AM, RMS *Carpathian* arrived on the scene in response to *Titanic's* earlier distress calls. Only 710 people were found alive and conveyed by *Carpathian* to New York; about 1500 people lost their lives.

How could such a magnificent ship built like a battleship be sunk by an iceberg which was not seen until the ship was virtually on top of it? One hundred years ago across the Atlantic, it was entirely the responsibility of the lookouts to spot an iceberg, and they could do so 9 miles ahead, providing at least 30 minutes for the ship to maneuver its course. The *Titanic* lookouts spotted the iceberg only 37 seconds before the starboard side of the ship hit it, opening up a 100-yard gash. At the time of the collision, it was a most unusual night—quite still, with innumerable stars in the sky. Although cold, it was thought to be a perfect night for spotting icebergs, although the danger of icebergs was recognized to be greater at night than during the day. The ship was going 22 knots per hour (25 miles per hour) because it wanted to make New York within 7 days as planned. If the speed had been reduced to 12 knots per hour, the disembarking in New York would have been delayed 2 days. When the ship collided with the iceberg, most passengers were in their rooms and few heard any disturbance or shock from the collision. Some had suggested that if the ship had hit the iceberg head on, the *Titanic* would have survived.

Nearly 100 years later, Tim Milton, a *Titanic* investigator for decades, asked the simple question: Why did the lookouts not see the iceberg until <1 minute before the collision and why did the *Californian* not come to the rescue when it was only 10 or so miles away? The answer apparently has to do with the night being *a mirage*, an optical phenomenon that creates the illusion of water, often with inverted reflections of distant objects. The mirage results from distortion of light by alternate layers of hot and cool air. As mentioned, on the night of the collision, the sky was clear but covered with stars. One passenger commented later that she had never seen so many stars in the sky. The lookouts, in other words, were unable to see the difference between an iceberg and a star in front of them since the stars came down essentially to water level. Likewise, the captain of the *Californian* was unable to see the huge *Titanic* because of confusion with the innumerable stars in the sky. The warm air suddenly mixing with the cold air also apparently played a prominent role.

The sinking of the *Titanic* led to many changes in maritime rules: to have adequate lifeboats for every passenger and crew member on every ship, to perform lifeboat drills on every passenger ship, to man wireless equipment on every passenger ship around the clock, and to set up an ice patrol to monitor the presence of icebergs in the North Atlantic.

WILLIAM CLIFFORD ROBERTS, MD
11 May 2012

1. Bell GD. *The Achievers: Six Styles of Personality and Leadership*. Chapel Hill, NC: Preston-Hill, 1973 (202 pp.).
2. Welch J, Welch S. What do great leaders have in common? They're authentic. *Fortune*, April 9, 2012.
3. Price C. Your body's mysteries solved. *Parade Magazine*, March 4, 2012.
4. Perrone M. Antibiotic use on farms is revisited. *Dallas Morning News*, March 24, 2012.
5. Houle D, Fleece J. Why one-third of hospitals will close by 2020. Available at http://www.kevinmd.com/blog/2012/03/onethird-hospitals-close-2020.html.
6. The American College of Cardiology releases list of commonly used—but not always necessary—tests or procedures. *Cardiosource.org*. Available at http://www.cardiosource.org/News-Media/Media-Center/News-Releases/2012/04/ChoosingWisely.aspx.
7. Belluck P. Prisons grapple with increasing dementia. *Dallas Morning News*, February 26, 2012.
8. Sudekum M. Tattoos warn of medical conditions. *Dallas Morning News*, February 28, 2012.
9. Jayson S. Birthrate for teens is lowest in history. *USA Today*, April 10, 2012.
10. Beresini E. The doctor won't see you now. *Outside Magazine*, April 2012.
11. Rimstidt A. Amazing athletes over age 40. *Saturday Evening Post*, May/June 2012.
12. Shellenbarger S. Safe over 70: drivers keep the keys. *Wall Street Journal*, February 29, 2012.
13. Rice D. Deadly avalanche highlights airbag. *USA Today*, February 19, 2012.
14. Nieland K. The unluckiest year. *Chicago Tribune*, February 12, 2012.
15. Associated Press. Texas drought losses soar. *Dallas Morning News*, March 22, 2012.
16. Foster M. 19,000 dead, 325,000 can't go home. *Dallas Morning News*, March 11, 2012.
17. Nassauer S. Leftovers: tasty or trash? *Wall Street Journal*, March 21, 2012.
18. Rosales C. Long-distance swimmer to take on Pacific. *Dallas Morning News*, March 24, 2012.

19. Rentilly J. Page churner. *AA/Americanway*, April 1, 2012.

20. Thomas SG. The gray divorcés. *Wall Street Journal*, March 3–4, 2012.

21. Meyers J. In the White House—haves and have-nots. *Dallas Morning News*, April 15, 2012.

22. The world's billionaires: top 100. *Forbes*, March 26, 2012.

23. Landers J. In terms of 'cool,' Dallas is lukewarm. *Dallas Morning News*, April 10, 2012.

24. Marsh B. America's grand hotels. *Saturday Evening Post*, May/June 2012.

25. Rozelle R. *My Boys and Girls Are in There: The 1937 New London School Explosion*. College Station, TX: Texas A&M University Press, 2012 (168 pp.).

26. Brown DM, Wereschagin M. *Gone at 3:17. The Untold Story of the Worst School Disaster in American History*. Dulles, VA: Potomac Books, 2012 (328 pp.).

27. Beesley L. *The Loss of the S. S. Titanic: Its Story and Its Lessons*. Fairfield, IA: Akasha Publishing, 2008 (135 pp.).

Chapter 8

October 2012

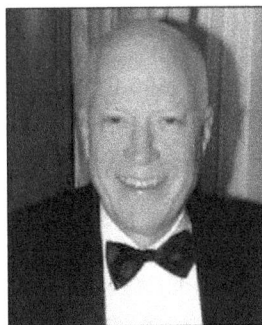
William C. Roberts, MD.

AFFORDABLE CARE ACT

Is it affordable? Is it desired by Americans? The nonpartisan Congressional Budget Office predicts that "Obamacare will reduce the nation's labor supply by 800,000 workers" (1). Some private economists predict a nationwide loss of up to 2 million jobs. A recent Chamber of Commerce survey indicated that 74% of small businesses say the law makes it more difficult to hire new workers. The law contains $813 billion of new taxes and is estimated to cost almost $2 trillion. The law takes $500 billion from Medicare. It creates a panel of 15 unselected bureaucrats—the Independent Payment Advisory Board—and empowers it to effectively ration health care to seniors. Its decisions can only be overturned by an act of Congress. This board is only one of 159 new federal boards, commissions, and programs that will soon be inserted between Americans and their physicians, not to mention the current 12,000 pages of new rules and mandates. Granting the federal government power over private medical decisions will have many ramifications. The 2700-page bill provides no reform of medical liability. It is estimated that 20% of all health care dispensed is defensive medicine due to fear of litigation, not medical necessity. The bill does not allow Americans the opportunity to buy health insurance across state lines. Today, the same policy for the same individual can cost twice as much depending upon the state in which he or she resides. The bill does not allow seniors the option of choosing their own Medicare policy through a premium-support system, a bipartisan idea. Our medical system certainly can be improved. So can our legal system; so can our educational system, etc. There is doubt whether the Affordable Care Act is the way to do it.

OBESITY CAMPAIGN

Gary Taubes, the author of *Why We Get Fat*, in a recent piece in *Newsweek* described how the government is going about its campaign to prevent obesity by stressing the wrong message—that we get fat because we eat too much and exercise too little (2). Taubes begins by pointing out that the very first childhood obesity clinic in the US was founded in late 1930 at Columbia University by a young German physician, Hilde Bruch, who had arrived in New York City in 1934 and was "startled" by the number of fat kids she saw—really fat ones, not only in clinics but on the streets and subways and in schools. And the year she arrived was the worst year of the Great Depression, an era of bread lines and soup kitchens, when 6 in 10 Americans were living in poverty. Taubes emphasizes that the most important item to prevent obesity is to decrease the quantities of sugar we take in: *sucrose*, the white granulated stuff that is metabolized by nearly every cell in the body, and *high fructose syrup*, which is metabolized by liver cells and is converted into fat. He stresses that the single most important way to lose weight or to prevent weight gain is to stop drinking sugar-sweetened beverages.

The other item Taubes presses is the myth that physical activity plays a meaningful role in keeping off pounds. We need to remember that we have to walk 35 miles to lose 1 pound, assuming we do not stop at one of the fast food chains during the walk. One reason Taubes likes the hormonal thesis of obesity is that it explains the fat kids in the Depression era in New York City. The problem could not have been that they ate too much because they didn't have enough food available. The problem then, as now, across the USA is the prevalence of sugars, refined flour, and starches in their diets. These are the least expensive calories and they can be plenty tasty without a lot of preparation and preservation. They make us fat while other foods (fruits, proteins, and green leafy vegetables) do not. I would also suggest the use of the drug Xenical 120 mg per day with the heaviest meal. (It has been withdrawn in the USA and now can be obtained via Internet from Canada.)

LORCASERIN HYDROCHLORIDE

The Endocrinologic and Metabolic Drugs Advisory Committee of the US Food and Drug Administration (FDA) approved a new drug application for lorcaserin hydrochloride, a selective serotonin 2c receptor agonist indicated for weight management in obese patients (body mass index ≥30 or ≥27 kg/m² if accompanied by weight-related comorbidities) (3). The recommended clinical dose is 10 mg twice daily.

AMERICAN DIETARY HABITS SPREADING

In the 1930s when Stalin enforced a drive toward collective farms, the czarist tradition of breeding meat cattle was lost (4).

Subsequently, Russia has mainly slaughtered retired dairy cows for meat, and those dairy cows yielded tough and thin portions, not something that beef lovers desire. When the Soviet Union fell in the 1990s, Russia started importing beef from New Zealand, Argentina, and the US, and soon the Russians acquired a taste for better cuts. In 2011, Russia purchased 1.1 million tons of beef and veal from abroad, the equivalent of about 3.3 million fattened steers. Beef imports in 2011 were valued at $2.6 billion, making up about 33% of domestic consumption. Putin is now on a campaign to provide more good beef for his expanding middle class, and he has imported several Texas cattle experts to help expand beef production in Russia. The 10 US ranchers employed by the Russians are teaching them ways to handle livestock, different methods of feeding, and signs of different illnesses and injuries. Thus, the US is engaged in a process of worsening Russian health.

And our fast-food chains have moved into Kuwait. Now only 12% of Kuwaitis are at ideal body weight (body mass index 18.5 to 25 kg/m²), meaning that at least 88% of Kuwaitis are overweight (5). According to data from the World Health Organization, Kuwait is the second most obese nation in the world, behind the USA! The obesity boom in Kuwait can be traced to the build-up to the 1991 Gulf War. That was when hundreds of thousands of US troops descended on the Gulf nation, bringing with them Taco Bell, Hardee's, Baskin Robbins, and Nathan's Famous Hot Dogs, among other chains. When the American military went in, they wanted fast food, which means in actuality quick plaques. Although war introduced fast-food chains to Kuwait cities, peace made them a permanent fixture. Some 3400 US troops remained in Kuwait after the war enforcing the no-fly zone over Iraq. McDonald's first opened in Kuwait in 1994, 3 years after the war ended. Malls and food courts stocked with American franchises such as Burger King, Domino's, and Krispy Kreme Doughnuts have since proliferated in Kuwait. The high-end Manhattan burger chain Shake Shack opened one of its two international outposts in Kuwait City. The other is in Dubai.

As waistlines in Kuwait and across the Persian Gulf have expanded over the last 3 or 4 years, so too has bariatric surgery. Ten years ago, there were only two bariatric surgeons in Kuwait. Today there are 20. By 2015, it is predicted that there will be 40. At least five major hospitals in Kuwait now perform hundreds or even thousands of stomach-stapling procedures each year. Each operation at the Royale Hayat Hospital, a gleaming 5-star resort/wellness center, costs between $8000 and $12,000. For those willing to be operated on at a state-run hospital, the procedure is free, but patients have to pay for the staples, which usually cost between $2500 and $3600, and there is a 2- to 3-year wait. At least 5000 people in Kuwait underwent the procedure in 2011, compared with 3000 in Canada, which has more than 30 times the population of Kuwait.

Other obesity-related businesses are also sprouting across Kuwait, ranging from gyms and weight-loss camps to diet centers and personal caterers that specialize in low-calorie meals. An array of sporting equipment manufacturers, drug companies, medical clinics, and health spas are sprouting. The mostly Indian and Pakistani tailors who sew the white robes, or *dishdashas,* for men and black robes, or *abayas,* for women are constantly busy in Kuwait letting out or taking in their customers' clothes.

There are some disincentives to move and to eat less in Kuwait. In 2011, for example, the Kuwaiti government gave each of its 1.1 million citizens about $3600 in subsidized food. In 2012, it gave all state employees a 25% raise. This coddling apparently has encouraged lethargy. The temperature also adds to the lethargy. Summer temperatures of 110°F to 120°F from 10:00 AM to 4:00 PM hinder walking in the streets. All of this, I suspect, does not make Americans proud.

NEW FARM BILL

A recent *Bloomberg Business Week* carried a piece discussing the old and new Department of Agriculture Farm Bills (6). The past one expired September 2012, and the new one, like the old one, will last 5 years. The new Farm Bill is a 1000-page law which Karen Weise indicates will cost $500 billion. The first Farm Bill was passed during the Great Depression, and it propped up prices by paying strapped farmers not to plant. In the 2008 bill that just expired, the largest share of the budget went to food stamps ($189 billion), which were first added to the Farm Bill in 1973. In addition to the food stamps, that Farm Bill included $42 billion for commodities, $24 billion for land conservation, $22 billion for crop insurance, and just over $7 billion for miscellaneous items, for a total of $284 billion. The original Farm Bill in 1937 was for $335 million, and $324 million of that went to farmers not to plant crops.

In the 1980s, the US government began shifting toward agriculture subsidies that led to an explosion of cheap, bountiful carbohydrates and meat. As a consequence, Americans consume nearly 20% more calories a day now than they did in the early 1980s. Since 1934, the federal government has limited sugar imports to boost domestic prices, a perk the industry fiercely protects. In June 2012, sugar lobbyists successfully worked to kill a Senate amendment to end the support. Without it, it is estimated that sugar prices would have dropped as much as 34%. Corn was the king of US crops: in 2011, growers got $2 billion in direct government support. It is no wonder that Americans eat more of it than Europe and China combined—including 11 billion pounds of breakfast cereal a year. And soy is well supported by the government. The ink in newsprint is now soy-based. Permanent-press cotton is a result of soy research. When large subsidies for ethanol, made from corn, were inserted into the 2002 Farm Bill, they were sold as a way to promote clean fuel and reduce dependence on oil. Ethanol became a bonanza for corn farmers. Increased demand has helped fuel record prices.

The Senate version of the new Farm Bill doubles funding for energy programs, including ethanol, to $1.5 billion over 10 years. When the price of milk drops, the government steps in to pay farmers and even buy cheese and powdered milk (276 million pounds of it in fiscal year 2009) to drive daily prices back up. The 2008 Farm Bill required the US Department of Agriculture to crack down on anticompetitive contracts—a reform intended to make it harder for buyers to favor large ranchers while freezing out smaller independents. This year, beef lobbyists may convince the senators to reverse the rule. The

Senate version of the new bill adds $1.9 billion in disaster assistance for farmers whose animals or crops are wiped out by natural disasters, such as blizzards, wildfires, or droughts. And not just cows and chickens—bee keepers qualify for government cash if at least 17.5% of their insects die. Potatoes are not included in the Farm Bill, because they aren't commodity crops, i.e., traded on exchanges, and the Farm Bill promotes and protects markets. Like most fruits and vegetables, potatoes are considered specialty crops, eligible for grants but not direct subsidies. The new Farm Bill would eliminate $5 billion in yearly payments to corn farmers and replace them with subsidized insurance based on revenue. Sixty-three percent of the government's agricultural subsidies for domestic food products in recent history have directly and indirectly supported meat and dairy production. Less than 1% of these subsidies have gone to fruits and vegetables. I wonder how many of the representatives and senators read the 1000-page bill.

TWO OBSERVATIONS SUGGESTING THAT WE DIE IN VENTRICULAR SYSTOLE

Does it take more energy for the cardiac ventricles to contract or to relax? And if it takes more energy for the ventricles to relax than to contract, would it be reasonable to believe that we die in ventricular systole rather than in ventricular diastole?

Two observations suggest that we die in ventricular systole. One, as illustrated in the *Figure*, if the minute size of the left ventricular cavity represents ventricular diastole, what size could possibly represent ventricular systole? Two, the thickness of the left ventricular free wall at necropsy corresponds to the thickness measured during life by the echocardiogram during ventricular systole, not during ventricular diastole (7).

If the left ventricle is dilated during life, it will also be dilated after death, and therefore in these circumstances it is not possible to know at necropsy that death occurred during ventricular systole. When the left ventricular cavity is of normal size during life, however, the left ventricular cavity is small or minute after life.

VANISHING ANIMAL LABORATORIES IN MEDICAL SCHOOLS

Dr. Neal Barnard, president of the Physicians Committee for Responsible Medicine, for years has been trying to eliminate the use of nonhuman animals for teaching purposes in medical schools (8). I remember the physiology class in medical school where we did one or more procedures on dogs during each laboratory and put the dead dog in a bag at the end. Dr. Barnard has found other ways of teaching and learning. The number of medical schools with animal laboratories has drastically decreased since 1985. Dr. Barnard has been very successful with his endeavors.

DETERMINING THE QUANTITY OF ALCOHOL CONSUMED

Questioning patients about their consumption of alcohol (ethanol) is an important part of history taking. To determine the specific quantity, it is essential to understand how much alcohol is in a bottle of spirits or a bottle of wine or a bottle of beer and the container sizes in which they are consumed. I am

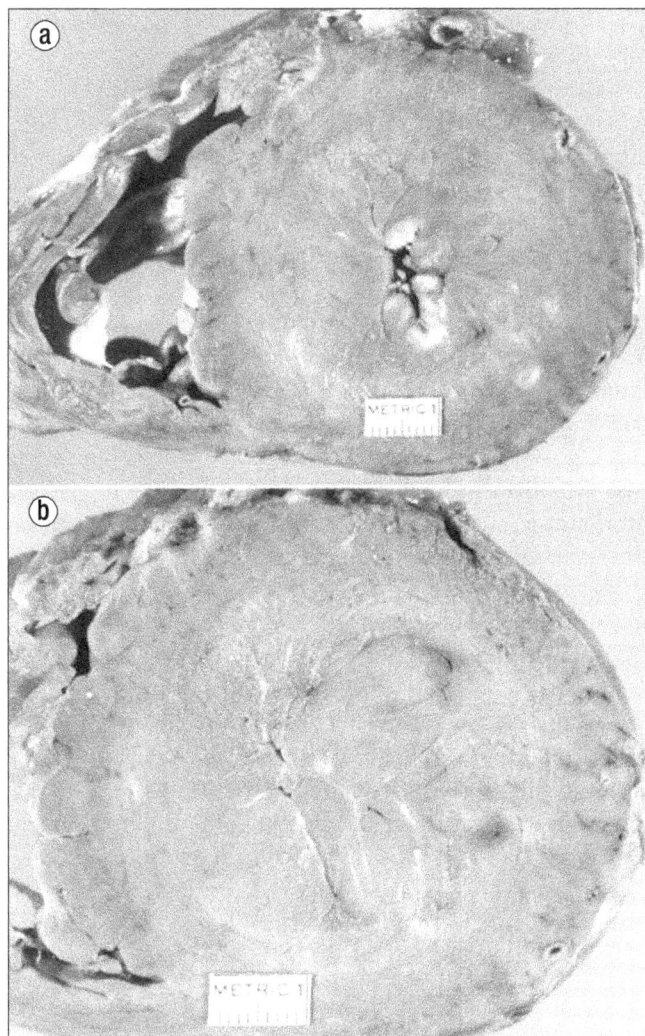

Figure. Cross-section of cardiac ventricles at the base showing **(a)** both ventricles and **(b)** a close-up of the left ventricle only in a 79-year-old man who died of a noncardiac nonvascular cause. The left ventricular cavity is minute.

reminded of the executive who asked his assistant to come into his office: "Aren't you proud of me?" he asked. "I am down to one cup of coffee a day." An enormous cup —probably holding 3000 mL—was sitting on his desk.

Spirits: The small container of spirits provided on commercial airline carriers to individual passengers contains 50 mL. Since the 50 mL generally contains 40% alcohol (80 proof), there is 20 mL (2/3 oz) of alcohol in each small bottle. The usual 750 mL bottle of spirits purchased in a store contains 40% alcohol or 300 mL of alcohol, an amount equal to 15 of the 50 mL bottles of spirits.

Wine: The small bottles of wine provided on commercial airline carriers to individual passengers contain 187 mL, and since they consist usually of about 13.5% alcohol, those containers provide 25 mL of alcohol. The usual bottle of wine purchased in a store contains 750 mL, the same quantity as the usual bottle of spirits, but the alcohol content is usually about 13.5%. Thus, the quantity of alcohol in a 750-mL bottle of wine is approximately 100 mL, such that consuming an entire bottle of wine provides essentially the same quantity of alcohol as consuming five 50-mL bottles of spirits. Four of the 187-mL–sized bottles of wine are equivalent to the 750-mL sized bottle.

Beer: The alcoholic content of beer varies, but usually in the US it is about 5% by volume. Thus, a 12-fl oz (355-mL) bottle or can contains 18 mL of ethanol, such that the alcohol content of five beers roughly equals drinking a full 750-mL bottle of wine or a third of a 750-mL bottle of spirits.

Alcohol equivalence: In general, drinking 12 oz of beer equals drinking 5 oz of wine or 1.5 oz of spirits. Or, 285 mL of beer equals 120 mL of wine or 30 mL (single jigger) of spirits. It is easier to keep track of beers than wine or spirits, particularly in homes or at parties. Wine glasses are often refilled before they are emptied, and wine glasses vary considerably in size (4, 5, 8, 12, 16, and 20 oz). The glasses are generally filled higher with red wine than with white wine. Becoming savvy to glass size obviously is important. Some hosts and party providers measure spirits before glasses are filled, and others do not. Thus, knowing glass sizes and watching the servers is helpful in estimating the quantity of alcohol consumed.

Calories in alcohol: They amount to 7 calories per mL or gram of alcohol. Thus, the 50-mL bottle of spirits with 40% by volume alcohol (80 proof; 20 mL of alcohol) provides 140 calories, and most spirit pourers provide at least this amount per cocktail. An ounce of 80-proof (40% alcohol) whiskey, gin, vodka, rum, tequila, and brandy contains 65 calories. Liqueurs (Drambuie, Cointreau, Kahlua) contain about 125 calories/ oz. A 5-oz glass of red or dry white wine, sherry, or champagne contains about 100 calories. A regular 12-oz (355-mL) bottle or can of beer contains 150 calories and "light" beer, 110 calories. And beer and wine also provide calories in the nonalcoholic portions of those drinks. Thus, although a little alcohol may be useful for our coronary arteries, lots of alcohol is bad for our brains, livers, and bellies.

DRUG ABUSE—OPANA

Prescription drug abuse is the nation's fastest-growing drug problem (9). The Centers for Disease Control and Prevention has classified the misuse of these powerful painkillers as an epidemic, with 1.3 million emergency room visits in 2010, a 115% increase from 2004. Overdose deaths on opioid pain relievers surpassed deaths from heroin and cocaine for the first time in 2008. The rise of Opana, whose active ingredient is oxymorphone, illustrates the adaptability of drug addicts and the never-ending challenge facing law enforcement authorities, addiction specialists, and pharmaceutical companies.

For years, drug abusers favored an extended-release version of OxyContin, a narcotic painkiller, for a powerful high. They would crush or dissolve the pill's time-release coating to get the full punch of the opioid oxycodone. But oxycodone's manufacturer reformulated it in August 2010, making it nearly impossible to crush, dissolve, and inject. By the beginning of 2011, more than 95% of prescriptions were being filled with reformulated OxyContin. As the supply of the old formulation dwindled, panicked drug abusers flooded Internet chat rooms in an attempt to find ways to outsmart the new technology, from pounding it with hammers to soaking it in acid.

Opana ER, an extended-release painkiller containing oxymorphone, came on the market in 2006. Although the manufacturer had completed development of a crush-resistant pill in 2010, approval from the FDA was delayed until late 2011. In the meantime, the old Opana formulation proliferated and its oxymorphone became one of the most common drugs found in the blood of overdose victims. The old formulation of Opana was not removed from the market until June 2012.

MILITARY SUICIDES

They are rising, as Mark Thompson and Nancy Gibbs point out (10). More US soldiers have killed themselves than have died in the Afghan war. Military suicides are at record levels. At the current pace, there will be 186 suicides in the army, 73 in the air force, 62 in the navy, and 45 in the marines in 2012. From 2001 to July 2012, 4486 US troops have died in Iraq, 1950 have died in Afghanistan, and 2676 have died by suicide. Of the suicides, 83% occurred in the US, 10% in Iraq or Afghanistan, and 7% in other sites; 38% of those who died had been deployed to Iraq or Afghanistan, 11% had had some combat experience, and 6% had witnessed killing in combat. Further, 26% had histories of substance abuse, 7% of major depression, 5% of posttraumatic stress syndrome, and 3% of traumatic brain injury.

The causes of death in the military in 2011 were as follows: combat, 26%; suicide, 20%; transport accidents, 17%; other accidents, 8%; cancer, 6%; heart disease, 5%; and other, 18%. The 20% suicide rate in the military compares to a 7% rate among civilian men aged 17 to 60 years. Active duty US troops die by their own hand at an average rate of 1 a day. Among all veterans, the rate is 1 every 80 minutes. So sad.

FIRST TEST-TUBE BABY

Leslie Brown, the mother of the world's first "test-tube baby," died June 6, 2012, in Bristol, UK (11). She was 64 years old. She is survived by her two daughters and three grandchildren. Her husband, John Brown, died in 2007 at age 64.

The in vitro fertilization technique that produced her daughter, Louise, was developed by Mr. Robert Edwards and Dr. Patrick Steptoe. Although in vitro fertilization is an established treatment now, it had a long, slow, and rocky start. The research by Mr. Edwards, a biologist, and Dr. Steptoe, a gynecologist, had gone on for 10 years, and the treatment had failed in about 60 couples by the mid 1970s. It had produced only one pregnancy, and that was ectopic and had to be aborted. Then, Leslie Brown and her husband, John, came along. She was a homemaker; he, a railroad employee. They had been trying for 9 years to conceive a child.

In vitro fertilization at the time was "an incredible leap into the unknown." Even if a pregnancy did result, would the baby be healthy? Critics predicted that the treatment could lead to terrible abnormalities. Ms. Brown became pregnant on the first try. Once the news got out, public fascination with her case was unrelenting. She was a quiet woman and the attention stunned her. Louise was born on July 25, 1978, and her birth was an instant global sensation and a turning point in the treatment of infertility. After Louise's birth, the Browns went home from the hospital to find reporters camped out on their street. For months, Leslie Brown could not leave the house without being chased, so the family moved to another house with a backyard allowing her to take Louise outside in peace. Four years later they had another daughter, Natalie, also conceived by in vitro fertilization, also on the first try.

It took time for in vitro fertilization to gain acceptance. Fears that it could harm mothers and children lingered, and there are still some religious objections. But overall, the technique has proved safe, and success rates have climbed to rival those of natural conception. About 5 million babies worldwide have been born through in vitro fertilization. In some developed countries, those methods now lead to 3% of all live births. In 2010, about 59,000 births in the US resulted from in vitro procedures. In 2010, at age 85, Mr. Edwards received the Nobel Prize in physiology/medicine. Unfortunately, his health had declined mentally and he was not in a position to understand the honor.

REDUCING SALT INTAKE

High salt intake has a direct relationship to blood pressure: the higher the salt intake, the higher the blood pressure. The higher the blood pressure, the higher the frequency of stroke, kidney disease, and aortic dissection. A 2000–2001 survey found that the mean estimated salt intake in adults in the UK was 9.5 g per day (12). In 2003, the British government committed to a nationwide salt reduction initiative to reduce the average salt intake to 6 g per day. To achieve that target by 2010, in 2006 their Food Standard Agency introduced voluntary salt reduction targets for the food industry for 85 categories of food. Publication of the UK dietary sodium excretion survey in 2008 showed that the average estimated salt intake for adults in the UK was 8.6 g per day, a 10% reduction compared to the 2000–2001 survey. Since that time further reductions have been targeted. The 2011 study aimed to collect usable 24-hour urine samples from 600 participants, aged 19 to 64 years, living in private households in the UK. The results of this latest survey were announced in June 2012: salt intake had fallen in adults in the UK from 9.5 g to 8.1 g per day, an approximate 1.5 g per-person per-day fall. This level is now the lowest salt intake of any developed country in the world. The British investigators estimated that this 1.5 g reduction in average daily salt intake, through the reduction it has on blood pressure, would prevent approximately 20,000 strokes, heart attacks, and heart failure, 850 of which would be fatal in the UK every year. This reduction provides huge cost savings. If the UK achieved the 6 g target, an estimated additional 17,000 lives a year would be saved. A successful policy depends on the rigorous setting of progressively lower salt targets, which are adopted voluntarily by the food industry. The US, Canada, and Australia now are beginning to follow the UK's lead in setting their own targets.

I had dinner recently with a prominent physician who after his plate appeared picked up the salt shaker and vigorously shook it over the food before he had a single bite. Although apparently only about 14% of the salt Americans take in each day comes from the salt shaker, there is no need to add additional salt at the table. It takes about one month to get used to eliminating the salt shaker. It is not impolite anymore to just pass the pepper shaker.

MANUFACTURING PROBLEMS OF DIETARY SUPPLEMENTS

In the last 4 years, the FDA has found violations of manufacturing rules in half of the nearly 450 dietary firms it has inspected (13). Some firms do not even have recipes, known as master manufacturing records, for their products. Others make their supplements in unsanitary factories. Others are unable to verify the identity of the ingredients that go into their products. The FDA began conducting inspections in 2008 to assess compliance with new regulations governing the manufacturing, packing, and holding of dietary supplements. One in four dietary supplement companies inspected by the agencies have received warning letters, considered a significant enforcement action. In 2012, FDA inspectors found violations of good manufacturing practices during two thirds of the 204 inspections they conducted in nearly 200 supplement facilities. Seventy of these inspections resulted in the agency's most serious rating. Some customers have suffered serious health problems linked to companies' poor manufacturing processes. In 2008, >200 people were poisoned by selenium after taking liquid multivitamin dietary supplements sold in health stores and by chiropractors. The products, called Total Body Formula and Total Body MegaFormula, contained an average of 41,000 micrograms of selenium per serving instead of 200.

ConsumerLab.com, an independent testing organization, has analyzed popular dietary supplements for about 12 years. The group says it has found a significant problem with about 1 in 4 products. Of 35 multivitamin products tested in 2011, 24 passed and 11 failed; of 22 fish oils tested, 16 passed and 6 failed; of 11 magnesium products tested in 2012, 9 passed and 2 failed; and of 11 ginseng products tested in 2010, 6 passed and 5 failed.

METAL-ON-METAL HIP REPLACEMENT DEVICES

During my first decade at the National Institutes of Health, I spent a good bit of time evaluating prosthetic heart valves. The 1960s was the first decade of successful cardiac valve replacement. During that 10-year period, there were many changes in the prosthetic valves. Each time a change was made, the manufacturer generally indicated that this change would prevent problems that occurred in the previously available prosthetic valves. That was unfortunately not always the case. For each new device, some time was required to determine whether the change was an improvement or not.

About 10 years ago, manufacturers of prosthetic hips went from plastic or ceramic to metal-on-metal hip sockets. The belief was that the new devices would be more resistant to wear and reduce the chances of dislocation. Recent data gathered in the UK appear to show just the opposite. In March 2012, British experts using the world's largest artificial joint registry advised physicians to stop using metal-on-metal hip replacements (14). They found that 3 times as many metal-on-metal hips have to be replaced within 5 years than the previously used prosthesis (6% vs. 2%). British regulators now recommend that people who have the implants get yearly blood tests to ensure no dangerous metals are seeping into their bodies as the components rub against each other. The FDA has not made recommendations for the estimated 500,000 American patients with the devices.

RETIREMENT LIVING

According to Kelly Greene (15), an estimated 733,000 people in the US live in an assisted-living facility as of 2010, the latest data available. Typically, assisted living consists of a small apartment with services that may or may not cost extra, such as medicine management, personal care, housekeeping and laundry, meals, activities, and transportation to doctors' appointments. A one-bedroom unit in an assisted-living facility costs as much as $9500 a month in 2011. Alternatives to assisted living exist:

Going offshore. Going abroad for long-term care is relatively new. For $3500 a month, a home can be rented in Costa Rica and shared with two other patients. The price includes a supervising nurse, three aides, a care coordinator, and a chauffeur.

Backyard MedCottage. So that older people can be with their families when they start to need help, several companies have developed separate living cottages in another's backyard. A MedCottage, which costs about $85,000, has a 12 × 24 living area with a handicap-accessible bathroom, kitchen, hospital bed, and living area and is outfitted so that the person living there can be monitored online. Building permits are getting easier to acquire.

Cohousing. This arrangement, which originated in Denver decades ago, was designed for those interested in living communally. In a cohousing development, residents live in private homes but share a central "common house" and other facilities. "Senior" cohousing is beginning to spread elsewhere (seniorcohousing.com). By 2020, there should be at least one cohousing community in every metro area in the US, and about one third are expected to serve older adults.

The permanent cruise. Dr. Lee Lindquist of Northwestern University's Fineberg School of Medicine was the first to compare living on a cruise ship to living in an assisted living facility on land. The cost of the two was fairly similar. On a cruise ship, a physician and nurses are available 24/7, while physicians are not always on site at an assisted-living facility. This particular choice appeals to me.

Spa living. Spa resorts increasingly are trying to expand into residential communities. Canyon Ranch's medical and wellness team in Miami Beach is one of these. Stay well.

LIVING 100 YEARS

In 1950, there were 2300 people in the US >100 years of age; by 2050, according to some estimates, that number could be 600,000 (16).

MEDICAL APPS

There are 40,000 medical applications for smart phones and tablets, and the market is in its infancy according to Jenny Gold of Kaiser Health News (17). Medical apps offer the opportunity to monitor health and encourage patient wellness moment to moment, instead of only during visits to the physician's office. Some apps even replace devices in hospitals and doctors' offices,

such as glucometers and the high-quality microscopes used by dermatologists to examine various skin lesions. So far the field has been unregulated. It is hard to know which apps live up to their claims or provide accurate information.

In 2011, the FDA released a first draft of guidelines that require developers making medical claims to apply for FDA approval, the same way new medical devices must be proven safe and effective before they can be sold. But there seems to be no way that the FDA can keep up. The Government Accountability Office says that the FDA takes 6 months to approve a device similar to an existing product, and 20 months to review a new one. Many developers apparently are not opposed to regulation, but they believe the FDA process does not fit the industry.

Some top-selling medical apps for iPhones:

1. Pregnancy++: Tracks the course of a woman's pregnancy, including weight, diet, and exercise. It also includes fetal pictures, a kick counter, and a contraction counter.
2. Pill Identifier: Allows the user to identify more than 10,000 over-the-counter and prescription pills based on their appearance.
3. Baby Connect: Tracks a baby's daily activities, including feeding, sleep, growth, health, and vaccines and creates graphical reports and trending charts. The information can be shared between parents, nannies, and health care providers.
4. Diagnosaurus DDx: Helps health care providers accurately diagnose patients quickly at the bedside. Providers can search >1000 diagnoses by organ system, symptom, and disease and use a special feature to consider alternative diagnoses when multiple conditions are possible.
5. Instant ECG: Teaches health care professionals the basics of reading electrocardiograms. The app offers video demonstrations of 30 arrhythmias to teach and then test a provider's ability to diagnose irregularities.

AIR-CONDITIONING

John Steele Gordon, the prominent business historian, recently described the development of air-conditioning (18). Before the Industrial Revolution, there were only two ways to stay cool in hot weather. One was to go to the ocean or mountains, and the other was to raise the rate of the evaporation of sweat by increasing air circulation across the skin. Thus, the fan, now 5000 years old, came into existence.

In 1758, Benjamin Franklin experimented with the rapid evaporation of volatile liquids, such as alcohol and ether, to cool water to a point below freezing. He was able to lower the temperature from 64° to 7°F. Franklin wrote to a friend: "One may see the possibility of freezing a man to death on a warm summer's day."

In 1828, Michael Faraday demonstrated that one could cool water by applying mechanical power to compress a volatile substance such as ammonia into a liquid and then by allowing it to rapidly evaporate.

In the 1830s, John Gorrie, a young physician living in Apalachicola, Florida, recognized that patients were more likely to survive an illness in cool weather than in hot. So, he rigged up pans full of ice near the ceiling in a hospital room. The ice would cool the air around it and because cold air is heavier than hot air would float downward over the patient and then out through holes in the room's floor. It was the first effective system of air-conditioning. Since ice was expensive in Apalachicola because it had to be imported by ship from the north, Gorrie began to experiment with making ice by mechanical means. In 1851, he was granted a patent on a machine that worked on Faraday's principle. He quit medicine to work on perfecting his invention but when his financial backer died, he was unable to carry on and died in poverty in 1855.

In the hot summer of 1881, President James Garfield lay dying of an assassin's bullet. To help keep him cool, naval engineers rigged up sheets of cloth soaked in iced water with a fan blowing air across them. The method kept his room 20 degrees cooler, but it used half a million pounds of ice over a 2-month period and did not lower the humidity, a crucial part of keeping both cool and comfortable.

In 1902, Willis Carrier, a young engineer in the Buffalo Forge Company in Buffalo, New York, invented the first modern air-conditioning to cool a printing plant. (High humidity could cause paper jams and prevent ink from drying quickly.) He used a compressor to liquefy ammonia and then evaporated it to cool water. Running the water through coils, he blew air across them, cooling the air and causing it to lose moisture through condensation on the coils. The air was then sent into the workplace via ducts. While useful for industrial purposes, the Carrier air-conditioning system was both large and dangerous, as ammonia is very toxic. But, by the early 1920s, he had developed a much more efficient compressor and started using a much safer refrigerant (Dielene) as the volatile. (Dupont invented Freon in 1928.)

In 1925, one of New York's movie theaters became the first to be air-conditioned, and it proved a huge hit with moviegoers. Other large theaters rapidly followed. So did department stores, which saw increased summer sales as a result. Office air-conditioning lagged behind, but when studies showed that productivity greatly increased when offices were cool, those buildings also became air-conditioned. The House of Representatives installed air-conditioning in 1928, and the Senate and White House soon followed.

Air-conditioners small enough to fit in a window and cool just one room became commercially available after World War II. In 1948, 74,000 units were sold; by 1953, over a million. The first automobile air-conditioner was offered in 1940; today, 99% of cars sold have air-conditioning.

And obviously air-conditioning had many profound results. Washington, DC, used to be nearly deserted in the summer because of the city's notorious heat and humidity. Today, the government runs year round. In the first half of the 20th century, the South was losing population; air-conditioning played a major role in changing that. When the present Parkland Hospital was built, it was not air-conditioned. That was inserted later at great expense.

STORM SHELTERS

The US Department of Housing and Urban Development and the Federal Emergency Management Agency (FEMA) encourage community shelters by awarding grants to help pay for them (19). Since 1999, FEMA has helped fund over 1300 community safe rooms in 20 cities, including 235 in 2011, up from 124 in 2010. The shelters hold anywhere from 50 to 300 people and some many more. Sounds like a good idea in view of the recent leveling tornadoes and hurricanes.

JUNE 2012 WEATHER

In June 2012 >2 million acres were burned in massive wildfires in much of the West, >110 million people were living under extreme heat advisories, and more than two thirds of the country was experiencing drought (20). In June 2012, 3215 daily high-temperature records were set nationwide. (In March 2012, 15,000 new records were set!) The 12 months ending in June were the warmest 12 continuous months on record in the US. Is all this evidence of global warming? In a report released on July 10, 2012, the National Climatic Data Center concluded that the odds that the unusual heat of the past 13 months was random were 1 in 1.6 million. Bryan Walsh in a piece in *Time* concluded that "climate change is real, and it's happening now. We can argue about what causes it, how to handle it and how to balance the cost of that action against the risk of doing nothing. . . . We're living in an igloo this summer and the ice is melting all around us."

WAGES OF US WORKERS

The number of workers earning wages in the private sector was 131 million during the fourth quarter of 2011, the latest data available (21). Of those, 10.6 million were employed in Texas. Nationally, the average weekly wage was $955, down 1.7% from 12 months earlier. The average weekly wage in Texas was $973. Wages for some occupations in the Dallas–Fort Worth–Arlington metropolitan area were as follows (numbers rounded off): chief executive, $194,000; dentist, $183,000; surgeon, $169,000; airline pilot, $165,000; family practitioner, $164,000; lawyer, $139,000; air traffic controller, $135,000; pharmacist, $112,000; dental hygienist, $73,000; registered nurse, $68,000; secondary schoolteacher, $58,000; chiropractor, $52,000; flight attendant, $47,000; substance abuse counselor, $35,000; and home health aide, $22,000.

AMERICA'S HOUSEHOLD WEALTH

According to the Federal Reserve Survey of Consumer Finances, the median net worth of American families was lower in 2010 than in 1989 (22). For all families, median net worth fell 39% from 2007 to 2010. The drop would have been bigger if measured at the market's 2009 bottom.

FASTEST-GROWING US CITIES

The latest numbers from the US Census Bureau show that 8 of the 15 fastest-growing large cities in the USA were located in Texas *(Table 1)* (23).

Table 1. The 15 fastest-growing large US cities by percentage increase from April 1, 2010, to July 1, 2011

	Percent increase	2011 total population
1. New Orleans, LA	4.9	360,740
2. Round Rock, TX	4.8	104,664
3. Austin, TX	3.8	820,611
4. Plano, TX	3.8	269,776
5. McKinney, TX	3.8	136,067
6. Frisco, TX	3.8	121,387
7. Denton, TX	3.4	117,187
8. Denver, CO	3.3	619,968
9. Cary, NC	3.2	139,633
10. Raleigh, NC	3.1	416,468
11. Alexandria, VA	3.1	144,301
12. Tampa, FL	3.1	346,037
13. McAllen, TX	3.0	133,742
14. Carrollton, TX	3.0	122,640
15. Atlanta, GA	3.0	432,427

*From the US Census Bureau: http://www.census.gov/newsroom/releases/archives/population/cb12-117.html

US TRAFFIC

According to *The Washington Post,* the cities that waste the most hours for drivers each year on average are the following (listed by city and followed by the number of hours wasted yearly in traffic): Honolulu, 58; New York, 57; Los Angeles, 56; San Francisco, 48; Bridgeport, CT, 45; Boston, 35; Seattle, 33; Chicago, 32.8; and Austin, 30 (24, 25).

RAISING CHILDREN

A recently released government report found that middle-income families (those with incomes from $60,000 to $103,000 yearly) with a child born in 2011 will spend about $235,000 in child-related expenses from birth through age 17 (26). Housing is the single largest expense, averaging $70,000, or 30% of the total cost, with the Northeast and urban West being the most expensive. The estimate also includes the cost of transportation, child care, education, food, clothing, health care, and miscellaneous expenses. In 1960, it was estimated that the cost of raising a child was just over $24,000 for middle-income families. (That would be $192,000 today when adjusted for inflation.) Child care is the second largest expense. Higher-earning families spend more on their children. Families with three or more children spend 22% less per child than those with two children. The savings result from hand-me-down clothes and toys, shared bedrooms, and buying food in larger quantities.

WHAT NORTH KOREAN CHILDREN LEARN ABOUT THE USA

A framed poster on the wall of a kindergarten classroom in North Korea shows children using rifles and bayonets to attack a helpless American soldier, his face bandaged and blood spurting from his mouth (27). Another poster depicts an American with a noose around his neck. For North Koreans, this systematic in-doctrination of anti-Americanism starts as early as kindergarten and is as much a part of the curriculum as learning to count. Toy pistols, rifles, and tanks sit lined up in neat rows on shelves. A favorite school-year game is to throw stones at a dummy of an American soldier with a beaked nose and straw-colored hair. The students in North Korea learn that their country has two main enemies: the Japanese who colonized Korea from 1910 to 1945 and the US, which fought against North Korea from 1950 to 1953. The students are told that North Korea's defense against outside forces remains the backbone of the country's foreign policy. The population is bred to seek revenge, even as the government professes to want peace. They are taught that the American imperialists started the war. The tragedy emerged by which the nation was divided into two parts. Nevertheless, when the rare American is seen in Pyong-Yang, the littlest North Koreans invariably wave and call out "hello" in English, showing fascination rather than fear.

PROLIFIC DIEGO

A Galapagos island is the home to Diego, a prolific, bossy reptile (28). He has sired hundreds of offspring and has been central to bringing the Espanola Island type of tortoise back from near extinction. Diego was plucked from Espanola by expeditioners between 1900 and 1930 and wound up in the San Diego Zoo in California. When the zoo returned him to the Galapagos in 1975, the only other known living members of his species were 2 males and 12 females. His species—*Chelonoidis hoodensis*—had all but been destroyed, mostly by domestic animals (introduced by humans) who ate their eggs. So, Diego and the others were placed in a corral at the park's breeding center on Santa Cruz, the main island in the isolated archipelago, whose unique flora and fauna helped inspire Charles Darwin's work on evolution. Diego was so dominant and aggressive, bullying other males with bites and shoves, that he had to be moved 8 years later to his own pen with five of the females. The reptiles are not monogamous. Diego apparently became the most sexually active of the bunch because he is the biggest and the oldest of the males, being nearly 3 feet long and weighing 175 pounds. The herpetologist for the Galapagos Conservancy, Linda Cayot, estimates that Diego is the father of 40% to 45% of the 1781 tortoises born in the breeding program and placed on Espanola Island.

At least 14 species of giant tortoises originally inhabited the islands, which are 620 miles off of Ecuador's Pacific coast, and 10 survived. Espanola, which encompasses 50 square miles, is arid, and in order to reach vegetation high enough off the ground, the tortoises developed the longest legs and necks of any of the species in the archipelago. Before humans arrived in the Galapagos, the six islands were home to tens of thousands of giant tortoises. The numbers were down to about 3000 in 1974, but the recovery program run by the National Park and the Charles Darwin Foundation has succeeded in increasing the overall population to about 20,000.

LIFE IN THE US IN 1776

Thomas Fleming's book, *What America Was Really Like in 1776,* recently appeared (29). He indicates that Americans at that time had the highest per capita income in the civilized world. They also paid the lowest taxes. By 1776, the 13 American colonies had been in existence for over 150 years—more than enough time for the talented and ambitious to acquire money and land. At the top of the South's earners were large planters such as George Washington. In the North, Southern incomes were more than matched by merchants such as John Hancock and Robert Morris. Next came lawyers such as John Adams, followed by tavern keepers, who often cleared 1000 pounds a year, or about $100,000 in today's money. Physicians were paid comparatively little, as were dentists, who were almost nonexistent.

In the Northern colonies, the top 10% of the population owned about 45% of the wealth. In some parts of the South, 10% owned 75% of the wealth. Unlike most other countries, America in 1776 had a thriving middle class. Well-to-do farmers shipped tons of corn, wheat, and rice to the West Indies and Europe, using the profits to send their children to private schools and buy their wives expensive gowns and carriages. Artisans, tailors, carpenters, and other skilled workmen also prospered, as did shop owners who dealt in a variety of goods.

Several hundred miles inland was the "back country," and at the time of the Revolution few people went there by choice. Most who went were poor and landless—younger sons, for example, whose older brothers had inherited the family's property. Life on the outskirts of civilization was hard and often violent. Morals on the Western frontier were often much more relaxed than they were in the civilized East.

America in 1776 was also a diverse nation. The first census, taken in 1790, revealed that only about 60% of the people came from England. The rest were German, Irish, Dutch, Scottish, Swedish, and African.

Men wore clothes that were as colorful as the ladies' garb. Women regularly spent a half day getting their hair "permanented" for a ball. Ladies seeking to preserve the sheen of youth spent a fortune on "paints" from China and lip salves from India.

Another American tradition beginning to take root was female independence. Although "domestic felicity" was considered vital to everyone's peace of mind, and although divorce was legal, it was rare. Money played a part in marriage among the more affluent, but family life was often full of affection.

By 1776, the Atlantic Ocean had become what one historian called "an information highway" across which poured books, magazines, newspapers, and copies of the debates in Parliament. The latter were read by John Adams, George Washington, Robert Morris, and other politically minded men. They concluded that the British were planning to tax the Americans into the kind of humiliation that Great Britain had inflicted on Ireland. Dr. Benjamin Rush, the Pennsylvanian who signed the Declaration of Independence, wrote that the 8-year war for independence was only the first step in the Revolution's destiny to transform America and the world. History confirmed his intuition.

THE GATE RULE

In one of Peggy Noonan's recent columns, she described the Gate Rule (30): People are either lined up at the gate trying to get out of a country or lined up trying to get in. In the US they are lined up to get in. Compared with many other countries, the US economy isn't in such bad shape. As Peggy Noonan says, "People don't want to come to a place when they know they will be treated badly. They don't want to call your home, their home unless they know you will make room for them in more than economic ways." The American friendliness, openness, and lack of old hatred are generally welcomed around the world.

SCOTT GORDON JUREK: ULTRAMARATHONER AND VEGETARIAN

Scott Jurek was born on October 26, 1973 (31). He began running long distance as a sophomore in high school to prepare for Nordic skiing. He disliked running at first but after spending summers running on trails with ski poles, he found a passion for trail running. On a challenge from his training partner, Scott ran the Minnesota Voyageur 50-Mile in 1994, placing second in his first attempt at an ultramarathon, without even having run a marathon. Scott was the valedictorian of his high school class and attended the College of St. Scholastica in Duluth, Minnesota, graduating with a master's degree in physical therapy in 1998. During his college years, he competed in a number of ultramarathon races and won many of them. In 1998, he began competing nationally and won two 50-mile runs and placed second in his first 100-mile run. He won his first 100-mile Western States Endurance Run on his first attempt and won it six more times continuously. He achieved the new course record of 15 hours and 36 minutes in 2004. During the next 5 years he notched a number of 50-mile and 100-mile wins. In 2006, he won his first of three consecutive victories in the Spartathlon, a 153-mile race between Athens and Sparta in Greece. Jurek is the only North American to ever win that race. In 2007, he won the Hardrock Hundred, setting a new course record at the time. In 2006, Jurek with a group of runners raced against the Tarahumara in Copper Canyon, Mexico. Jurek narrowly lost to the fastest Tarahumara runner, but in 2007 he won the race. In 2010, Jurek broke the USA Track and Field all-surface record distance run by an American in 24 hours with 165.7 miles.

Jurek became a vegetarian in 1998 and is an advocate of plant-based eating for health and ethical/environmental reasons (32). He cites his diet as the key to his superior athletic performance and recovery. He became a vegan in 1999. When Jurek was very young his mother was diagnosed with multiple sclerosis. Her struggles taught him to persevere in difficult circumstances, and he credits her memory as his major source of strength. He has won at least twenty-five 50-mile, 100-mile, and 152-mile races and holds the US record for 24-hour distance on all-surfaces (165.7 miles). In 2012, his book, *Eat and Run: My Unlikely Journey to Ultramarathon Greatness*, appeared.

FEMALE VERSUS MALE OLYMPIANS

When the US Olympic Committee unveiled its 2012 530-member team, women outnumbered men for the first time: 269 vs. 261 (33). The increasing presence of female Olympians on the US team is attributed to the growth of opportunities since the passage of Title IV, the 1972 gender-equality law. (For the 1972 US Olympic team, only 21% were female: 84 of 400.)

SPORTS OF PRESIDENTS

The sporting activities of the 20th and 21st century presidents are listed in *Table 2* (34). Theodore Roosevelt and George W. Bush appear to be the most physically fit during most of their lives. William Howard Taft, at 300 pounds, was the least fit. Woodrow Wilson was the starting centerfielder for Davidson College in North Carolina but didn't make the cut at Princeton. He played a record 1000-plus rounds of golf as president. Herbert Hoover served as student manager of Stanford's football and baseball teams. Dwight Eisenhower was dubbed the "Kansas Cyclone." He was linebacker and running back at West

Point back when the academy was a football powerhouse. He played >800 rounds of golf as president and was the first president to score a hole in one. John F. Kennedy was a member of Harvard's junior varsity golf, swimming, and football squads and was on the varsity team in sailing. Lyndon Baines Johnson was a fisherman. He was said to have a long drive in golf but could not break 100. Nixon played basketball at Whittier College but mostly rode the bench on the gridiron. He loved bowling in the White House. Gerald Ford was the best athlete of them all. He was an all-American center on Michigan's national football teams and he could have played in the National Football League but instead went to Yale Law School, where he also coached football. Jimmy Carter was a big-time runner in track and cross-country for the Naval Academy. Ronald Reagan was a football player at Eureka College. George H. W. Bush was a star first-baseman and captain of Yale's baseball team. Bill Clinton installed a jogging track on the White House lawn. He cheated big time in golf. George W. Bush is a fitness fanatic. He was the first president to have run a marathon and he still loves mountain biking. Barack Obama was nicknamed "Barry O'Bomber" as a high school basketball player. He is an average golfer at best and is said to have played over 100 rounds of golf during his first 3 years as president.

MISPLACED VALUES

Long-term contracts have become common in major league baseball. Over time, players who land long-term, big money deals often prove poor investments (35). A few examples: *Alex Rodriquez*, $275 million for 10 years (expires 2017); *Troy Tulowitzki*, $157 million for 10 years (expires 2020); Albert Pujols, $252 million for 10 years (expires 2021); *Prince Fielder*, $214 million for 9 years (expires 2020); *Mark Teixeira*, $180 million for 8 years (expires 2016); *Adrian Gonzalez*, $154 million for 7 years (expires 2018); *Joey Votto*, $240 million for 10 years (expires 2023); *Joe Mauer*, $184 million for 8 years (expires 2018); *C. C. Sabathia*, $161 million for 7 years (expires 2015); and *Miguel Cabrera*, $152 million for 8 years (expires 2015).

CELL PHONE OBSESSION

On June 29, 2007, the first iPhone went on sale (36). The Apple device cost $600 and had no physical keyboard, limited email options, and no copy and paste. In hindsight, it wasn't so hot. Since that date Apple has sold >220 million iPhones worldwide and sparked a commercial, cultural, and behavioral revolution. According to a study of medical workers at Bay State Medical Center in Springfield, Massachusetts, 76% say they have experienced "phantom vibration," that insistent buzz from an imagined text or phone call, possibly the result of random nerves firing, biochemical noise that our brains easily turn out until they were reconditioned by the iPhone. According to Larry Rosen, a psychologist and author of *iDisorder: Understanding Our Obsession with Technology and Overcoming Its Hold on Us*, nearly 30% of people born after 1980 are anxious if they can't check Facebook every few minutes. Others repeatedly pat their pockets to make sure their smart phone is still there.

Table 2. Sporting activities of US presidents

President	College athlete	Recreational sports
Theodore Roosevelt	+ Boxing Wrestling	Polo Exploring Hunting
William Howard Taft	+ Baseball	Golf
Warren G. Harding	0	Golf
Calvin Coolidge	0	Fishing Horseback riding
Herbert Hoover	0	Fishing
Franklin D. Roosevelt	0	0
Harry S Truman	0*	0
Dwight Eisenhower	+ Football	Golf
John F. Kennedy	+ Golf Swimming Football Sailing	Golf Sailing
Lyndon Baines Johnson	0	Fishing Golf
Richard Nixon	Basketball Football	Bowling
Gerald Ford	+ Football	Golf Skiing
Jimmy Carter	+ Track	Running
Ronald Reagan	+ Football	
George H. W. Bush	+ Baseball	Golf Boating Horseshoes
William J. Clinton	0	Jogging Golf
George W. Bush	0	Running Mountain biking
Barack Obama	0	Golf Basketball

*Did not attend college.

This obsession, of course, has been good for Apple. The company's annual revenue climbed from $24 billion in 2007 to $108 billion in 2011, and its stock price is up almost 400% over the same period. According to Rosen: "The great thing about the iPhone is that we carry it with us all day long. The bad part is that we carry it with us all day long." That makes people lab rats in a real-time psychological experiment that's altering behavior at lightning speed. By 2016, there may be more mobile devices than people. Thanks to the ubiquity of smartphones, many museum-goers "skip the step of actually looking at the artwork and move straight to photographing," says Elizabeth Broun, director of the Smithsonian American Art Museum in Washington, DC. Is the iPhone a crutch that does too much of our thinking and increasingly takes the place of real human connections?

WILLIAM CLIFFORD ROBERTS, MD
20 July 2012

1. Hensarling J. 'Obamacare' undermines economy, patient care. *Dallas Morning News*, June 29, 2012.
2. Taubes G. Why our obesity crisis is getting worse. *Newsweek*, May 7, 2012.
3. Costa S. New drug application for obesity gets OK from FDA advisory panel. *Cardiology Today*, June 2012.
4. Khrennikov I, Sysoyeva M. Beef: the new opiate of the Russian masses? *Bloomberg Businessweek*, June 25–July 1, 2012.
5. Savodnik P. The other Gulf War syndrome. *Bloomberg Businessweek*, June 25–July 1, 2012.
6. Bjerga A. The fight over half a trillion. *Bloomberg Businessweek*, July 2–8, 2012.
7. Maron BJ, Henry WL, Roberts WC, Epstein SE. Comparison of echocardiographic and necropsy measurements of ventricular wall thicknesses in patients with and without disproportionate septal thickening. *Circulation* 1977;55(2):341–346.
8. Barnard ND. Saving my first patient. *Good Medicine* 2012;3 (Summer):2.
9. Leger DL. Opana: the new OxyContin. *USA Today*, July 11, 2012.
10. Thompson M, Gibbs N. More U.S. soldiers have killed themselves than have died in the Afghan war. Why can't the army win the war on suicide? *Time*, July 23, 2012.
11. Grady D. Mother of first test-tube baby brought hope to millions. *Dallas Morning News*, June 24, 2012.
12. Sadler K, Nicholson S, Steer T, Gill V, Bates B, Tipping S, Cox L, Lennox A, Prentice A. WASH (World Action on Salt & Health) National Diet and Nutrition Survey—assessment of dietary sodium in adults (aged 19 to 64 years) in England, 2011. June 21, 2012.
13. Tsouderos T. It's downright scary. Major problems found at firms making dietary supplements. *Dallas Morning News*, July 8, 2012.
14. Perrone M. FDA takes new look at metal hips. *Dallas Morning News*, June 24, 2012.
15. Greene K. The new retirement resorts. *Wall Street Journal*, March 17–18, 2012.
16. Older and wiser. *Smithsonian.com*, February 2012.
17. Gold J. Medical apps bump up against regulators. *USA Today*, July 3, 2012.
18. Gordon JS. Air conditioning, blessed invention. *Wall Street Journal*, July 11, 2012.
19. Keen J. Communities construct storm shelters. *USA Today*, June 22, 2012.
20. Walsh B. Endless summer: the record heat is a taste of how climate change can play out. *Time*, July 23, 2012.
21. Bowen B. A cut above the rest. *Dallas Morning News*, July 9, 2012.
22. Coy P. America's vanishing household wealth. *Bloomberg Businessweek*, July 2–8, 2012.
23. Young ME. Texas cities fill map of fastest-growing areas. *Dallas Morning News*, June 29, 2012.
24. Kane S. The worst traffic in America? It's not Los Angeles. *Washington Post*, May 25, 2012.
25. US Department of Commerce, US Census Bureau. INRIX national traffic scorecard report (May 2012). Available at http://www.inrix.com/scorecard/default.asp.
26. Hananel S. Bringing up baby? It's pricey. *Dallas Morning News*, June 24, 2012.
27. Lee JH. Today's lesson: Why N. Korea hates U.S. *Dallas Morning News*, June 24, 2012.
28. Solano G. Tortoise a bully—and prolific. *Dallas Morning News*, July 4, 2012.
29. Fleming T. *What America Was Really Like in 1776*. Boston: New Word City.
30. Noonan P. Is that allowed? It is here. *Wall Street Journal*, July 7–8, 2012.
31. 10 questions about Scott Jurek. *Time*, July 23, 2012.
32. Bittman M. Diet and exercise to the extremes. *New York Times*, May 12, 2010.
33. Whiteside K. Women majority on Team USA. *USA Today*, July 11, 2012.
34. Benning T. Who's the ultimate jock-in-chief? *Dallas Morning News*, March 18, 2012.
35. Cowlishaw T. First-class baggage. *Dallas Morning News*, June 26, 2012.
36. Burrows P. The first five years of iPhone mass obsession. *Bloomberg BusinessWeek*, June 21, 2012.

Chapter 9

January 2013

HYDROPHOBIA

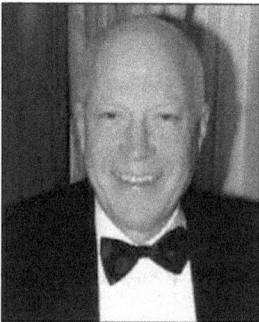

William C. Roberts, MD.

Few diseases bring as much gut-wrenching ancient fear as rabies. Infection from the bite of a slavering animal means death unless the individual is vaccinated early. The husband-and-wife team of Bill Wasik, a writer, and Monica Murphy, a veterinarian, have written a well-researched tale of the war against the world's most diabolical virus (1). The rabies virus is the most fatal one in the world. It kills nearly 100% of its hosts in most species. The virus is shaped like a bullet, a cylindrical shell of glycoprotein and lipids that carries in its rounded tip a malevolent payload of helical RNA. On entering a living thing, it eschews the bloodstream. Instead, unlike almost any other virus, rabies courses through the nervous system, creeping upstream at 1 or 2 cm per day (on average) through the axoplasm, the transmission lines that conduct electrical impulses to and from the brain. Once inside the brain, the virus works slowly but fatally to warp the mind, suppressing the rational and stimulating the animal. Aggression rises to fever pitch; inhibitions melt away; salivation increases. The infected creature now has only days to live, and these will likely be spent on the attack, foaming at the mouth, chasing and lunging and biting in the throes of madness because the demon, as Wasik and Murphy write, that possesses him seeks more hosts. The rabid bite is the visible symbol of the animal infecting the human.

Wasik and Murphy write that about 60% of our diseases are zoonotic, that is, they originate in the nonhuman animal population: swine flu, AIDS, West Nile, Ebola, rabies. Nothing, they write, has made humans sicker than our association with nonhuman animals. Not only our emerging diseases today but the major killers throughout the ages—smallpox, tuberculosis, malaria, and influenza—evolved from similar diseases in nonhuman animals. This is what Jared Diamond has called "the lethal gift of livestock," a major shaper of human destiny.

Yet until the 20th century, humans had no idea that so many of their illnesses derived from nonhuman hosts. There was the Black Death or bubonic plague, which spreads to humans via fleas living on the backs of rats and other rodents.

Scholars blamed nearly everything else, from demonic forces in bad air to astronomical happenings and even human malefactors. For centuries, rabies was the only illness in which the animalistic transfer, or more like a transformation, was evident. A mad animal bit; a bad man appeared; each would die a terrible death. The madness could lurk within any mammal, even in—especially in—the most domesticated and loyal of all, the dog. As the lone visible instance of animal-to-human infection, rabies has always shaded into something more supernatural: into bestial metamorphoses, into monstrous hybridities. As Susan Sonntag wrote, "That infection transforms people into madden animals."

During the 20th century, after Pasteur's invention of a rabies vaccine provided a near-foolproof means of preventing its fatality in humans, our fascination with rabies seemed only to swell. The vaccine itself became as mythologized as the bug, such that even today many Americans believe that treatment requires some 20 or 30 shots, delivered with a foot-long syringe into the stomach. (In fact, today's vaccine entails four shots into the arm that are not particularly deep.) Even as vaccination of dogs in the USA was reducing the infection rate in that species to negligible levels, a generation of children learned to scrutinize their pet pooches for the slightest sign of madness.

Every year about 55,000 persons, according to the World Health Organization, die of rabies. Few of these deaths, however, occur in the USA or Western Europe. The deaths are mainly in Asia and Africa, from countries where vaccination is too expensive or too difficult to procure.

The sequence of horrors faced by a typical rabies patient today is hardly different from those experienced by the man who was probably the most eminent rabies victim in history: *Charles Lennox*, fourth Duke of Richmond, who for 2 years leading up to his death in 1819 served as governor-general of Canada, the top post in what was then still a colonial government. The duke was a lover of dogs. Ironically, it was not a dog but rather a fox, the ostensibly tame pet of a soldier whose garrison the duke had occasion to inspect in Quebec, whose jaws were to blame for his demise. When the fox tangled with the duke's own dog, Lennox naturally stepped in to separate the two. The mad fox seized this chance to insult the visiting dignitary, chomping down hard on the base of his thumb. After a bite, the rabies virus binds quickly into the peripheral nerves but then makes its course with almost impossible sloth, usually requiring at least 3 weeks and often as long as 3 months to arrive at and penetrate the brain. On rare occasions, a full year, or even 5 years, can elapse before the onset of symptoms. During this time, the wound will heal and the victim may even forget about his scrape with a snarling beast. But healed or not, as the virus enters the brain, the wound will usually return with some odd sensation occurring at the site, such as stabbing pain or numbness, burning or unnatural cold, tingling or itching, or even a tremor. At roughly the same time these soon-to-be-doomed patients typically display general signs of influenza, with fever and perhaps a sore throat or nausea. In the case of the Duke of Richmond, symptoms began with shoulder pains and a sore throat and then progressed the following day to insomnia and fatigue.

All this is merely prelude to its most notable symptom in humans, unique to rabies among all diseases: a terrifying condition called *hydrophobia*, a fear of water, though the word "fear" does not do justice to the eerie and fully physical manner in which it manifests. Present the hydrophobic patient with a cup of water, and, desperately though he wants to drink it, his entire body rebels against the consummation of this act. The outstretched arm jerks away just as it is about to bring the water to the parched lips. Other times the entire body convulses at the thought. Just beholding the water can make the diaphragm involuntarily contract, causing patients to gag and retch. During the course of his illness, the Duke of Richmond finally lost all desire to drink any liquids. He could not even accept his customary shave, so repelled was he by the water in the basin. They tried to put him in a boat but he jumped back to the shore. Taken to the closest house, he begged to be moved further inland. The sound of running water became unbearable to him.

Fever spikes high during the final phase of the disease. The mouth salivates profusely. Tears stream from the eyes. Goosebumps break out on the skin. Cries of agony can produce the impression of an almost animal bark. In the throes of their convulsions, patients have even been known to bite. They also hallucinate. Not uncommonly, male patients succumb to an even more lurid sort of abandon. The virus's action on the limbic system of the brain can cause them to exhibit hypersexual behavior: increased desire, involuntary erections, and even orgasms, sometimes occurring at a rate of once per hour. Some cases have reported up to 30 ejaculations in a single day. And yet, despite all the horrors of hydrophobia, the attacks often subside, for a time allowing sufferers periods of poignant lucidity. They are given the opportunity to fully contemplate what their condition portends. Before his death, the duke dictated a lengthy letter to his oldest daughter, giving instruction that his beloved dog be handed over to her.

Lewis Pasteur and his assistants, to develop their vaccine, had to corral dogs at the apex of their madness and extract deadly slather from their snarling jaws. Pasteur once performed this trick with a glass tube held in his mouth as two assistants with gloved hands penned down a rabid bulldog.

Diagnosing rabies for veterinarians today is a gruesome affair. Vets do not use a blood test for rabies in animals. It is not a pinprick and wait-and-see affair. Only a sampling from the brain will suffice. Therefore, the animal must be killed with its head removed and shipped off to authorities for study.

Despite a thorough investigation using all the tools of the Pasteur laboratory, no combination of methods and media available to Pasteur and his assistants would yield a microbial cause for rabies. Even as Pasteur's team discovered that the infectious principle for rabies resided in both the central nervous system and the salivary glands, they failed to culture a pathogen from either location. Thanks largely to the work of Pasteur himself, it was by this time a basic tenet of medical science that infectious diseases are caused by specific demonstrable microorganisms. Robert Koch's famous "postulates," first articulated in 1880, had made clear the relation between microorganisms and disease, defining a disease-causing microbe as one that appears exclusively in diseased individuals; that can be isolated and cultured from a disease host; that will cause disease when next introduced into a susceptible host; and that can be subsequently recovered from the experimental host and shown to be identical in culture to the microbe originally isolated. For rabies, not a single one of these conditions had been met. Koch's precepts have often been summed up with the phrase "one disease, one microbe," and Pasteur concurred with this view, but his vision saw a third term in this equation: one vaccine. He believed every disease-causing microbe, once isolated, could be attenuated so as to safely confer immunity on a potential host. But it was hard to see how this equation could hold true unless a pathogen could be isolated, identified, trapped under glass, and then tamed.

Pasteur referred to the unseen—apparently unseeable— agent of rabies as a virus. The word *virus* had until that point been associated with a darkly mysterious etiology. Rabies behaved as though it were a microbiotic contagion, and so Pasteur maintained absolute faith that it was one, even though he could neither culture it in broth nor observe it under the microscope. The word *virus* conveyed his uncertainty about rabies' specific form and characteristics. It was not until 1898 that a virus was scientifically defined as a microbe that is invisible under the light microscope and can pass through a filter designed to trap bacteria; it was not until 1903 that it was experimentally demonstrated that the agent of rabies fit within that category.

Despite the confounding invincibility of rabies, despite the fact that it seemed to violate the scientific principles of the day to do so, Pasteur persevered in his work on the vaccine. He concluded early on that trying to cultivate the agent of rabies using existing laboratory methods would be fruitless. Instead, he refocused his attention and that of his assistants on inducing immunity in animals and eventually humans, to what would remain an obscure, intangible foe.

There occurred in 1880 in Paris a surge of rabies such that the Pasteur laboratory had no trouble obtaining infectious material. They got it from kennels of the National Veterinary School and from private veterinary offices around the city. Because rabies could not be cultured on a plate or in a vial, it had to be maintained in living tissue. In the 1880s, this meant within the corporeal cells of a living afflicted animal. The maintenance of rabid animals within the modest rooms and basement of the

Pasteur laboratory was discomforting to the personnel. There was the ever-present risk of contracting rabies.

To create and test a vaccine against rabies, the Pasteur team first had to develop a strain of rabies that behaved more reliably than the natural infection. The crude method of one animal's biting another, followed by an anxious wait over weeks or longer to see whether infection had been transmitted, was unsatisfactory. The technique involved the dangerous collection of saliva from a raging animal. They soon found that rabies could be as readily communicated with material from the affected animal's brain stem as with its saliva. Thus, they were able to improve the infection rate and shorten the incubation period by administering chloroform anesthesia to the recipient animal, trepanning a hole in its skull, and then inoculating the rabid nervous tissue into the dura mater. The trepanation technique allowed successful transfer of the rabies to the healthy animal in every case attempted. Signs of disease were apparent in the inoculated animal in <2 weeks, and death occurred within a month. Canine rabies was thereby passed to a rabbit and from one rabbit to another rabbit, and from that rabbit to still another rabbit, and so on in successive passages. The incubation period became reliably shorter. Once 21 passages had been made, brain to brain, one rabbit to another, the incubation period had decreased to 8 days and there it became fixed. The shortened incubation period was associated with increased virulence.

The next step would be attenuation: the deliberate weakening of the virus to induce immunity without causing disease. If the infection inhabited the brain before protective immunity had taken hold, the patient's death from rabies would be as certain as ever. Pasteur created his highly immunogenic but determinately safe rabies vaccine strain through a two-stage process: a first stage to hone the virulence of the virus and a second to deliberately blunt it. Both stages relied on manipulation of postmortem nervous tissue from rabid animals. Soon they were able to demonstrate the powerful effectiveness of their attenuated-virulent strain as a vaccine.

The first patient to receive the Pasteur vaccine was Joseph Meister, a 9-year-old boy who had received 14 penetrating wounds to his legs and hand by a vicious dog while walking to school. After receiving approval from two prominent pediatricians (Louis Pasteur had never been trained as a physician nor did he have a medical license), Meister received his first injection on July 6, 1885, 60 hours after the bites of July 4. He received, in a syringe, portions of the spinal cord from a rabbit dead of rabies on June 21, 1885. The cord had been kept in a flask of dry air for 15 days. The full 10-day treatment consisted of 13 inoculations, all delivering postmortem spinal tissue from a rabid rabbit. Each successive injection would contain a section of cord that had been exposed to air for a shorter time than the one before it so that as the series proceeded the vaccine would become less attenuated. On July 16, Meister received his final inoculation, the most virulent tissue of all: rabid spinal cord from a dog that had been infected with a strain of rabies virus maximally strengthened by serial passage in the rabbit and harvested only 1 day prior to injection.

The boy remained free of rabies symptoms. Pasteur's modest laboratory was immediately transformed into a clinic and dispensary. People terrified of rabies arrived in droves to receive inoculations. By December 1885, 80 courses of treatment had been completed or were in progress in Pasteur's bustling lab.

In December 1885, four children from New Jersey bitten by rabid dogs were en route to Paris to receive Pasteur's now internationally famous cure. These four children also were cured, and that announcement led to a profound change in the way Americans thought about science and medicine. It reversed the assumption that older doctors and older medicines were better than new ones. It created a new expectation that medicine can and should change, that progress was to be expected, that the new advances would come from laboratory experiments on animals, and that specific injections would be a major tool of the new medicine. By the year 1900, there were at least six clinics in the USA devoted to administering rabies vaccines. Pasteur had a fundraising campaign in several countries to expand his laboratory, which in 1888 became known as the Institut Pasteur.

US DRUG SHORTAGES

An editorial by Sharmila Devi (2) in *Lancet* suggests that severe shortages of drugs, such as sterile injectables, in the USA will continue for several more years. Around 280 drugs, almost all manufactured in the USA, remain in short supply because of several factors: a dwindling number of makers of some drugs, deteriorating conditions in factories, and low prices for generics, leading to a lack of investment to upgrade plants. According to Devi, the shortages have led to delays in surgery and cancer treatments, left patients in pain, and forced hospitals to prescribe less effective substitutes. The US Food and Drug Administration (FDA) is at the forefront of an increasingly complex battle to ensure that the US retains access to critical drugs. President Obama issued an executive order in October 2011 requiring drug companies to report to the FDA when critical supplies were threatened. New legislation that would make it mandatory for companies to notify the FDA of supply problems and give the agency extra powers languishes in Congress.

SHORTENING MEDICAL TRAINING

Currently, it takes an average of 14 years of college, medical school, residency, and fellowship to train a subspecialty physician. Emanuel and Fuchs (3) from the University of Pennsylvania and Stanford University suggest that this period could easily be reduced to 10 years, or by approximately 30%. The time wasted by some of our most highly educated and talented people is improper. Future efforts to reduce the Medicare budget will likely be accompanied by a reduction in the federal government's support of graduate medical education. Streamlining residencies will save money for academic health centers because they would have to spend less on training that now is compensated by federal support. Additionally, shortening the length of training would benefit medical students and trainees. With one less year of medical school they would have lower debts. The average medical student graduates today with $160,000 in debt.

Changing the structure of training might force medical leaders to eliminate unnecessary and repetitive material.

This shortening is already occurring. According to Emanuel and Fuchs, >30 medical schools now operate 6- or 7-year medical programs in which premedical training is reduced from the typical 4 years of college to 2 or 3 years. Most medical schools in the UK and Europe have 6 years of medical school training after graduation from high school.

Why is medical school 4 years in length? The answer probably has to do with the Flexner Report's recommendation in 1910 for 2 years of premedical science training followed by 2 years of clinical training. Yet, most physicians could be trained in significantly less time. Since 1997, the University of Pennsylvania has had only 1.5 years of preclinical science training. Duke University medical students focus on the basic sciences in the first year, complete core clerkships during the second year, and devote the third and fourth years to research and electives.

The important patient care skills can be obtained in <2 years of clinical training. Harvard Medical School requires students to complete only 15 months of clinical rotations. Eliminating one-half year of preclinical and one-half year of clinical training can be done without adversely affecting academic performance. Clinical training of 1.5 years still gives students sufficient exposure to a wide range of specialties. Texas Tech School of Medicine and two Canadian medical schools now offer 3-year medical school programs.

It is also possible to reduce residency training by 1 year. For internal medicine, pediatrics, and similar 3-year residencies, the third year is not essential to ensure competency. Many trainees already are permitted to short-track into subspecialty fellowships, reducing their residency from 3 to 2 years. Shortening training in an era of workweek limits will force hospitals to reengineer programs to ensure residents' clinical competence.

Many surgical training programs include a year of research. The most important factor, however, in becoming a competent surgeon is high volume—performing specific procedures multiple times. A research year, of course, does not add to surgical volume and usually does not improve surgical skills.

REDUCING HEALTH CARE COSTS

One way is to shift health care responsibility away from physicians and hospitals to each of us. Most of us know what good health habits are. The challenge is to do them so that we stay healthy. The top of the list in my view is *to maintain an ideal body weight*. Doing so tends to keep the blood pressure and blood glucose down so our chances of developing hypertension and diabetes mellitus decrease considerably. Exercise keeps us more mentally alert as well as providing us with more energy and pep. There is nothing better than good home scales: weighing every day and not letting those pounds accumulate. Learning to use a blood pressure cuff at home and recording the number is useful. Daily flossing of our teeth yields healthy gums and decreases dental expenses. The health care system in the USA is broken, and each of us needs to do our part to keep illness away.

MILK ALTERNATIVES

In recent times I have switched from skim milk to milk substitutes, including soy, almond, coconut, flax, or rice. Sales of these nondairy milk beverages reached $1.3 billion in 2011, a jump of more than 10% from 2009 (4). These milk substitutes have fewer calories, less fat, and less protein than whole milk. One cup of whole milk has approximately 150 calories, nearly 8 grams of fat, and 8 grams of protein. Soy milk, in contrast, has 90 calories, 3.5 grams of fat, and 6 grams of protein. Flax milk has no protein, and almond, rice, and coconut milk have only 1 gram. These milk substitutes last much longer in the refrigerator than regular milk. The alternative milks can be expensive, however, sometimes $5 to $6 for a gallon compared with about $3.50 for regular milk.

COFFEE DRINKING AND MORTALITY

Freedman and colleagues (5) from Rockville, Maryland, and Washington, DC, examined the association of coffee drinking with subsequent total and cause-specific mortality among 229,119 men and 173,141 women in the National Institutes of Health–AARP Diet and Health Study. All were 50 to 71 years of age at baseline. Participants with cancer, heart disease, and stroke were excluded. Coffee consumption was assessed once at baseline. During 5,148,760 person-years of follow up between 1995 and 2008, a total of 33,731 men and 18,784 women died. The risk of death was increased among coffee drinkers. Coffee drinkers, however, were also more likely to smoke, and after adjustment for tobacco-smoking status and other potential confounders, there was a significant inverse association between coffee consumption and mortality. Adjusted hazard ratios for death among men who drank coffee as compared with those who did not were as follows: 0.99 for drinking <1 cup per day, 0.94 for 1 cup, 0.90 for 2 or 3 cups, 0.88 for 4 or 5 cups, and 0.90 for ≥6 cups of coffee per day. The respective hazard ratios among women were 1.01, 0.95, 0.87, 0.84, and 0.85. Inverse associations were observed for deaths due to heart disease, respiratory disease, stroke, injuries and accidents, diabetes mellitus, and infections, but not for deaths due to cancer. Thus, coffee consumption was associated with less total and cause-specific mortality. Thank goodness!

SITTING TIME AND MORTALITY RISKS

Investigators from Sydney, Australia, examined questionnaire data in New South Wales from 220,497 individuals aged 45 or older. During 621,695 person-years of follow-up (mean follow-up 2.8 years), 5405 deaths were registered (6). All-cause mortality hazard ratios were 1.02, 1.15, and 1.40 for 4 to <8 hours, 8 to <11 hours, and ≥11 hours per day of sitting, respectively, compared with <4 hours per day adjusting for physical activity and other confounders. The association between sitting and all-cause mortality was consistent across the sexes, age groups, body mass index categories, and physical activity levels, and for healthy participants as well as participants with preexisting cardiovascular disease or diabetes mellitus. Thus, prolonged sitting is a risk factor for all-cause mortality, independent of physical activity! Get up and move.

SEVERE OBESITY

Severe obesity is usually defined as a body mass index ≥40 kg/m², or roughly 100 or more pounds overweight. In 2010, 6.6% of US adults, roughly 15.5 million people, had a body mass index ≥40 (7). Severe obesity is approximately 50% higher among women than men and is twice as high among blacks as Hispanics and whites. The percentage of severely obese under age 40 is similar to those who are over age 40 years. It is difficult to be healthy if one weighs too much.

HOSPITAL CALORIES

Mayor Michael Bloomberg, in my view, has done much for the health of New York City dwellers. His latest health campaign is aimed at banishing sugary and fatty foods from both public and private hospitals (8). In recent years the city's 15 public hospitals have cut calories in patients' meals and restricted the sale of sugary drinks and unhealthy snacks at vending machines. Now the city is tackling hospital cafeteria food, and the Healthy Hospital Food Initiative is expanding its reach to 16 private hospitals. The hospital cafeteria crackdown will ban deep fryers, make leafy green salads a mandatory option, and allow only healthy snacks to be stocked near the cafeteria entrance and at cash registers. At least half of all sandwiches and salads must be made or served with whole grains. Half-sized sandwich portions must be available for sale. Most hospitals have already overhauled their vending machines by allowing only two types of 12-oz high-calorie beverages at each vending machine, and most also have swapped out most baked goods for snacks such as granola bars and nuts. Mayor Bloomberg has a strong podium, and he is using it well.

SMOKING AND THE FEDERAL CIGARETTE TAX

The Federal Cigarette Tax jumped from $0.39 to $1.01 per pack on April 1, 2009, to finance expanded health care for children (9). The change has brought in more than $30 billion in new revenue. The tax increase lifted prices 22% overnight, more than all state and local tax hikes combined over the past 10 years when adjusted for inflation. Tobacco companies have raised their prices to make money off of fewer customers. Consumer spending on tobacco rose from $80 billion in 2008 to $98 billion in 2011 in inflation-adjusted dollars, even though the amount of tobacco purchased fell 11%. Higher taxes accounted for about half that spending increase. Today, taxes and fees make up 55% of Marlboro's retail price.

The tax hike helped restart a long-term decline in smoking that had stalled in recent years. The federal tax hike helped push tobacco use down 19% in 2011, the lowest level on record according to surveys from the Centers for Disease Control and Prevention. Overall, about 3 million fewer people smoked in 2011 than in 2009, despite a larger population. The tax is hardest on families who make <$50,000 a year, and this group accounts for two thirds of smokers. Teen smoking immediately fell about 12% when the tax hike took effect. Higher taxes, however, are not the only reason smoking has fallen dramatically among adults since the early 1980s and among teens since the mid 1990s. Health concerns,

smoke-free buildings, and marketing restrictions have played a role.

Even smokers who do not quit smoke less. In the 1990s, one of every 20 high school students smoked 10 or more cigarettes a day; today, one in 71 students smoke that much. The elderly and Hispanics cut smoking most dramatically, each down more than 15% from 2008 to 2011. More women than men have quit smoking. Least affected were middle-aged men, down just 1%. About 1 million adults on Medicaid quit smoking.

50TH ANNIVERSARY OF THE CORONARY CARE UNIT CONCEPT

In 1937, my father had an acute myocardial infarction (AMI) at age 57 and was hospitalized at Emory University Hospital for 1 month. He then was placed in bed at home for another 2 months. From months 4 through 6, his movements were limited to the house and its immediate environs, and then from months 7 to 12 he was able to get out into the community. His partners paid him for a full year while he was resting from the heart attack. In 1939, just 2 years later, Mallory and associates (10) from Boston, Massachusetts, asked the simple question: How long does it take to heal an AMI? They found that it takes 2 months to heal a large AMI and about 6 weeks to heal a small AMI. Thus, my father was out of work 10 months unnecessarily. In 1941, at age 61, he had a second AMI. As a cardiologist himself, he decided this time that he would stay home, and a few days later that is where he died.

When I interned in medicine at Boston City Hospital in 1958, the site where Mallory et al demonstrated the length of time it takes to heal an AMI, patients with AMI were placed in the general ward, and the mortality rate during the hospitalization was approximately 35%.

In a beautiful piece by Dr. W. Bruce Fye, cardiologist and renowned medical historian, the history of the coronary care unit (CCU) is beautifully presented (11). The concept of the CCU, as Fye writes, was first described in North America in an abstract in *Circulation* in October 1961 by Los Angeles cardiologist Morris Wilburne, who outlined a technology-inspired extension of the intensive care unit model that had been developed during the previous decade. There was a crucial difference, as Fye describes. The intensive care unit was a place to care for acutely ill patients with a broad range of surgical and medical problems. The CCU, in contrast, was conceived as a program of care that targeted a specific group of patients: those at risk of sudden death in the context of an AMI. Such patients were admitted to a special space staffed by nurses trained to use new electronic technologies for the rapid diagnosis and treatment of life-threatening arrhythmias and to perform cardiopulmonary resuscitation. On October 14, 1961, almost the same day that *Circulation* published Wilburne's abstract, *Lancet* published Desmond Julian's long article, "Treatment of cardiac arrest and acute myocardial ischemia and infarction" (12). Julian called closed-chest massage an "outstanding advance" and recommended combining it with artificial respiration and transthoracic defibrillation. In his beautiful article, Fye published Wilburne's abstract in full and described early CCUs developed in a number of US hospitals. The CCU rapidly decreased mortality rates during AMI, which are now about 5%. This is a gem of an article.

FREDERICK NOVY AND THE RAT VIRUS

Frederick Novy (1864–1957), a US physician, medical researcher, and influential microbiologist of the early 20th century, devised culture techniques to visualize anaerobic bacteria, parasites, and spirochetes (13). In 1909, he began investigating the cause of unexplained deaths in his laboratory rats. In 1918, the test tubes he had been using for these experiments vanished from his laboratory. His dream of finding a virus as the likely cause of the mysterious deaths of his rats apparently was lost. Novy retired in 1935. Thirty-three years later, in 1951, a box containing the test tubes was discovered by chance during clean up in preparation for a laboratory move. Novy's curiosity had not waned with time. Notified of the find and 16 years into his retirement, he returned to his laboratory at the age of 88 to continue the experiments he had begun >40 years earlier. He completed his investigations in 1953 and published his findings. A virus was indeed the unidentified organism that had swiftly killed his laboratory rats in 1909.

WARREN BUFFETT'S PHILANTHROPIC HERO

At the Forbes 400 Summit on Philanthropy, which was held at the iconic main branch of the New York Public Library, Warren Buffett, worth $50 billion, brought a well-worn hardcover copy of *I Remember*, the 1940 autobiography of Abraham Flexner (14). Buffett stated, "Abraham Flexner probably influenced philanthropy as much as any individual in the country . . . not in terms of the money he used but of what he brought to the game" (15).

Abraham Flexner from Louisville, Kentucky, first attracted public attention in 1908 for his book *The American College,* which condemned higher education for its reliance on lectures vs small classes and hands-on teaching. His prescient analysis attracted the attention of Andrew Carnegie, who was keen to reform medical schools. In 1910, The Carnegie Foundation published *The Flexner Report*, which for the first time set national standards for physician training. Within 2 years of publication of the report by Flexner, a nonphysician, 50% of the US medical schools had closed. Thus, Flexner drastically changed medical education. In 1930, Flexner, backed by Louis Bamberger, with Princeton's Institute for Advanced Study, recruited the likes of Albert Einstein and Jay Robert Oppenheimer.

Buffett indicated that Flexner had studied what both the people with the money do, and what the people who are implementing the ideas do with the money. Buffett indicated that Carnegie did not go out and visit all the medical schools himself. He got Flexner to do it. George Eastman wanted to start a great medical school in Rochester and didn't know how to do it. He called Flexner and said, "Tell me how to do it." Buffett said he believed in getting things done through other people. Buffett recalled a *New York Times* editorial about Flexner when Flexner died in 1959: "No other American of his time has contributed more to the welfare of this country and humanity in general." Buffett has set himself up for a similar epitaph.

DOCTOR VISITS

Americans reduced the number of times they visited physicians during the past 10 years, a time when the cost of health insurance, deductibles, and copays soared (16, 17). Among people aged 18 to 64, the average number of visits to physicians and hospitals decreased from 4.8 visits in 2001 to 3.9 in 2010, according to a Census Bureau report released in October 2012. The report also found that people reporting "poor," "fair," or "good" health were more likely to be uninsured than those reporting "excellent" or "very good" health. Insurance status is a very strong predictor of health. Nearly 39% of people living in poverty did not visit a medical provider in 2010. The percentage of the uninsured who received routine checkups decreased from 13.5% in 2001 to 11.7% in 2010. Most Americans consider themselves very healthy. Nearly 66% reported their health as "excellent" or "very good." An additional 24% said their health was "good." A slightly greater percentage of men reported excellent health than women (33.9% vs 31.6%). Just over 92% of the US population in 2011 did not spend a night in the hospital. Nearly 57% of the population took no prescription medicines in 2011. Age is strongly related to prescription medication use; 80% of older adults reported regular prescription use compared with 12.5% of children.

PATIENTS READING THEIR DOCTORS' NOTES

Delbanco and colleagues (18) from Boston, Massachusetts, evaluated the effect on physicians and patients of facilitating patient access to visit notes over secure Internet portals. Of 13,564 patients with visit notes available, 11,797 opened at least one note and nearly half of them completed a postintervention survey. Just over 80% reported that open notes helped them feel more in control of their care; about 70% of those taking medications reported increased medication adherence; about 30% had privacy concerns; about 5% reported that the notes caused confusion, worry, or offense; and about 30% reported sharing notes with others. The volume of electronic messages from patients to physicians did not change. After the intervention, few physicians reported longer visits or more time addressing patients' questions outside of visits with little effect on practice size. About 20% of the physicians reported changing documentation content, and about 10% reported taking more time writing notes. About 60% of patients believe they should be able to add comments to a physician's note. One of three patients believe they should be able to approve the notes' content, but about 90% of physicians did not agree. At the end of the experimental period, 99% of patients wanted open notes to continue, and no physician elected to stop.

TRANSPARENCY AND ACCOUNTABLITY IN MEDICINE

Dr. Marty Makary, a surgeon at The Johns Hopkins Hospital and lead developer of the surgical checklist adopted by the World Health Organization, is the author of *Unaccountable: What Hospitals Won't Tell You and How Transparency Can Revolutionize Healthcare,* published in September 2012. He summarized his points in a recent piece in the *Wall Street Journal* (19). He suggested five ways to make health care safer:

1. *Online dashboards.* He recommends that every hospital have an online informational "dashboard" that includes its rates of infection, readmission, surgical complications, and "never event" errors (mistakes that should never occur, like leaving a surgical sponge inside a patient). The dashboard also should list the hospital's annual volume for each type of surgery and patient satisfaction scores.

2. *Safety culture scores.* The people who work in hospitals know whether their institutions are safe or not. Makary, with a colleague at The Johns Hopkins Hospital, J. Byron Sexton, administered an anonymous survey of physicians, nurses, technicians, and other employees at 60 US hospitals. They found that one third of them believed that teamwork at their hospital was bad. They opined that care at hospitals where teamwork is poor is unsafe. The hospitals that had good teamwork had lower infection rates and better patient outcomes. Good teamwork meant safer care.

3. *Cameras.* Cameras, of course, are used frequently in health care, but usually no video is made. Reviewing tapes of cardiac catheterization procedures, arthroscopic surgery, and other procedures could be used for peer-based quality improvement. One physician investigator analyzed videotapes of colonoscopy procedures and after he announced that he was going to do so, the average length of the procedures increased by 50% and the quality scores increased by 30%. The physicians performed better when they knew someone was checking their work. The same sort of intervention has been used for hand washing. Some patients have requested copies of their procedure videos and were willing to pay for them. Patients are hungry for transparency.

4. *Open notes.* He suggests that patients be permitted to examine the notes taken by their physicians. Makary switched from taking notes in the presence of patients to dictating the notes in their presence. He found that patients would remember something while he was dictating that they had not mentioned earlier.

5. *No more gagging.* Although there are many signs that health care is moving toward increased transparency, there is also some movement backwards. Increasingly, patients checking in to see physicians are being asked to sign a gag order, promising never to say anything negative about their physician online or elsewhere. Additionally, victims of a medical mistake are being asked by hospital lawyers to never speak publicly about the injury, a condition of any settlement. These types of gag orders would be best banned. As he states, "They are utterly contrary to a patient's right to know and to the concept of learning from our errors."

Transparency can also help to restore the public's trust. Many Americans believe that medicine has become an increasingly secretive, even arrogant industry. With more transparency—and the accountability that it brings—we can address the cost crisis, deliver safer care, and improve how we are seen by the communities we serve.

ILLICIT DRUG USE AND PRESCRIPTION DRUG ABUSE

The Mental Health Services Administration interviewed 67,500 people aged 12 and older in 2011 and found that 22.5 million Americans, nearly 9% of the population, said they regularly used illicit drugs (such as marijuana, cocaine, hallucinogens, and inhalants) or abused prescription drugs (such as pain relievers, tranquilizers, stimulants, and sedatives) (20). In 2011, 6.1 million people in the US abused narcotic pain pills, tranquilizers, stimulants, and sedatives, down from 7 million in 2010. Pain pill abuse dropped from 2.1% of the population in 2009 to 1.7% in 2011. Still, the number of people addicted to pain relievers grew from 936,000 in 2002 to 1.4 million in 2011. About one third of the addicts were 18 to 25 years of age. While cocaine abuse has dropped from 2.4 million regular users in 2006 to 1.4 million in 2011, heroin abuse is rising, growing from 161,000 in 2007 to 281,000 in 2011. Marijuana remains the most commonly abused drug at all ages. Among youth, drinking alcohol and smoking cigarettes declined, but marijuana use has increased steadily since 2008. The study found that 12.4% of 8th and 10th graders had used marijuana in the previous month, the highest rate since 2003. Most states now operate prescription drug monitoring programs, which can identify physicians who prescribe excessive doses of the drugs and patients who seek multiple prescriptions from different physicians.

LANCE ARMSTRONG

Did he win those seven Tour de France jerseys or not? In Europe he passed 137 drug tests but in the US he was convicted (21, 22). Was he racing against other substance abuse users or were they clean and he was the only one impure? I suspect there were very few racers in the Tour de France who weren't on some kind of "dope." Could Lance Armstrong have won any, much less all seven of those races, without some kind of performance boost? I doubt it because all the others were doing the same thing. That does not mean that Lance Armstrong or any of the others were right. I hope the performance enhancers are out of his system and out of the systems of all racers in the Tour de France. He still came in first in seven Tour de France races. Whether first means he won or not is a question that remains. Armstrong beat cancer and founded a fine foundation. He was one of the most talented athletes in the world. Armstrong broke the rules of the "official" system by submitting to the operative system's rules. The how-it-really-works system of competitive cycling virtually required him to drug and to lie about it if he was to be a success. His competitors went down the same path. Not only should Armstrong bear the weight of responsibility for his actions, but the entire world of competitive cycling should not have looked the other way so often when cyclists have drugged.

OLDER DRIVERS

Today, nearly 34 million drivers in the USA are 65 years of age or older (23). By 2030, about 57 million, about one quarter of all licensed US drivers, will be ≥65 years of age. The oldest drivers have the highest rates of fatal crashes, often because they are too frail to survive their injuries. The *Figure* shows the frequency of fatal crashes per 100 million miles traveled by age group. Texas, 29 other states, and the District of Columbia

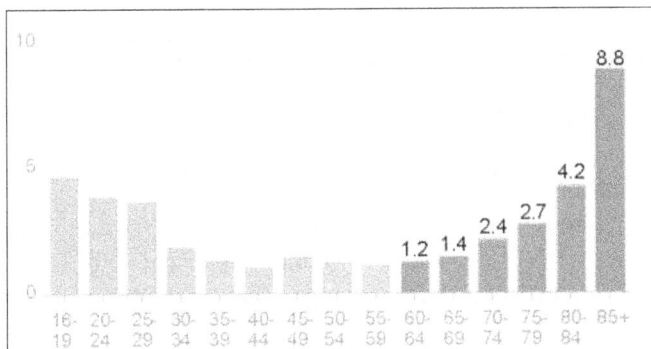

Figure. Fatal crashes per 100 million miles traveled, by age. The oldest drivers have the highest rate of deadly crashes, often because they are too frail to survive their injuries. Source: National Highway Traffic Safety Administration. Reprinted with permission from Associated Press.

have some special license requirements for older drivers, ranging from more vision testing to more frequent renewing of their licenses. Starting at age 79, Texas drivers must renew their license in person rather than by mail or online and get a vision test. Starting at age 85, drivers must renew their licenses every 2 years, instead of every 6. These requirements began in 2007, a result of "Katie's law," after a 2006 Dallas-area crash in which a 90-year-old driver ran a stoplight and killed a 17-year-old who was driving to school.

Some helpful hints: The University of Michigan developed an online self-test to help drivers detect safety changes: http://www.um-saferdriving.org. AAA and AARP offer websites with similar tools and links to driving courses: http://www.seniordriving.aaa.com and http://www.aarp.org/home-garden/transportation/driver_safety/.

ROAD KILLERS

The Federal Aid Highway Act of 1956 started the planet's largest public works: the 42,795-mile national system of interstate and defense highways. Ginger Strand, in a book entitled *Killer on the Road,* describes what happened as these highways came about (24). The expressways, the nation's first limited-access divided highways, produced the *highway killer,* variously known as the "Hitcher," the "Freeway Killer," the "Interstate Killer," the "Killer on the Road," the "I-5 Killer," and the "Beltway Sniper." Highways and violence quickly became intertwined. By the 1980s, when the interstate network was completed, highways were considered a dangerous place, not just because of accidents, but also because of hitchhiking, breakdowns, rest areas, truck stops, and aggressive drivers. The book by Strand provides brief biographies of some of these road killers. After graduating from college in 1954 from Southern Methodist University, I hitchhiked to Idaho to work in the forest service. That would be unwise to do today.

The highways were developed for several reasons. Eisenhower, president at the time, had seen Germany's autobahns during the war and wanted Americans to have the same thing. Ike was looking for a stimulus program. He and his economic advisors believed road building would be an effective way to "prime the pump" of the economy and avoid recession. The highway program was thus first and foremost an attempt to counter

recession. Defense was only added to the interstate network's name after the highway bill failed to be approved the first time it went to Congress. The highways thus became part of the Cold War drive to heighten the nation's civil defenses. The roads were designed to evacuate cities and move military troops and tanks. One mile in every five had to be straight so that airplanes could land on the interstate in a war emergency. The defense part, however, was mainly a myth. The main reason was economic stimulus. By the time the bill was passed, defense was so far from anyone's mind that no one even thought to ask the military to weigh in on highway standards. Highways fostered mobility and mobility represented prosperity, connection, growth. It meant growth for the economy, and the nation needed to grow its auto industry. Since one in every 7 workers in the USA directly or indirectly built or serviced the automobile, the roads were built in a way to induce Americans to buy cars.

Teenagers across the country saw cars as a route to everything good: adulthood, self-determination, achievement, sex. Almost as soon as they were invented, cars became a key element in the American dream and the open road soon joined it. Selling more cars meant manufacturing more cars; manufacturing more cars meant creating more jobs; creating more jobs meant more people to buy more cars—and on and on it went. Although it was sold to the public as a program for jobs and civil defense, the interstate highway program was driven by the principle of growth, the last of the big New Deal programs.

The large-scale economic effect of highway building was to drive up inflation and intensify economic upswings and downswings—exactly the opposite of what Ike had hoped. The highway bill would do little for the real economic losers.

PLAY

My mother was not particularly good at it. She worked all the time. Although I have met and befriended masters of play, I'm not particularly good at it either. Stuart Brown, a 79-year-old physician in California, and Christopher Vaughan have written a book entitled *Play: How it Shapes the Brain, Opens the Imagination, and Invigorates the Soul* (25). They share case studies that show how incorporating play—whatever it is people love to do—makes them better at everything, from work to relationships.

TATTOOS

According to a piece by Kim Painter in *USA Today,* 23% of women and 19% of men in the USA have one or more tattoos (26). According to a Harris Poll, most people like their tattoos but at least 15% regret they have them. Bencini and colleagues (27) in Milan and Bergamo, Italy, treated 352 people from 1995 to 2010 and described factors that make some tattoos harder to remove than others. The physicians used repeated laser treatments spaced several weeks apart. The devices used, called Q-switched lasers, removed tattoos from 47% of patients in 10 sessions and from nearly 75% in 15 sessions. (In the US, a laser session costs $200 to $600.) Tattoos were harder to remove if they were >12 inches in diameter, had colors other than black or red, had been in place for >3 years old, were on feet or legs, and were on smokers. Smoking apparently impairs the natural healing procedures that help clear ink after treatment.

RESILIENCE

It is of course the ability to bounce or spring back, the ability to recover strength, spirits, good humor, etc., quickly, and buoyancy. Jane McGonigal, the inventor of the game SuperBetter and the author of *Reality is Broken: Why Games Make Us Better and How They Can Change the World,* recently had a piece in the *Dallas Morning News* entitled "The Productive Value of Wasting Time" (28). Worldwide we spend 7 billion hours a week playing video games and 300 million minutes a day on Angry Birds. She suggests that engaging in some activities we assume to be nonproductive—as tiny exercises—may actually be a smart way to spend time, especially at work. These practices, she spins, can make people more resourceful problem solvers, more collaborative, and less likely to give up when the going gets tough. In other words, they make people more resilient. Her personal goal is to waste at least 4 minutes every hour.

There are four aspects to the ability to snap back and go on after a hit—physical, mental, emotional, and social—and each can be developed with activities that appear to fritter away time. *Physical resilience,* she writes, is crucial because it allows our heart, lungs, and brain to react efficiently to stressful situations. A sedentary lifestyle is the number one obstacle to being able to endure and bounce back. Willpower gets stronger the more we exercise it. Tackling pointless but mildly challenging tasks, such as snapping one's fingers exactly 50 times or counting backward from 100 by sevens, she states, is a scientifically backed way to improve focus and determination and thus *mental resilience. Emotional resilience* has to do with being less afraid of failure and more open to using different strategies. We should try to experience, on average, three positive emotions for every one negative emotion over the course of a day. And *social resilience* is about the relationships that help us find resources when we need them. Gratitude and touch help us develop habits that connect us to others. Greater resilience, she emphasizes, will make us more capable.

ALGORITHMS

Christopher Steiner, a former reporter for *Forbes* magazine and currently an Internet entrepreneur, writes that the first known algorithm dates back to 2500 BC and was found on clay tablets near Baghdad. It recorded Sumerian instructions for how to equally divide grain harvests between varying numbers of men. In his book, *Automate This: How Algorithms Came to Rule Our World,* the 10 chapters explore different sorts of contemporary algorithms and their uses, from their embrace by record labels to their potential to transform health care (29). Algorithmic trading, whereby traders recede into the background and leave it to the algorithms to identify and act on arbitrage opportunities, has taken over Wall Street in the past 3 decades. But Wall Street is not the driving force behind the culture-wide algorithmic fetish. Steiner has qualms with the proliferation of algorithmic decision-making. Although he believes that we

need to accept our algorithmic overlords, before doing so we should vigorously and transparently debate the rules they will impose. The real question isn't whether to live with algorithms, but how to live with them.

LIVING ALONE

About 32 million Americans live by themselves, comprising about 28% of the nation's 115 million households (30). The 7.9 million women aged ≥65 years who live alone make up almost half of all women living solo; about 3.3 million men ≥65 years live alone. In 1960, only 13% of US households had only one occupant; by 2011, 28% of US households had a single occupant, including 10% of those ≥65.

DIMINISHING INCOME

In January 2009, the median household income in the USA was nearly $55,000 (31). By June 2012, it had fallen to $51,000, adjusted for inflation. That's $4019 in lost real income, nearly a month's income every year. The real median household income in 2000 in the USA was $55,500. Some of the decline is due to smaller family size, lower fertility rates, and more Americans living alone. But some was also due to the subpar economic growth across the 2000s. Real income for middle-income households rose by roughly 30% from 1983 to 2005, according to the Congressional Budget Office.

So what explains the falling real incomes? Slow growth is certainly one explanation, but another culprit has been rising prices, especially for food, gasoline, medical procedures, and college tuition. Rising health care costs have also forced employers to take money that used to go into higher wages to pay higher premiums. During the last nearly 4 years, black Americans have had real income fall by more than 11%. Every age group except the elderly has seen a decline in income. Those aged 65 to 75 saw an average 6.5% gain in income, though most were not working and collected Medicare and Social Security. The last time incomes fell this fast was during the late 1970s.

ONLINE MANNERS

Elizabeth Bernstein (32), writing in the *Wall Street Journal,* recently asked, "Why are we so nasty to each other online? Whether on Facebook, Twitter, message boards or websites, we say things to each other that we would never say face-to-face." Bernstein suggests that anonymity is a powerful force. "Hiding behind a fake screen name makes us feel invincible, as well as invisible." But there is no anonymity on Facebook. She argues that even when we reveal our real identities we still misbehave online. Some have argued that browsing Facebook lowers our self-control. She goes on to write that "most of us present an enhanced image of ourselves on Facebook. This positive image—and the encouragement we get . . . boost our self-esteem. And when we have an inflated sense of self we tend to exhibit poor self-control."

FEMALES OVERTAKING MALES

The following observations are from a recent editorial by David Brooks (33). In elementary and high school, male academic performance is lagging. Boys earn three quarters of the D's and F's. By college, men are clearly behind. Only 40% of bachelor's degrees and master's degrees go to men. Because of their lower skills, men are dropping out of the labor force. In 1954, 96% of American men between ages 25 and 54 worked; today, that number is 80%, an all-time low participation of the male labor force. Millions of men are collecting disability. Even many of those who do have a job are doing poorly. Annual earnings for prime-aged men have dropped 28% over the past 40 years. Men still dominate at the top of the corporate ladder, probably because many women take time off to raise children, but women lead or are gaining nearly everywhere else. Women in their 20s outearn men in their 20s, and 12 of the 15 fastest-growing professions are dominated by women.

To succeed today, one has to be able to sit still and focus in school at an early age, to be emotionally sensitive and aware of context, and to communicate smoothly. For genetic and cultural reasons, many men do poorly at these tasks.

David Brooks took his information from the new book, *The End of Men* by Hanna Rosin. Rosin's view is a bit different from Brooks'. And it has to do with adaptability. Women, Rosin argues, are like immigrants who have moved to a new country. They see a new social context and they flexibly adapt to new circumstances. Men are like immigrants who have physically moved to a new country but who have kept their minds in the old country. They speak the old language, follow the old mores, and are more likely to be rigid; women are more fluid. This theory has less to do with innate traits and more to do with social position. When there is a big social change, the people who are on the top of the old order are bound to cling to the old ways. The people who are on the bottom are bound to experience a burst of energy. Rosin in essence says that women are adapting to today's economy more flexibly and resiliently than men.

A study by the National Federation of Independent Businesses found that small businesses owned by women outperformed male-owned small businesses as during the last recession. In finance, women who switched firms were more likely to see their performance improve, whereas men were more likely to see theirs decline. There is also evidence that women are better able to adjust to divorce. Today, more women than men see their incomes rise by 25% after a marital breakup. Four years ago men and women adhered to certain ideologies, what it meant to be a man or a woman. Young women today, Rosin argues, are more like clean slates, having abandoned both feminist and prefeminist preconceptions. Men still adhere to the masculinity rules, which limit their vision and their movement.

BIRTHS IN WOMEN IN THEIR TEENS AND TWENTIES

The number of US births has been falling since 2007, when it peaked at 4.3 million, just before the worst economic downturn since the 1930s (34). The 2011 data from the National Center for Health Statistics show that the number of births to girls aged 15 to 19 years dropped 20% to just fewer than 330,000, the lowest since 1946. Teen birth rates fell 8% to 31 per 100,000, the lowest recorded since 1940. The rate has fallen more than 3% a year since 1991. The number of births to women aged 20 to 24 declined 3%, and the birth rate dropped 5% to 85 per 1000, the lowest ever recorded in the USA. For ages 25 to 29, the birth rate of 107 per 1000 women was the lowest since 1976. Although the recession may have led women in their 20s to postpone starting a family, the economy usually does not affect teens, whose births are largely unintended and unplanned. Good news!

BALDNESS

According to a piece in *The Wall Street Journal,* men with shaved heads are perceived to be more masculine, dominant, and, in some cases, to have greater leadership potential than those with longer locks or those with thinning hair, according to a recent study from the University of Pennsylvania Wharton School (35). That finding may explain why the "buzz look" has caught on among business leaders in recent years. Some executives say the style makes them appear younger or at least makes their age less evident and gives them more confidence than a comb-over or monk-like pate.

The study was carried out by Albert Mannes, who tested people's perception of men with shaved heads. In one experiment he showed photos of 344 men in two versions: one showing the man with hair and the other showing him with his hair digitally removed so his head appeared shaved. The subjects reported finding the men with shaved heads more dominant than their hirsute counterparts. Men with shorn heads were even perceived as an inch taller and about 13% stronger than those with fuller manes. The study found that men with thinning hair were viewed as the least attractive and least powerful of the bunch, a finding that tracks with other studies showing that people perceive men with typical male-pattern baldness, which affects roughly 35 million Americans, as older and less attractive. Dr. Mannes indicated that he was inspired to conduct the research after noticing that people treated him differently when he shaved off his own thinning hair.

The look is catching on. A 2010 study from razor maker Gillette found that 13% of respondents said they shave their heads, citing reasons as varied as fashion, sports, and already thinning hair. Another investigator at the University of Louisville indicates that a bare scalp "is nature's way of telling the rest of the world that you are a survivor." He adds that the deliberate shaved head look conveys aggressiveness and competitiveness and shows a "willingness to stand against social norms."

Other features that signal dominance include narrow eyes and lips and broad faces and square jaws. For women, the equation is trickier. Dominant features may be less helpful at work than youthful, feminine features, which are deemed more attractive.

POPULATION REPRESENTED BY EACH MEMBER OF THE HOUSE OF REPRESENTATIVES

The House of Representatives consists of 435 members, and each represents an average of 711,000 persons (36). In 1839, the House included 242 members. After the 1910 Census, with the population just over 92 million, the number of House members was increased to 435 from 394, with the average district then including just over 210,000 people. In 1929, Congress permanently fixed the number of representatives at 435, where it remains today, even though our population is now 315 million persons. Each representative today has over 710,000 constituents. By comparison, many other countries with representative governments have larger representative bodies with more favorable ratios: the United Kingdom has 62 million people and 650 members of Parliament, one for every 95,000 residents; Japan's 127 million people elect 480 representatives, one for every 264,000; France's National Assembly has 577 members, each representing 118,000 people. Since 1998, the reelection rate for US House incumbents has been nearly 95%.

WILLIAM CLIFFORD ROBERTS, MD
31 October 2012

1. Wasik B, Murphy M. *Rabid: A Cultural History of the World's Most Diabolical Virus.* New York: Penguin Group, 2012 (275 pp.).
2. Devi S. US drug shortages could continue for years. *Lancet* 2012;379 (9820):990–991.
3. Emanuel EJ, Fuchs VR. Shortening medical training by 30%. *JAMA* 2012;307(11):1143–1144.
4. Kinosian J. Udder chaos. *AARP The Magazine*, August/September 2012.
5. Freedman ND, Park Y, Abnet CC, Hollenbeck AR, Sinha R. Association of coffee drinking with total and cause-specific mortality. *N Engl J Med* 2012;366(20):1891–1904.
6. van der Ploeg HP, Chey T, Korda RJ, Banks E, Bauman A. Sitting time and all-cause mortality risk in 222 497 Australian adults. *Arch Intern Med* 2012;172(6):494–500.
7. Hellmich N. Percentage of severely obese adults skyrockets. *USA Today*, October 2, 2012.
8. Barr M, Dobnik V. Hospital snacks are new target in NYC. *Dallas Morning News,* September 25, 2012.
9. Cauchon D. Big tax increase reduces smoking. *USA Today*, September 11, 2012.
10. Mallory GK, White PD, Salcedo-Salgar J. The speed of healing of myocardial infarction. A study of the pathologic anatomy in seventy-two cases. *Am Heart J* 1939;18:647–671.
11. Fye WB. Resuscitating a *Circulation* abstract to celebrate the 50th anniversary of the coronary care unit concept. *Circulation* 2011;124(17):1886–1893.
12. Julian DG. Treatment of cardiac arrest in acute myocardial ischaemia and infarction. *Lancet* 1961;2(7207):840–844.
13. Kazanjian P. Lifelong curiosity: Frederick Novy and the rat virus. *Ann Intern Med* 2012;156(3):234–237.
14. Flexner A. *I Remember: the Autobiography of Abraham Flexner.* New York: Simon and Schuster, 1940 (414 pp.).
15. Lane R. Warren Buffett's philanthropic hero. *Forbes*, October 8, 2012.
16. Lloyd J. Doctor's visits down; are we healthier or cutting costs? *USA Today*, October 2, 2012.
17. Tavernise S. Working-age Americans going to doctor less often. *Dallas Morning News*, October 2, 2012.
18. Delbanco T, Walker J, Bell SK, Darer JD, Elmore JG, Farag N, Feldman HJ, Mejilla R, Ngo L, Ralston JD, Ross SE, Trivedi N, Vodicka E, Leveille SG. Inviting patients to read their doctors' notes: a quasi-experimental study and a look ahead. *Ann Intern Med* 2012;157(7):461–470.
19. Makary M. How to stop hospitals from killing us. *Wall Street Journal*, September 22–23, 2012.
20. Leinwand Leger D. Painkiller abuse declines in 2011. *USA Today*, September 25, 2012.
21. Minora L, Townsend B. His cause still lives strong. *Dallas Morning News*, October 21, 2012.
22. Rigby C. How are we to view Lance Armstrong? *Dallas Morning News*, October 21, 2012.
23. Neergaard L. States' rules for older drivers all over the map, reflect safety fears. *Dallas Morning News*, September 18, 2012.
24. Strand G. *Killer on the Road: Violence and the American Interstate.* Austin, TX: University of Texas Press, 2012 (252 pp.).
25. Brown S, Vaughan C. *Play: How it Shapes the Brain, Opens the Imagination, and Invigorates the Soul.* New York: Penguin Group, 2009 (240 pp.).
26. Painter K. Can you lose that tattoo? Maybe. *USA Today*, September 20, 2012.
27. Bencini PL, Cazzaniga S, Tourlaki A, Galimberti MG, Naldi L. Removal of tattoos by Q-switched laser: variables influencing outcome and sequelae in a large cohort of treated patients. *Arch Dermatol* 2012 Sep 17 [Epub ahead of print].
28. McGonigal J. The productive value of wasting time. *Dallas Morning News*, October 20, 2012.
29. Steiner C. *Automate This: How Algorithms Came to Rule Our World.* New York: Portfolio Penguin, 2012 (256 pp.).
30. El Nasser H, Overberg P. In USA, more choose to live alone. *USA Today*, October 11, 2012.
31. Tavernise S. Rich got richer, poor stayed the same in 2011. *Dallas Morning News*, September 13, 2012.
32. Bernstein E. Why we are so rude online. *Wall Street Journal*, October 2, 2012.
33. Brooks D. Men in decline. *Dallas Morning News*, September 12, 2012.
34. Jayson S. Births in teens, 20s hit new lows. *USA Today*, October 3, 2012.
35. Silverman RE. Bald is powerful. *Wall Street Journal*, October 3, 2012.
36. Watkins WJ. Who cares about Congress? *USA Today*, October 11, 2012.

Chapter 10

April 2013

US HEALTH

An expert panel appointed by the US Institute of Medicine reported their findings in January 2013 (1, 2). We in the US live shorter lives than any of 16 peer nations, including Australia, Canada, Japan, and 13 European countries *(Figure 1)*. Swiss men live nearly 4 years longer than American men, and Japanese women live >5 years longer than American women. Americans get their health care in a less coordinated system than in any of the 16 other nations, and we in the US pay more for it. The cost of care in the US in 2011 was $2.7 trillion, or $8680 for each American. The closest among the other 16 nations was Switzerland, which spent $5489 per person. Americans are more reckless than those in the other 16 countries. Only Italians wear seatbelts less often. Nowhere else do motorcyclists go without helmets as often. Americans die more often in traffic accidents linked to alcohol consumption, and they own far more guns (89 per 100 people compared with 46 per 100 people in Switzerland, the peer group country with the next highest rate of gun ownership).

Far fewer Americans than in the past use tobacco, and only the Swedes now smoke fewer cigarettes than Americans. This is a reversal of the situation in the 1950s, when Americans smoked the most. Nevertheless, in 2003, smoking accounted for 1 in 5 deaths among Americans >50 years of age. But, smoking-related deaths are expected to decline further in the USA with the drop in the number of smokers and the rise in countries like France, where 46% of adults smoke.

The panel pointed out, of course, that what we eat is a major factor in the lower US lifespan. Americans eat, on average, 3770 calories a day. That's 1100 more calories than the average adult male needs, and 1700 more calories than an average woman should consume. Between 1999 and 2001, Austrians, Belgians, and Italians ate more but, by 2007, Americans were well ahead of anyone else. The average Swede consumes 17% fewer calories daily than the average American.

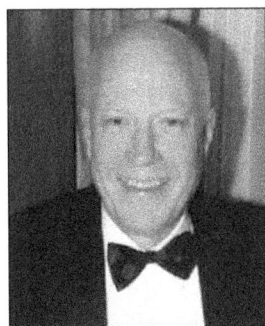

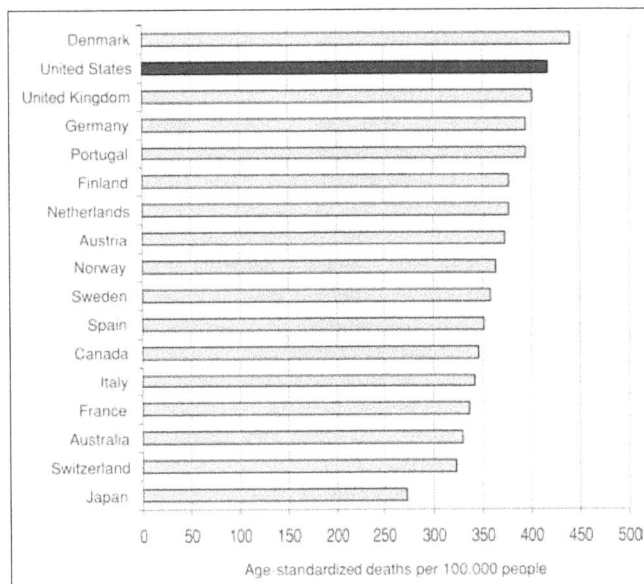

William C. Roberts, MD.

Figure 1. Mortality from noncommunicable diseases in 17 peer countries, 2008. Reprinted with permission from National Academies Press.

GLOBAL OBESITY

Overweight and obese people now outnumber the malnourished by nearly 2 to 1. According to the World Health Organization (WHO), in 2010, 80% of American adult men and 77% of women were overweight (3). Obesity costs at least $150 billion a year in American health care spending. But obesity is spreading rapidly in other parts of the world. Saudi Arabia and other Arab states and many Pacific Island nations are fatter than in the USA. Most of the adult population of Samoa is obese; in 2008, 46% of Egyptian women were obese. Mexican women are heavier than US women, and Mexican men will soon eclipse US men in poundage. These changes in part reflect advances in public health. In 1900, pneumonia, tuberculosis, and childhood diarrhea were the leading killers of Americans. Now, the top causes of death are noninfectious diseases, mainly atherosclerosis, hypertension, and cancer. In 2008, 63% of deaths around the world were caused by noncommunicable diseases and 80% of them occurred in low- and middle-income countries.

Many countries are trying to come to grips with this major shift in public health. Japanese companies require employees to undergo annual physicals that include waistline measurements.

Measurements of over 33.5 inches in men and over 35.4 inches in women count against the company. If too many fail the test, the firm has to increase its contribution to public health care for the elderly. Several countries tax soft drinks and other sugared beverages. Mexican legislators introduced a bill in December 2012 that would add a 20% tax to the cost of such drinks. In 2011, the average Mexican adult consumed 728 servings of Coca-Cola; the average American, 403 servings. The China Health Ministry has asked Dr. Kenneth Cooper of Dallas, founder and chairman of Cooper Aerobics, to explore the introduction of Fitness Gram Testing among its schoolchildren. Cooper indicated that Ross Perot contributed $2 million to help pay for a computer system to aggregate the results. Ten years ago there was hardly any obesity in China, according to Cooper. WHO estimates that 45% of Chinese men and 32% of Chinese women are now overweight or obese. The fast-food chains are rapidly expanding in China. Yum Brands, which owns Pizza Hut, KFC, and Taco Bell restaurants, has 38,000 restaurants globally, including 740 Pizza Huts and 4,043 KFC establishments in China.

Business groups complain that taxes, regulations, and unfair trade practices hurt their international competitiveness. Now, we can add body weight to that list. The Organization for Economic Cooperation and Development (OECD) in 2012 updated an obesity epidemic watch among its 34 country members (usually described as the wealthier developed countries) and found that the average rate of obesity across the OECD was 17% (4); in the USA, 34%; in Korea, 4%; in Germany, nearly 15%; in the UK, 23%; and in Mexico, 30%. In 19 of the 34 OECD countries, most of the population is now either obese or overweight. In the US and in Texas, more than two thirds of the population is either obese or overweight (*Figure 2*). Texas comptroller Susan Combs has estimated that obesity costs Texas employers nearly $10 billion in 2009.

BODY WEIGHT AND LEADERSHIP ABILITY

New research suggests that extra pounds or enlarged waistlines affect an executive's perceived leadership ability as well as stamina on the job (5). Leadership experts and executive recruiters say that staying trim is now virtually required for anyone on track for the CEO corner office. Executives with larger waistlines and higher body mass indexes tend to be perceived as less effective both in performance and interpersonal relationships. While weight remains a taboo conversation topic in the workplace, heavy executives are judged to be less capable because of assumptions about how weight affects health and stamina. A business school professor recently stated that he could not name a single overweight Fortune 500 CEO.

SODA CONSUMPTION

In the USA, soda consumption is declining (6). Per capita consumption of carbonated soft drinks in 2005 was over 50 gallons, and by 2012, 42 gallons. Soda companies raised prices in 2011 and again in 2012 and volumes kept falling. The sugary bubbles are simply unhealthy. Sodas' traditional target market, namely youth, is often now turning to water, energy drinks, and coffee instead. This of course is good news unless you happen to be an investor in Coca-Cola, PepsiCo, or Dr. Pepper/Snapple, which I avoid.

US MILK CONSUMPTION

In 1975, the US milk consumption per capita was 28.6 gallons and by 2011 it had fallen to 20.2 gallons (7). This decline is good news. Cows are the biggest source of our cholesterol, including their muscle, milk, butter, and cheese, and also our biggest source of saturated fat.

RELATION OF PHYSICAL ACTIVITY AND SEDENTARY BEHAVIOR TO SERUM PROSTATE-SPECIFIC ANTIGEN

A recent piece in the *Mayo Clinic Proceedings* (8) involving 1672 men found that for every 1-hour increase in sedentary behavior, the participants were 16% more likely to have an elevated prostate-specific antigen (PSA) concentration, and for every 1-hour increase in light physical activity, participants were 18% less likely to have an elevated PSA concentration. We men sit on our prostate gland. Get up and keep moving.

FASTING VS NONFASTING MEASUREMENTS OF BLOOD LIPIDS

Current guidelines recommend that total lipids and lipid subclass levels be measured with a patient in a fasting state

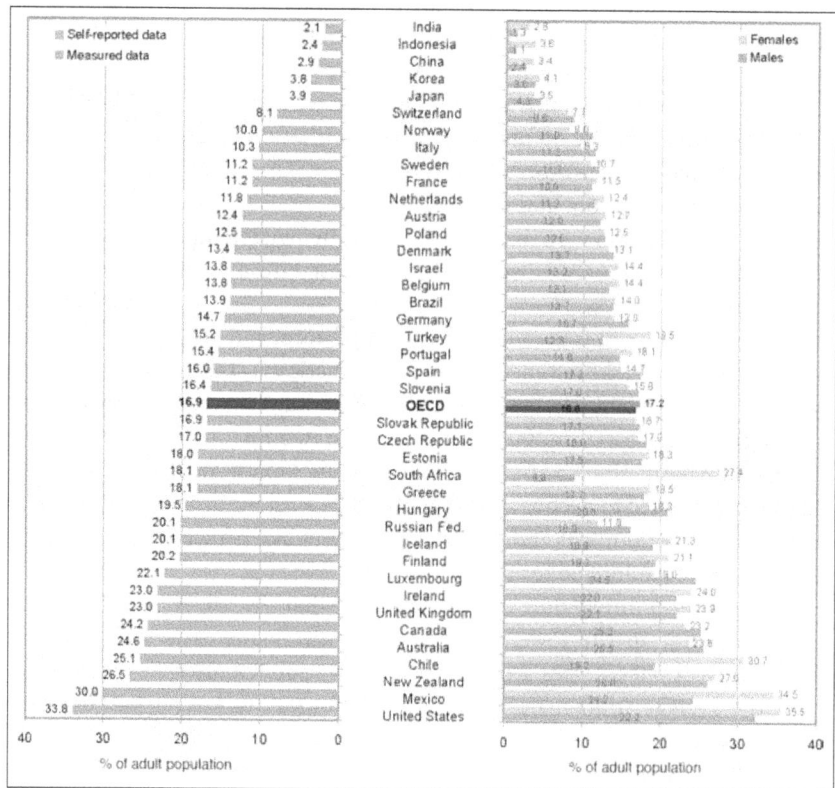

Figure 2. Prevalence of obesity among adults, 2009 (or nearest year). Reprinted with permission from OECD (2011), "Overweight and obesity among adults," in *Health at a Glance 2011: OECD Indicators*, OECD Publishing. http://dx.doi.org/10.1787/health_glance-2011-18-en

(>8 hours after the last meal). Fasting recommendations were originally introduced to decrease variability and achieve consistency in the metabolic states of patients at the time of sample collection. Several studies, however, suggest that measurement of lipid subclasses in a nonfasting state is an acceptable alternative, with some nonfasting markers being better at predicting the risk of cardiac events. Sidhu and Naugler (9) measured various lipid levels with fasting intervals varying from 1 to >16 hours in 209,180 individuals. The mean levels of total cholesterol and high-density lipoprotein cholesterol differed little among individuals with various fasting times. The mean calculated low-density lipoprotein cholesterol levels showed up to 10% variation among groups of patients with differing fasting intervals. The mean triglyceride levels showed variations of up to 20%.

MORE ON TATTOOS

Tattoos have become increasingly popular in recent years. In the USA, in 2012, an estimated 21% of adults had tattoos, up from 14% in 2008. The process of tattooing exposes the recipient to risks of infections, some of which are serious and difficult to treat. Historically, as LeBlanc and colleagues (10) emphasize, the control of tattoo-associated dermatologic infections has focused on ensuring safe tattooing practices and preventing contamination of ink used in the tattoo parlors—a regulatory task overseen by state and local authorities. In 2012, several outbreaks of nontuberculous microbacterial infections associated with contaminated tattoo ink raised questions about the adequacy of prevention efforts implemented at the tattoo-parlor level. The Food and Drug Administration (FDA) began reaching out to health care providers, public health officials, consumers, and the tattoo industry to develop more effective measures for tattoo ink-related public health problems. Some reports of tattoo-related nontuberculous microbacterial infections suggested that tap water or distilled water used to dilute inks at tattoo parlors was a likely source of contamination. Findings from more recent outbreaks suggested that the inks were contaminated before distribution.

Under the Federal Food, Drug, and Cosmetic Act, tattoo inks are considered to be cosmetics, whereas the pigments used in the inks are color additives that require premarketing approval. This law requires that cosmetics and their ingredients not be adulterated or misbranded, which means, among other things, that they cannot contain poisonous or deleterious substances or unproved color additives, be manufactured or held in unsanitary conditions, or be falsely labeled. Furthermore, cosmetic manufacturers are supposed to ensure the safety of a product before marketing it. But, the FDA does not have the authority to require premarketing submission of safety data from manufacturers, distributors, or marketers of cosmetic products, with the exception of most color additives (dyes, pigments, or other substances used to impart color). The FDA, however, can conduct investigations, request that a manufacturer recall volatile products, issue advisory letters, and request that the Department of Justice conduct seizures, enjoin a firm or person from manufacturing or distributing products, or file criminal charges against a firm or responsible persons on behalf of the FDA.

It is particularly important to increase awareness about certain types of tattoo ink–related infections because of several features of nontuberculous microbacteria. They may be difficult to diagnose and treat. It can take up to 6 weeks to identify the organism. A special culture medium and a skin biopsy may be required. Antibiotic choices are limited by the susceptibility profile of the organism, and prolonged treatment may be necessary to clear the infection. Moreover, complications such as co-infections with pathogens such as methicillin-resistant *Staphylococcus aureus* may pose additional challenges. Beware of tattoos.

RENAL SYMPATHETIC DENERVATION FOR DRUG-RESISTANT HYPERTENSION

Esler and colleagues (11) for the Symplicity HTN-2 investigators indicate that among the 7 billion people residing on Planet Earth, nearly 1 billion adults have high blood pressure. Despite the availability of numerous effective antihypertensive medicines, hypertension remains uncontrolled for various reasons, including inadequate treatment. Among hypertensive patients receiving treatment, the estimated proportion of patients with blood pressure uncontrolled (>140/90 mm Hg) ranges from 45% to 85% in Europe and North America. Furthermore, a subset of patients who adhere to a prescribed pharmaceutical regimen of ≥3 drugs, including a diuretic, continue to have uncontrolled or resistant hypertension. In the US, estimates of resistant hypertension prevalence range from 10% to 30% of adults receiving drug treatment for hypertension. These numbers reflect a serious health challenge because every 20/10 mm Hg increase in blood pressure leads to a doubling of cardiovascular mortality.

The sympathetic nervous system plays an important role in hypertension. Catheterization-based renal denervation is a minimally invasive procedure involving the application of radiofrequency energy in short bursts along the length of the main renal arteries to ablate the renal nerves that lie within and just beyond the artery's adventitia.

The Symplicity HTN-2 trial randomized patients with resistant hypertension to either renal denervation or to no renal denervation, with both groups maintained for 6 months on antihypertensive medications. The primary endpoint, change in office-based systolic blood pressure at 6-month follow-up, demonstrated a significant difference in systolic blood pressure between the treatment and control groups. Patients in the control group then had the option to receive the renal denervation procedure. The 1-year results of this second trial, which included 6-month outcomes for the control group who were treated with renal denervation, resulted in a significant drop in blood pressure similar to that observed in patients receiving immediate denervation. Thus, renal denervation appears to provide a safe and sustained reduction of blood pressure to 1 year in patients with previous resistant hypertension.

WHY PATIENTS VISIT DOCTORS

St. Sauver and colleagues (12) from the Mayo Clinic analyzed medical records of 142,377 patients in the county in which the Mayo Clinic is located to learn of the various conditions that prompted patients to visit their physicians during a 5-year period (2005–2009). Fifty-three percent of the patients were female. The 20 most common conditions among these individuals were as follows: skin disorders, 43%; osteoarthritis and joint disorders, 34%; back problems, 24%; disorders of lipid metabolism, 22%; upper respiratory disease (excluding asthma), 22%; anxiety, depression, and bipolar disorders, 20%; chronic neurologic disorders, 20%; hypertension, 18%; headaches, including migraine, 14%; diabetes mellitus, 14%; arrhythmias, 13%; esophageal disorders, 10%; asthma, 9%; thyroid disorders, 9%; iron deficiency and other anemia, 9%; bowel disorders, 9%; cancer, 8%; biliary and liver disorders, 8%; obstructive pulmonary disorders, 8%; and coronary heart disease, 8%. Ten of the 15 most prevalent disease groups were more common in women in almost all age groups, whereas disorders of lipid metabolism, hypertension, and diabetes were more common in men. The prevalence of 7 of the 10 most common groups increased with advancing age. Prevalence also varied across ethnic groups (whites, blacks, and Asians).

BEDBUGS AND SNIFFING DOGS

Canines trained to detect bedbugs did big business in Dallas during the summer of 2012 (13), and that infestation may be back this summer. Bedbugs are resilient and can travel on everything. As someone said, "It's basically a hitchhiker. It goes on suitcases and people spread it to other people. And once they make their way into a home, getting rid of them can cost several thousand dollars." Apparently there is a pheromone in the bedbugs that dogs can smell. Dogs are about 97% accurate in finding the bugs, while humans are only about 30% accurate.

GRAPHOLOGY

I have kept a visitor's book in my office for years and request a signature and address from all those willing to provide it. A number of years ago, while visiting The Greenbrier in West Virginia, I took a class on graphology. The teacher talked about letters leaning to the left or right, whether or not the long letters touched the top line or the lower letters went below the lower line, and whether or not there were lively movements in the top one and flamboyant swirls in the lower ones and what they meant. She recommended that potential spouses before marriage have a couple of paragraphs of their handwriting analyzed by a graphologist.

Sherlock Holmes asked Dr. Watson in *The Sign of Four,* "What do you make of this fellow's scribble?" (14). "Look at his long letters," he said. "They hardly arise above the common herd. That *d* might be an *a*, and that *l* an *e*. Men of character always differentiate their long letters, however illegibly they may write. There is vacillation in his *k*'s and self-esteem in his capitals."

THE LEAST HEART-HEALTHY STATE IN THE USA

The official state meal of Oklahoma—designated by the legislature in 1988—includes barbecue pork, chicken-fried steak, sausage, biscuit and gravy, fried okra and squash, strawberries, black-eyed peas, grits, corn, cornbread, and pecan pie. A survey by the Centers for Disease Control and Prevention (CDC), published in 2012, indicates that only 1% of adults in Oklahoma are free from risk factors for or behaviors increasing the risk for heart disease—the highest rate for any state in the nation (15). Oklahomans also are less likely to report eating 5 or more servings of fruits and vegetables a day, and they are the most likely to be overweight.

DROWSY DRIVING

According to a study by the CDC, one in 24 motorists admitted to falling asleep behind the wheel in the past month (16, 17). The problem is more common in men than women and in drivers aged 25 to 34 compared to older drivers. According to Angie Wheaton, the lead author of the CDC study, approximately 2.5% of all fatal motor vehicle crashes (around 730 in 2009) involved drowsy drivers, as did 2% of crashes that resulted in nonfatal injuries (around 30,000 in 2009). They also found that around 4% of respondents fell asleep while driving in the previous year. The government estimated that approximately 3% of fatal traffic crashes involve drowsy drivers, but some studies have put that estimate as high as 33%. Brief moments of nodding off can be extremely dangerous, particularly when traveling 60 miles per hour. A single second translates to moving 90 feet, the length of 2 school buses. According to Dr. Kingman Strohl, a pulmonologist in Cleveland, a typical driver makes about 1000 decisions a minute. If a person has not slept for 18 consecutive hours, his or her impairment on those decision-making tasks is similar to that of someone above the legal alcohol limit. Everyone knows about driving and alcohol drinking, but there is much less emphasis on the importance of sleep before driving.

FALLING TELEVISIONS

According to Kim Painter, falling TV sets have killed >200 children since 2000 (18). The Consumer Products Safety Commission showed that 29 people in the US, most of them children, were killed by falling TVs in 2011 alone, and 18,000 people a year in the US, most of them children, are treated for injuries from falling TVs. That is happening despite the widespread switch to lighter flat-screens. Safety experts say the switch may actually be making the problem worse, because consumers often take old, heavy sets out of their family rooms and put them atop unstable bedroom dressers and playroom shelves. Children climb up on furniture to turn the TV on and there goes the heavy television as well as the piece of furniture. The 50- to 100-pound TVs can crush a child. The TVs often are on shelves never designed to hold the heavy weight. Flat-screen TVs also fall on kids because parents do not install them in the safest way. Let's secure these TVs, and if anchoring is not an option, place the TV on a low sturdy base and remove any items from the top that might attract children.

GUNS

The US has about 315 million people and about 290 million guns. Germany has about 80 million people and 5.5 million guns (19). Germany has recently initiated a large registry that details every legal gun owner in the country, along with information about all of their firearms. The new gun database, which went into service January 1, 2013, allows law enforcement officials to scroll through lists of owners and their guns in seconds on their computers. And the gun owners did not resist the establishment of this registry. Many gun advocates in Germany say that if cars can be registered and regulated, so can weapons. It's not quite that way in the USA, but the US has about 50 times as many guns as are present in Germany.

In the US it is easy to acquire any number of weapons and unlimited amounts of ammunition. Those who pass laws make it possible. The National Rifle Association traditionally muzzles any congressional attempts at gun control laws. Surely there is a relation between the number of people killed with guns and the number of guns available.

VIRGINIA TECH, FORT HOOD, AURORA, SANDY HOOK . . .

Using news accounts and records from the Federal Bureau of Investigation (FBI) from 2006 through 2010, the most recent years for which complete records were available, *USA Today* identified 156 murders that met the FBI definition of mass killings, in which 4 or more people are killed by the attacker (20). The attacks killed 774 people, including at least 161 children aged 12 or younger. Mass killers, in other words, target Americans once every 2 weeks on average, in attacks that range from robberies to horrific public shooting sprees like the massacre in Newtown, Connecticut. The *USA Today* review did not include murders in 2011 or 2012, both of which were marked by a series of high-profile public shootings. The 2006 to 2010 killings offer a portrait of mass murder that in many ways belies the stereotype of a lone gunman targeting strangers: lone gunmen, such as the one who terrorized Sandy Hook Elementary School, account for fewer than half of the nation's mass killers. About one quarter of mass murderers involved 2 or more killers. A third of mass killings did not involve guns. Mass murderers tend to be older than other killers, an average of nearly 32 years of age. Like all killers, they are overwhelmingly men. The mass killings during those 5 years accounted for about 1% of all murders during that time in the USA.

DALLAS CRIME

Despite increases in some major areas—rape, robbery, and murder—overall reported crime in Dallas dropped nearly 11% in 2012 compared to 2011, a record ninth consecutive year crime has fallen in the city (21, 22). The drop is in line with what is happening nationally and was driven by significant decreases in every area of property crime, which had about 7600 fewer offenses in 2012 than the previous year. Twenty percent more thieves were arrested in 2012 than in 2011 through the help of a task force that targets rings that buy and sell stolen property. Police Chief David Brown indicated that the longer a thief is in jail, the better the stats are going to be. Murders in Dallas in 2012 numbered 151, an increase from 133 the previous year. In comparison, Chicago had 506 murders in 2012, nearly twice as many killed than US troops in Afghanistan.

MILITARY SUICIDES

Suicides in the US military surged to a record 349 in 2012, far exceeding American combat deaths in Afghanistan (n = 295 Americans), and up from 301 in 2001 (23). Defense Secretary Leon Panetta and others have called the problem an epidemic. The problem appears to reflect severe strains on military personnel burdened with more than a decade of combat in Afghanistan and Iraq, complicated by anxiety over being forced out of a shrinking workforce. The 349 total in 2012 was the highest since the Pentagon began tracking suicides in 2001. The army, by far the largest of the military services, had the highest number of suicides among active-duty troops in 2012 at 182. The Marine Corps had the highest percentage increase—a 50% jump to 48. The Air Force had 59, and the Navy, 60 suicides, an increase in each of about 15% over the previous year.

GENDERCIDE

There are too many examples of global violence against women. Beverly Hill, who is founder and president of the Gendercide Awareness Project, calls it *gendercide*—the elimination of females, both young and old, through sex-selective abortion, infanticide, gross neglect, and in the case of older women (particularly widows), lack of access to food and shelter (24). The United Nations Population Fund, which tracks this problem, has estimated that 117 million women are missing in the world because of these practices. "Missing," as Ms. Hill indicates, equals death. That's more deaths than World War I and World War II combined. She indicates that it is no exaggeration to say that gendercide is an atrocity as colossal as any the world has seen. East Asia, South Asia, West Asia, the Middle East, Africa, and Southeastern Europe are all ravaged by gendercide. Every year, according to Ms. Hill, we lose 2 million baby girls to sex-selective abortion and infanticide alone. That equates to 4 girls every minute.

The United Nations reports that China has the greatest sex imbalance in the world, with 10% of its female population eliminated; India and Afghanistan follow with 7%. These sex imbalances lead to a host of social problems. Contrary to popular belief, the status of women does not improve when females are in short supply. In fact, just the opposite occurs. Sex trafficking increases, as does the buying and selling of brides. Aging bachelors, unable to find women of appropriate age, marry ever younger girls. These child brides leave school and begin bearing children. Maternal death rates are high. Ms. Hill goes on to indicate that there is a strong correlation between sex imbalance and crime. Sex ratios apparently are the best predictors of murder rates in India—better predictors than poverty, illiteracy, or urbanization. Crime spiked in the Chinese regions where sex-selective technology first became available. And finally, Ms. Hill writes: "Gendercide proceeds from the belief that female life is disposable. Gendercide devastates the hopes of women everywhere. It is unworthy of us as human beings. It is time to end this slaughter."

WOMEN IN CONGRESS

Of the 100 US Senators, 20 (20%) are women and of the 435 House Representatives, 78 (18%) are women; both of these are records (25).

FIBRONACCI NUMBERS

By definition, the first 2 numbers of the Fibronacci sequence are 0 and 1. Each subsequent number is the sum of the previous two (26). The Fibronacci sequence is:

0, 1, 1, 2, 3, 5, 8, 13, 21, 34, 55, 89, 144, etc.

The ratio of any two consecutive numbers eventually approaches the "golden ratio" of 0.618.

1/1 1/2 2/3 3/5 5/8 8/13 13/21 21/34 34/55 55/89 89/144

1.00 .500 .667 0.600 .625 0.615 0.619 0.618 0.618 0.618 0.618

The sequence made its first appearance in the West in the book *Liber Abaci* (1202) by Leonardo of Pisa, also known as Fibronacci. (The sequence first appeared in Indian literature centuries before.) The Fibronacci sequence is important in nature: it describes the branching in trees, the arrangement of leaves on a stem, the fruitlets of a pineapple, the flowering of an artichoke, the uncurling of a fern, and the arrangement of a pine cone. Fibronacci numbers are truly fascinating. They have many implications for mathematicians.

PUBLIC HIGH SCHOOL GRADUATION RATES

The percentage of students at public high schools who graduate on time has reached its highest level in nearly 40 years (27). The public high school graduation rate, i.e., students earning a diploma within 4 years of starting high school, reached 78% for the class of 2010, the highest rate since 1974. Graduation rates improved for every race and ethnicity in 2010. The student graduation rates were as follows: Asians, 93%; Whites, 83%; Hispanics, 74%; American Indians and Alaskan natives, 69%; African Americans, 66%. In 2010, 38 states had higher graduation rates, while rates for the other 12 states were flat.

SMART DEVICES WINNING

Using a cellphone during class used to mean possible confiscation and perhaps detention for students (28). Now, a growing number of schools are turning to the smart phones students bring to school as an instructional device that can augment classroom learning. Teachers ask students to use their smart phones to look up vocabulary words, take photos of an assignment written on the board, or text themselves homework reminders. Teachers use countless apps to better connect students with coursework on a platform they are familiar with. The Verizon Foundation chose 12 schools in 2012 and 24 in 2013 to receive up to $50,000 in grant funding to bring laptops, tablets, and mobile phones to class. The focus is on science, math, and technology studies. The apps offer an easy way to do research, solve problems quickly, and motivate students.

IQ

The average American in 1900 had an IQ that by today's standards would measure about 67 (29). Since the traditional definition of mental retardation was an IQ < 70, that leads to the remarkable conclusion that most Americans at the beginning of the 20th century would today be considered "intellectually disabled." The trend of rising intelligence is known as the Flynn effect, named for James R. Flynn, the New Zealander who pioneered this area of research. The average American IQ has been rising steadily by 3 points a decade. Spaniards gained 19 points over 28 years, and the Dutch, 20 points over 30 years. Kenyan children gained nearly 1 point a year. These figures are from Flynn's new book entitled *Are We Getting Smarter?* It's an uplifting tale, a reminder that human capacity is on the upswing. The country that tops the IQ charts is Singapore, at 108. Singaporeans have great respect for learning and an outstanding school system. Flynn argues that IQ is rising because in industrialized societies we give our brains a constant mental workout, much greater than when we were mostly living on isolated farms. Modern TV shows and other entertainment can be cognitively demanding, and video games require more thought that Solitaire. It appears that talent is universal but opportunity is not. Our public school budgets are being slashed. According to Nicholas Kristof, some 61 million children in the world still don't attend primary school. The cost of a single F-35 fighter could pay for more than 4 years of the Reading Is Fundamental program in the entire USA.

DEGREES AND INCOMES OF US ETHNIC GROUPS

As reported by Siegel (30), in 2010, the percentages of Americans aged 25 and older with at least a bachelor's degree were as follows: all US, 28%; Asians, 49%; Whites, 31%; Blacks, 18%; and Hispanics, 13%. The median household income in the US in 2010 was as follows: all US, $49,800; Asians, $66,000; Whites, $54,000; Hispanics, $40,000; and Blacks, $33,300.

TWO INTERESTING HERBIVORES

My friend, Dr. Vince Friedewald in Austin, sent me the following information on camels and kangaroos (31). Camels can live where food and water are scarce. They have an amazing ability to conserve water. When dehydrated, a camel can drink as much as 120 liters (32 gallons) in 15 minutes. To conserve water, camels can regulate their body temperature so that they hardly sweat, their kidneys can concentrate the urine, and they store a lot of water in their erythrocytes, which have the ability to swell to over twice their normal size without bursting. The camel's hump functions as a reservoir of adipose tissue that they can metabolize to provide emergency energy. As the fat is depleted, the hump wilts and flops to one side. The fatty humps also help keep the animal cool, as fat conducts the sun's heat relatively slowly and their woolly covering provides extra insulation. Thus, camels can go for weeks with little or no water or food.

Kangaroos in Australia have the ability to cross vast distances in search of food and water, keys to their survival. Capable of an 8-meter (25-foot) single bound across level ground, the red kangaroo is one of the world's greatest long jumpers. Thanks to large feet and strong legs, it can travel at over 50 kilometers (30 miles) per hour for hours. While a kangaroo's hind legs are big and powerful, they can't work independently of each other, and so kangaroos have to hop on two feet. The hind leg tendons are strong and elastic. With every hop, elastic energy is recaptured in the tendons ready for the next jump. The kangaroos use their long tail for balance and counterbalance. It swings up as the animal leaves the ground and down as the legs swing back with every bounce to help propel the kangaroo. A kangaroo's big toes are in the center of the other toes, not to one side like in humans, and are thus in line with their leg bones, enabling them to push off with great force. The kangaroo has a pouch to carry the newborn for about 10 months after birth. To win the Olympics a human has to jump further than a kangaroo (to nearly 9 meters). The best jumper of all is the snow leopard, who can leap 15 meters.

THE AVALANCHE OF UNFUNDED DEBT

Mortimer B. Zuckerman, the editor of *U.S. News & World Report* and the publisher of *The New York Daily News,* in a December 2012 column paints the picture well (32, 33): "A sound in the mountain range. . . . It's the sound made by an avalanche, the trillions of dollars of debt that's heading our way, gathering speed and mass. For most people, it's out of earshot." Liabilities are not set out by our government in accordance with well-established norms of the private sector, where our overhang of liabilities would set off alarm bells in the markets, with boards of directors in emergency sessions. We have gone from being the world's largest creditor nation, with no foreign debt at the end of World War II, to the world's largest debtor, with half of our public debt held by foreign countries. During the last 4 years alone, our national debt has grown by more than $5 trillion to over $16 trillion. Although the Federal Reserve is keeping borrowing rates historically low, the cost of paying interest on the debt for fiscal year 2012 was just under $360,000,000,000!

Despite our huge annual deficit, the greatest fiscal challenge to the US government, opines Zuckerman, is its total liabilities. Our federal balance sheet, he indicates, does not include the unfunded obligations of Medicare, Social Security, and the future retirement benefits of federal employees. The estimated unfunded total of these commitments is more than $87 trillion, or 550% of our gross domestic product. And the debt per household is more than 10 times the median family income! The real *annual* accrued expense of Medicare and Social Security is $7 trillion. The government's balance sheet does not include any of these obligations but focuses on the current year deficits and the accumulated national debt. The annual budget deficit, however, is only about one fifth of the more accurate figure! Zuckerman argues that if Americans saw our financial statements in the same way that public companies report their pension liabilities, these liabilities would require borrowing on a scale that would not only bankrupt the programs themselves but would bankrupt the entire government. Zuckerman adds that the Social Security programs and other mandatory programs are not subject to an annual spending limit. Today, <40% of our budget is actually decided by Congress and the president, down from 62% 40 years ago. Our liabilities are so huge and are multiplying so fast that eventually they cannot be honored. Today, all payroll taxes for Social Security and Medicare are spent in the year that they

are collected, leaving no leftovers for the unfunded obligations! And this does not take into account other risks such as the fact that the Federal Housing Authority confronts a $16.3 billion net deficit after its latest audit that may force a taxpayer bailout for the first time in its 78-year history. And, by 2016, the Disability Insurance Trust Fund will be fully depleted.

US TAX RATES

Taking into account all taxes on earnings and consumer spending—including federal, state, and local income taxes, Social Security and Medicare payroll taxes, excise taxes, and state and local sales taxes—the US average effective tax rate is around 40%. High tax rates—on labor, income, and consumption, as indicated by Prescott and Ohanian (34)—reduce the incentive to work by making consumption more expensive relative to leisure. The incentive to produce goods for the market is particularly depressed when the tax revenue is returned to households either as government transfers or transfers in kind—such as public schooling, police and fire protection, food stamps, and health care—that substitute for private consumption. In the 1950s, when European tax rates were low, many Western Europeans, including the French and Germans, worked more hours per capita than did Americans. Over time, tax rates that affect earnings and consumption rose substantially in Western Europe and have accounted for much of the nearly 30% decline in work hours in several European countries—to 1000 per adult per year today from around 1400 in the 1950s. The average American today works just over 1300 hours per year, the same as Japan, which has the same tax rate essentially as does America.

OBAMACARE'S INDEPENDENT PAYMENT ADVISORY BOARD

The Independent Payment Advisory Board (IPAB) is a government-appointed panel to help slow the growth of Medicare spending (35). The 15-person IPAB will propose Medicare cuts if the growth in the program's spending exceeds inflationary targets. Some fear that their decisions will lead to rationing. The law, however, gives the panel no authority to ration care or cut benefits for Medicare recipients. It can't touch reimbursement to hospitals until 2020. Instead, it is expected to find savings by eliminating fraud and reducing payments to private insurance companies that work with Medicare and prescription drug providers. And, it can only do that if the government is projected to spend more than it's supposed to. Each spring, the Office of the Actuary of the Centers for Medicare and Medicaid Services forecasts how much the programs will cost 2 years in the future. On April 30, 2013, the panel will issue its per capita estimates for 2015. The actuary also will release a spending target, based on predictions about the pace of health care inflation. If the increase in expected Medicare costs exceeds the spending target, the IPAB steps in to propose cuts. It will take a 60% Senate vote to reject its recommendations, and then legislators must find alternate cuts that achieve the same savings. The law allows them to debate the IPAB's proposal for 30 hours maximum, making it filibuster proof.

How will the White House recruit the board members? So far no IPAB members have been appointed, even though the board is supposed to get to work by April 2013. The law requires the panel to be made up of prominent physicians, economists, hospital executives, and insurance industry representatives. Candidates are subject to Senate approval, which means that they must endure potentially hostile public hearings. Board members willing to go through all that must also agree to serve for 6 years, full time; they have to quit their current jobs because of conflict of interest concerns. The annual salary for each board member is $165,300. And, the life of an IPAB member may be rather dull since its powers kick in only if spending is surging. It's no wonder that Obama has yet to announce his candidates. If there is no IPAB in place by the time its services are needed, the law allows the secretary of the US Department of Health and Human Services to do its job until the panel is up and running. I can't imagine who would want to be one of the 15 on that panel!

WATER

When the headline of the *Dallas Morning News* reads "The word on water: Conserve," we have a problem (36). The state is running out of water, as shown in *Figure 3*. The projected Texas population in the next 50 years is expected to grow from 25 million to about 46 million (54%↑) and the projected need for additional water from 3.62 to 8.33 million acre-feet per year (43%↑). Get ready. Life with limited water will not be the same. Quick showers, low-flush toilets, and irrigation restrictions will be the norm. San Antonio, Texas, apparently is already in the swing of water conservation, and we must follow in Dallas.

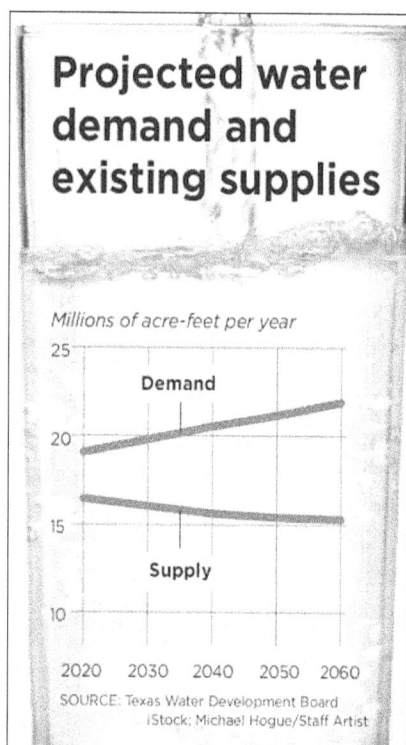

Figure 3. The supply and demand for water in Texas. Reprinted with permission from *The Dallas Morning News*.

US OIL BOOM

It's really unbelievable, at least to me. The US oil output is surging so fast that the USA could soon overtake Saudi Arabia as the world's biggest producer (37). Driven by high prices and new drilling methods, US production of crude and other liquid hydrocarbons rose approximately 7% in 2012 to an average of just under 11 million barrels per day. This is the fourth straight year of crude increases and the biggest single year since 1951. The Energy Department forecast that US production of crude and other liquid hydrocarbons, which include biofuels, will average 11.4 million barrels per day in 2013. That would be a record for the US and just below Saudi Arabia's output of 11.6 million barrels per day. The production is forecast to reach 13 to 15 million barrels per day in the US by 2020, helping to make North America "the new Middle East." I used to think that making the US "energy independent" was a joke, but it is great to see that it isn't.

BALLPOINT PEN

We all use them. Peter Pesic summarized the book *Ballpoint* written by Hungarian author György Muldova (38, 39). The Hungarians are astonishingly creative. Eleven won the Nobel Prize during the 20th century, far more per capita than from other nations. There were other Hungarian geniuses, including mathematician *John Von Neumann* and physicists *Leo Szilard* and *Edward Teller*. Talented students flourished in some Budapest schools until the 1920s when the government began limiting university admissions to those "who are completely reputable in respect of their national allegiance," effectively excluding Jews, who thereafter emigrated when they could.

One of the Jewish beneficiaries of those Budapest schools was *László Biró* (1899–1985), a journalist and artist in the 1930s who noted that the ink used for newspapers dried relatively quickly compared with the ink for fountain pens. Handwritten papers had to be carefully blotted or set aside until the ink dried. Biró tried using quick-drying ink in a fountain pen, but the fluid was too thick to flow down to the nib and simply clogged the reservoir. He solved the problem of how to deliver thick, quick-drying ink to a paper surface without requiring the ink to flow by closing the end of the pen instead of using a nib, leaving an opening with just enough room for a tiny metal ball that would spin against the ink in the reservoir, distributing it to the paper. Through much trial and error and with the help of an early backer and business partner, Endor Goy (1896–1991), Biró developed a working ballpoint pen. The two men signed a contract to produce and market the pen in 1938. Biró kept refining the pen and experimenting with recipes for the ink paste essential for his concept while fleeing dangers in Europe and finally settling in Argentina. Though Biró faced the hardships of wartime immigration, he soon started up a pen-manufacturing operation in Argentina. Biró's story is relatively well known in much of the English-speaking world. "Biró" is synonymous with ballpoint pen. In Argentina, the pen is known as a "Birome," and Biró's birthday, September 29, is celebrated as "Inventor's Day" in Argentina. Thus, the ballpoint took its place alongside the zipper, the pencil, and the paperclip devised by inventors who long struggled to produce objects we now take for granted.

EPPIE AND POPO

These were their nicknames. They were identical twins, Esther Pauline Friedman Lederer and Pauline Esther Friedman Phillips, aka Abigail Van Buren, born in Sioux City, Iowa, on July 4, 1918. They shared a joint wedding and honeymoon trip. Esther was the first to become a columnist, taking over the *Chicago Sun-Times'* "Ann Landers" column in 1955. Pauline, living in California, started a replacement advice column for the *San Francisco Chronicle,* "Dear Abby," in 1956. She created her own byline, combining a biblical wise woman with the eighth president of the US. Within 2 years, both columns were in a combined 400 newspapers. Pauline's *Dear Abby* column at its peak appeared in 1400 papers. *Life* magazine in 1958 said the sisters were "the most widely read and most quoted women in the world." For a long time they did not speak to each other, but their differences were eventually patched up. Mother and daughter started sharing the byline in 2000, and Jeanne Phillips took over in 2002. Amazing (40).

SPORTS

Stan Musial: Years ago I was invited to give a talk in St. Louis by the son-in-law of Stan Musial, a physician, who brought me a baseball signed by Stan-the-Man. It is one of my favorite sport collectibles. When I was growing up, Musial was one of my baseball heroes. He played 22 years in the Major Leagues, all with St. Louis, in 3026 games. He had 10,972 at-bats and only struck out just over 600 times (41). He had 3630 hits, scored 1942 runs, had 6134 total bases, and hit 475 home runs. He won the National League batting title 7 times and participated in 24 all-star games. And all the time he was a great guy. He contributed to his community generously. He was 6 feet tall and weighed 175 pounds. Those also are my dimensions, but Musial had a much better eye for the ball.

Stacy Lewis: She is the first American to be named Player of the Year on the Ladies Professional Golf Association tour since 1994 (42). She had severe scoliosis and wore a back brace 18 hours a day for 7 years as a child. She had a steel rod with 5 screws installed in her spine just after getting her high school diploma. She didn't know at that time whether she could play golf again, but she certainly did.

Johnny Manzial: As a red-shirt freshman, "Johnny Football" won the Heisman Trophy Award for 2012 and shortly after doing so set the Cotton Bowl record for total offense with 516 yards (43, 44). Seven other college football players have played in the Cotton Bowl after receiving the Heisman Award, but none came close to doing what Johnny Manzial did in the January 2013 classic.

Golf: The average professional golfer takes 15,000 steps during an 18-hole round, walks 7 miles, and burns 2000 calories. The numbers when using a cart are unclear.

BODY WEIGHT IN THE NATIONAL FOOTBALL LEAGUE

Fran Tarkenton, a National Football League quarterback from 1961 to 1978 and member of the Pro Football Hall of Fame, in a recent piece in *The Wall Street Journal* discussed body weight of professional football players when he played

and subsequently (45). When Tarkenton entered pro football in 1961, every member of his offensive line weighed <250 pounds. During his last year, 1978, the biggest lineman on his team weighed 260 pounds. No Super Bowl–winning team had a 300 pounder on its roster until the 1982 Washington Redskins. Now, it is unusual for a team to have fewer than ten 300 pounders. This year's Super Bowl teams, the San Francisco 49ers and the Baltimore Ravens, had twenty-four 300 pounders between them.

Have players gotten bigger thanks to genetics, diet, and nutrition? Or is there something else going on? Shortly after retiring from football, Tarkenton learned from an owner of one of the biggest gym chains in the country that muscles can only get so big by weightlifting regimes alone. Huge muscles come from performance-enhancing drugs, which Tarkenton indicated were just starting to enter professional football during his time. The National Football League does not talk about steroids or human growth hormone, but these drugs make players bigger, faster, and stronger, and they are used widely in football. Why do so many former players look like miniature versions of themselves after they retire?

In their most recent collective-bargaining agreement, signed in 2011, the National Football League and the Player's Union agreed to start testing players for human growth hormone. Yet, two seasons later there still isn't any testing! (In contrast, Major League Baseball in recent years worked out a testing regime that includes human growth hormone.) At the college football level, meanwhile, testing looks almost exclusively for recreational drugs, with practically no attention to performance-enhancing ones.

Although everyone claims to care about player safety at all levels of the game, the use of performance-enhancing drugs, which have made current players bigger and stronger than ever, causes collisions to be more violent and players therefore to suffer worse injuries. These violent encounters on the field not only affect the safety of the players during games but they clearly affect long-term health—dementia, Alzheimer's disease, depression, suicide, and early death.

William C Roberts

WILLIAM CLIFFORD ROBERTS, MD
1 February 2013

1. Landers J. U.S. losing ground on health frontier. *Dallas Morning News*, January 15, 2013.
2. Tavernise S. Study: People living longer around world. *New York Times*, December 14, 2012.
3. Landers J. Obesity spreads in wider world. *Dallas Morning News*, January 20, 2013.
4. Landers J. Obesity weighs on U.S. productivity. *Dallas Morning News*, August 14, 2012.
5. Kwoh L. Want to be CEO? What's your BMI? *Wall Street Journal*, January 16, 2013.
6. Esteri M. Is this the end of the soft drink era? *Wall Street Journal*, January 19–20, 2013.

7. Berry I, Gee K. The U.S. milk business is in 'crisis.' *Wall Street Journal,* December 11, 2012.

8. Loprinzi PD, Kohli M. Effect of physical activity and sedentary behavior on serum prostate-specific antigen concentrations: results from the National Health and Nutrition Examination Survey (NHANES), 2003–2006. *Mayo Clin Proc* 2013;88(1):11–21.

9. Sidhu D, Naugler C. Fasting time and lipid levels in a community-based population: a cross-sectional study. *Arch Intern Med* 2012;172(22):1707–1710.

10. LeBlanc PM, Hollinger KA, Klontz KC. Tattoo ink-related infections—awareness, diagnosis, reporting, and prevention. *N Engl J Med* 2012;367(11):985–987.

11. Esler MD, Krum H, Schlaich M, Schmieder RE, Böhm M, Sobotka PA; Symplicity HTN-2 Investigators. Renal sympathetic denervation for treatment of drug-resistant hypertension: one-year results from the Symplicity HTN-2 randomized, controlled trial. *Circulation* 2012;126(25):2976–2782.

12. St Sauver JL, Warner DO, Yawn BP, Jacobson DJ, McGree ME, Pankratz JJ, Melton LJ 3rd, Roger VL, Ebbert JO, Rocca WA. Why patients visit their doctors: assessing the most prevalent conditions in a defined American population. *Mayo Clin Proc* 2013;88(1):56–67.

13. Lopez R. Business booming for dogs trained to sniff out bedbugs. *Dallas Morning News,* September 2, 2012.

14. Campbell J. The vacillation of his k's [Review of the book *The Missing Ink,* by P. Hensher, Faber, 270 pages]. *U.S. News & World Report,* December 2012.

15. Fang J, Yang Q, Hong Y, Loustalot F. Status of cardiovascular health among adult Americans in the 50 states and the District of Columbia, 2009. *J Am Heart Assoc* 2012;1(6):e005371.

16. Wheaton AG, Chapman DP, Presley-Cantrell LR, Croft JB, Roehler DR; Centers for Disease Control and Prevention (CDC). Drowsy driving—19 states and the District of Columbia, 2009–2010. *MMWR Morb Mortal Wkly Rep* 2013;61:1033–1037.

17. Strobbe M. 4% admit dozing while they drove. *Dallas Morning News,* January 4, 2013.

18. Painter K. Falling TVs can kill, but few parents are aware of the risk. *U.S. News & World Report,* December 13, 2012.

19. Birnbaum M. Germany begins gun registry. *Washington Post,* January 20, 2013.

20. Hoyer M, Heath B. Virginia Tech, Fort Hood, Aurora, Sandy Hook . . . names only hint at mass killings crisis: one every two weeks. *USA Today,* December 19, 2012.

21. Eiserer T. Crime stats down again. Property offenses lead drop in 2012, but rape, murder rise slightly. *Dallas Morning News,* January 15, 2013.

22. Eiserer T. '12 murder total up, still among lowest. *Dallas Morning News,* January 3, 2013.

23. Burns R. Suicides in military hit record in '12. *Dallas Morning News,* January 15, 2013.

24. Hill B. Females fall victim to 'gendercide.' *Dallas Morning News,* January 15, 2013.

25. Camia C. Record number of women in Congress. *USA Today,* January 4, 2013.

26. Doroghazi RM. Fibronacci numbers. *Physician Investor Newsletter,* May 14, 2012.

27. Layton L. More making it through high school. *Washington Post,* January 22, 2013.

28. Shane B. Smart devices make for smart kids. *USA Today,* December 28, 2012.

29. Kristof N. As long as IQs are climbing . . . *Dallas Morning News,* December 26, 2012.

30. Siegel L. Rise of the tiger nation. *Wall Street Journal,* October 27–28, 2012.

31. Why camels have the hump? Why are kangaroos expert jumpers? www.howitworksdaily.com, October 2009.

32. Zuckerman MB. Brace for an avalanche of unfunded debt. *U.S. News & World Report,* January 6, 2013.

33. Zuckerman MB. For the U.S. economy the news is bad and worse. *U.S. News & World Report,* January 6, 2013.

34. Prescott EC, Ohanian LE. Taxes are much higher than you think. *Wall Street Journal,* December 12, 2012.

35. Leonard D. The boring, awful life of a death panelist. *Bloomberg Businessweek,* January 21–27, 2013.

36. Shannon K. The word on water: conserve. *Dallas Morning News,* January 23, 2013.

37. Fahay J. U.S. sees oil output surge. *Dallas Morning News,* October 24, 2012.

38. Pesic P. The man who changed the way we write. *Wall Street Journal,* August 17, 2012.

39. Moldova G. *Ballpoint: A Tale of Genius and Grit, Perilous Times, and the Invention That Changed the Way We Write.* North Adams, MA: New Europe, 2012.

40. Miller S. Dear Abby columnist gave advice to millions. *Wall Street Journal,* January 18, 2013.

41. Nightengale B. "The Man" crush. *USA Today,* January 21, 2013.

42. DiMeglio S. Underdog Lewis now atop LPGA. *USA Today,* November 15, 2012.

43. Hairopoulos K. Aggies make loud statement. *Dallas Morning News,* January 5, 2013.

44. Sherrington K. Can't be beat. *Dallas Morning News,* January 5, 2013.

45. Tarkenton F. When it comes to doping, pro football punts. *Wall Street Journal,* January 31, 2013.

Chapter 11

July 2013

SIMPLIFY

In his book *Walden,* Henry David Thoreau made the case against the complexity of modern life as he saw it in the 19th century. "Our life is frittered away by detail. An honest man has hardly need to count more than his 10 fingers, or in extreme cases, he may add his 10 toes, and lump the rest. Simplicity, simplicity, simplicity!" he wrote. "Let your affairs be as two or three and not a hundred or a thousand; instead of a million count half a dozen, and keep your accounts on your thumb-nail. . . . Simplify, simplify." Alan Siegel and Irene Etzkorn have written a book entitled *Simple: Conquering the Crisis of Complexity* (1). They stress that "complexity is the coward's way out." There is nothing simple about simplicity, and achieving it requires following three major principles: *empathizing* (by perceiving others' needs and expectations), *distilling* (by reducing to its essence the substance of one's offer), and *clarifying* (by making the offering easier to understand or use). Empathy, they write, is the only way to truly shorten the distance between an organization providing services and the individual receiving them.

The Cleveland Clinic, they indicate, understands that empathizing with patients is critical, so it does not just focus on simplifying medical care but looks at everything the patient experiences: smells, sounds, greetings, hospital gowns, security, and appointment scheduling. It was not until staff members were wheeled through hallways lying in hospital beds that they realized how disconcerting and dizzying that experience can be. Preparing patients for the "thrill" ride is simply a gesture to allay fears. The clinic's guiding principle—patients first—is used as a mantra by chief executive *Delos Cosgrove*, who weaves patient experience stories into all of his presentations. Everyone at the hospital, regardless of his or her job, is called a "caretaker." Through this simple change in vocabulary, the Cleveland Clinic is able to send an important signal to everyone in the organization about what is expected.

What makes the biggest impression during a patient's stay in a hospital? The Cleveland Clinic staff found that it was the small details: how long it took a nurse to answer the call bell, the availability of food on request, whether staff members follow the "10-4 rule" ("when 10 feet away from a patient smile and make eye contact; when 4 feet away address the patient"). Borrowing from the hospitality industry, the Cleveland Clinic has even paid attention to the scent in the air. No antiseptic aroma; the air smells like a signature fragrance favored by 4-star hotel chains. Everything from the way physicians talk to patients (in plain English and with a willingness to answer questions until there are none left), to the hospital gowns (designed by Diane von Furstenberg to combine ease of access with a touch of dignity), to the clear, concise bills patients receive when checking out reflects a commitment to simplifying the interaction between a human being and a large complex medical establishment. The hospital has achieved simplicity through the elimination of "hassles" and the addition of clearer, more human communication.

One key to achieving empathy is feedback. The hospital gathers lots of it from patients and displays the data in patient experience "dashboards." For staff members eager to do well and for comparison with their peers, "bedside manner" becomes a measurable attribute, not an intangible quality.

Sometimes simplicity can be a matter of life and death. A decade ago, worried that confusing prescription labels threatened the health of her grandparents, *Deborah Adler* decided to do something about it. A graphic designer, she took on the challenge for her master's thesis. Rearranging the small type on the typical prescription label, Ms. Adler put the information in a logical order, giving prominence to the things that most people need to know at the moment they are reaching for their medicine. She divided the label into two parts, separated by a thick black line, and placed the critical information, such as the name and dosage of the medication, at the top, with everything else relegated to the bottom. Ms. Adler next considered the shape of the bottles. The wraparound labels on conventional round bottles were difficult to read, so she designed a flat tube-shaped container that stood upright on its cap with plenty of room for a large flat label that could be read easily at a glance. Also, by color-coding the bottles, she made it possible for family members to distinguish among their individual medications. Her simpler, clearer drug packaging has been adopted by Target Pharmacies nationwide.

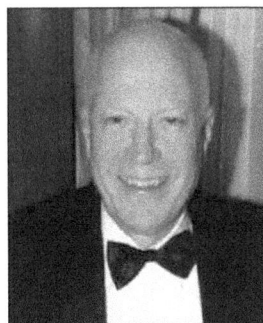

William C. Roberts, MD.

Siegel and Etzkorn go on to ask "What do we still need to simplify?" For ordinary personal and commercial transactions, they indicate we need brief online contracts with interactive features explaining key words, concepts, and computations. We need personal health records that can be easily used and updated by all health care providers. We need summaries of our home and automobile insurance that clearly explain how we will be reimbursed when the next storm hits; clear, 1-page hospital bills that will allow us to recognize each element in the care that we receive; and a simplified tax code that will eliminate the need for costly tax return preparation by professionals.

Simplicity may sound like a narrow standard, but it can winnow down unnecessary choices and clarify messages to customers, clients, patients, and citizens.

DEFINING A GOOD LIFE

George E. Vaillant has just published *Triumphs of Experience: The Men of the Harvard Grant Study* (2). The following comes from his book.

In 1938, *Dr. Arien V. Bock*, professor of hygiene and chief of Harvard Student Health Services, launched a study of 268 Harvard male sophomores, selected as the best and the brightest in the classes of 1939 through 1944. (John F. Kennedy was one of those selected.) The study was meant to last for 15 to 20 years and answer the question of what defines the best health possible, something, it was assumed, this highly privileged group would exemplify. Financial support originally came from William T. Grant, owner of a chain of "dime stores" who wanted to find out what makes a good store manager. Later, support came from other sources and eventually from the National Institutes of Health.

Despite the original intention to end the study after 2 decades and despite financial trouble after Grant pulled out in 1947, it continues to this day, still known as the Harvard Grant Study, although officially renamed the Harvard Study of Adult Development. The study's aim has grown broader to determine which early traits best predict a successful life. Most of the surviving men now are in their 90s. It is thus one of the longest prospective studies of adult development ever conducted and certainly the most exhaustively documented.

Over the course of the men's lives, a team of investigators collected a vast amount of information about them. They performed physical and psychiatric examinations, IQ tests, and various medical and lab tests and conducted repeated interviews with them as well as their parents and later their wives and children. At least every 2 years, the investigators used lengthy questionnaires to delve into everything from the men's daydreams to whether they like their subordinates at work. So frequent and intimate was the contact between the investigators and subjects that a bond formed between them, and except through death there were very few dropouts.

In 1954, when it looked as though the study would end for lack of funding, the Tobacco Industry Research Committee stepped in and provided most of the money for about a decade, ostensibly because it wanted to learn about the "positive reasons" people smoke. After that, funding came from several sources, including the National Institute on Alcohol Abuse and Alcoholism, which required the investigators to pay particular attention to alcoholism. The study is now supported by the National Institute on Aging.

During the 75 years of the study, there have been only four directors, and George Vaillant, MD, who served from 1972 to 2004, had the longest term by far. He is now 78 years old, with a string of papers and 3 books about the study to his credit, and the 2012 book is expected to be his final summary of the overall findings.

With no definition of what constitutes a good life and so many possible predictors, it has been difficult to draw unambiguous conclusions, except for a few major ones. During the early years it was thought that success was largely determined by physical constitution, so one of the criteria used to select men for the study in the first place was a muscular body build thought to be characteristic of men destined for success. By the time Vaillant, a psychiatrist, took over the directorship, the emphasis had shifted to the quality of personal relationships, particularly in childhood. Now, with a new director and new technology, there is renewed attention to physical findings—not muscles, but brains—as revealed by imaging studies.

In 2009, Vaillant attempted to define what constitutes a good life in men, aged 60 to 80, by devising what he called a "decathlon of flourishing." It consists of 10 variables, including being listed in *Who's Who in America*, earning income in the study's top quartile, and being in a good marriage. Using these variables, each man could be given a score ranging from 0 to 10. Vaillant then looked back at the data collected in earlier years to see what factors best correlated with a high score in late life. Vaillant concluded that since the quality of personal relationships (for example, a "warm childhood") was the strongest predictor of a high score, the "most important influence by far on a flourishing life is love." The "decathlon" includes few measures of feelings of usefulness to society at large or enjoyment, for example, of solitude.

There is nothing ambiguous about some of the study's findings. The men in the Harvard Grant Study were extraordinarily long lived; fully 30% of them survived into their 90s, compared with only 3% to 5% of men in the general population of that generation. We have long known that being affluent and well educated is the best possible insurer of good health. But the size of the effect in the study is startling. So strong is the correlation with education that the study men who went to graduate school lived even longer than those who didn't.

One of Vaillant's major themes is that adult development continues long after adolescence. In the Harvard Grant Study, the factors associated with flourishing changed with age, and those that were important in youth or middle age were not necessarily important in old age. In fact, many were so inconsistent that one has doubts about how much importance one can attach to them. In general, however, these men seemed more content with their lives as they aged and they reported happier marriages—whether it was a long first marriage or a recent second. Where they landed at about age 70 seemed to matter most.

Another of Vaillant's themes is the devastating effects of alcoholism. According to him, alcoholism was the cause, not the consequence, of unhappiness in these men. Most of the 62 divorces were associated with alcoholism, either in the men or their wives, as were professional setbacks and early death. Vaillant is absolutely certain that alcoholism is the horse, not the cart. The men did not drown their sorrows in alcohol, he believes, but inherited a vulnerability to alcohol which then caused their sorrows. There is no other study of lifetime alcohol abuse as long and as thorough as this one, and he believes that this aspect of the study is perhaps its greatest contribution.

The main strength of the Harvard Grant Study—namely, its long life—is also one of its main weaknesses. These men were dinosaurs in the sense that the world they inhabited for most of their lives is gone forever. Vaillant, for example, found that a warm childhood was a predictor of success, but that almost surely meant something different in the 1920s than it does today. Parents were stricter then than today's doting parents. Also, the household then probably revolved around the husband, not the children as today. Marriages were different too. Although Vaillant does not say, it is likely that nearly all the study men had wives who didn't work outside the home—something unlikely now. Thus, many of the findings are dated, and even when they provide unambiguous conclusions, they are unlikely to apply to people today.

Dr. Marsha Angell, the reviewer of the book in *The New York Review* (3), asked why the men in the Harvard Grant Study, despite all common sense expectations, seem to grow more content and not less content in old age. After all, by the time they were over 70, they were no doubt experiencing many of the physical limitations of age and they had to know that their time was running out, that any day they could become seriously ill and begin an inexorable decline to decrepitude and death. Why were they happier than they seemingly had any right to be? Maybe one answer, as Dr. Angell suggests, is that they had learned to live in the present, not the future, and in the present, most of them had acquired enough resources to live comfortably, yet didn't have to work anymore or work as hard if they didn't want to. So the tension of competing at work was relaxed; their children were probably married and self-supporting, and they had freedom. These were ambitious men who probably cared a great deal about professional advancement. (A quarter of each class became lawyers or physicians; 15% became teachers, mostly at the college level; 20% became businessmen; and the remaining 40% entered other fields. Four ran for the US Senate, one served in a presidential cabinet, one was a governor, and one was president [John F. Kennedy].)

After they retired, perhaps it was a relief not to be thinking ahead to the next professional goal and also not to experience gaps between career aspirations and achievements. They could find serenity in cultivating their garden—or taking up watercolors or carpentry or otherwise broadening their interests at leisure. And living in the present helps people not to think about the looming existential threats of illness and death.

The fact that marriages were happier after age 70 no doubt added to the contentment. But why were they happier? Was it simply a matter of having found the right partner (about a third of the happiest marriages were not the first) or perhaps having rubbed up against each other so long that the barnacles had worn away? There may be another reason, Dr. Angell questions, one that would have been particularly relevant for marriages that had taken place when men and women had sharply divided roles and men were dominant. As they age, women tend to become psychologically more independent for a variety of reasons, while men become more dependent, particularly when they retire and spend more time at home (the traditional woman's domain). As the men of the Harvard Grant Study and their wives became more equal and probably shared more interests by virtue of being together more, they probably became more companionable. Vaillant refers to "hormonal changes that 'feminize' husbands and 'masculinize' wives." He also believes the "empty nest is often more of a blessing than a burden." Angell speculates that old age takes many men almost by surprise; it sneaks up on them and is all the more disturbing for that. In contrast, women are all too aware of aging, starting with their first gray hair or wrinkle. By the time they are in their 50s they are well accustomed to the loss that comes with age. That may make them better able to help and support their husbands, as the men find that having been a master of the universe is no protection against old age.

But this happy outcome—more contentment and better marriages—depends crucially on having the means to live in comfort. Without that, it is hard to imagine such equanimity in the face of old age. If you don't know whether you can afford to heat your home next winter or pay your medical bills or hire a helper if you become disabled, old age is a particularly harsh time of life. Financial security is no doubt something that distinguished the study men from less privileged men. As the founders of the study intended, these were the most fortunate of men, and it is wrong to assume that others will age in the same gentle way. A golden old age also depends on remaining reasonably healthy, and they did well in this respect, too, although about a quarter of them who reached their 90s had dementia.

Dr. Marsha Angell, now also in her 70s, also finds many offsetting advantages of getting older. One of them is a sharper sense of what is important in life. She indicates that she has a clearer sense of what matters and what doesn't. Her sources of pleasure are different now and more varied. She indicates that, for example, she takes greater pleasure now in beautiful vistas. Ordinary daily activities, like reading the paper and discussing the news with her husband over breakfast, have taken on an added pleasure beyond the activities themselves just because of the ritual. Although she is still active professionally, she is less concerned with maintaining a professional presence. She looks forward to learning Italian, taking a course in astronomy, and finally reading *War and Peace*.

She has become much more pessimistic about the state of the world: the unsustainable population growth, potentially disastrous climate change, depletion of natural resources, pollution of the oceans, increasing inequality both within and across countries, and violent tribalism of all forms, national and religious.

Nearly everyone over a certain age observes that time seems to pass much more quickly. So extreme is the acceleration, says Angell, that she wonders whether it isn't a result of some physical law, not just a perception. Maybe it's akin to Einstein's discovery that as speed increases, time slows. Perhaps this is the reverse—as our bodies slow, time speeds up. In any case, the rush of her days is in stark contrast to the magically endless days of her childhood. She also finds it hard to remember that she is no longer younger despite the physical signs, since she is still the same person and in many ways has the same feelings. I feel the same way. It's particularly disquieting to recall that many people and places I knew no longer exist except in my memory. Still, she opines that although she dislikes the fact that her days are going so quickly, that's the way it is and she has had a good run like the men in the Harvard Grant Study.

ARE YOU WEALTHY?

Scott Burns (4) asked four questions to determine one's wealth: 1) *Do you make payments on your house or car?* If yes, one is not wealthy. 2) *Does your interest and/or dividend income exceed what you pay in interest?* The more income one has from sources that don't involve working, the closer you are to being wealthy. 3) *Can you keep what you have without actually working?* If losing your job means the repo guy will be visiting soon, you are not wealthy. 4) *When you are asked "What do you do?" do you reply by stating your occupation?* If so, you are not wealthy and may be a workaholic. Scott Burns suggested answering that question by saying "In the event of what?"

PHYSICIAN-PATIENT E-MAILING

According to Sumathi Reddy (5), just under one third of physicians reported e-mailing patients in 2012, up from 27% in 2007, according to annual studies of more than 3000 physicians conducted by Manhattan Research, a health care market research firm. Those texting rose from 12% in 2010 to 18% in 2012. Physicians who shun e-mail cite concerns ranging from privacy and security issues to liability, inconvenience, and the risk of miscommunication of important medical information. Also, time spent e-mailing patients is unpaid. Few physicians charge for the service. Those who do e-mail say it is a convenient way to communicate with patients without the hassle of playing phone tag and that it can keep patients from relying on Google searches that can sometimes lead to inaccurate information. Patients tend to love the access. Some physicians give every patient a business card that includes their e-mail address, but others give it only when asked. E-mailing with patients apparently generates good will. One physician indicated it improved his reputation and his online ratings. A physician in Manhattan apparently ends each new patient visit by asking if the patient would like to communicate via e-mail. If so, he asks the patient to sign a form agreeing to communicate electronically about health matters and giving him authority to discuss medical issues over e-mail. The form ensures that he is compliant with the Health Insurance Portability and Accountability Act, commonly referred to as HIPAA, designed to protect the privacy of health information. HIPAA compliance is a major concern

raised by physicians who do not e-mail. The law requires that electronic communication related to an individual's health is protected and secure.

As part of the federal government's Stimulus Act, physicians are being encouraged through financial incentives to use electronic medical records. One part of that effort includes the use of secure messaging to share health information with patients through, say, an online portal. Opinions on this matter would be welcomed by readers.

DESIGNER DRUGS

These are synthetic drugs that duplicate the experiences of LSD, marijuana, cocaine, ecstasy, and amphetamines (6). Because laboratory-created compounds differ slightly in chemical structure from the illegal drug they mimic, consumers of the drugs can claim that their purchases from websites or head shops are legal. Many national governments have declared some of the new compounds illegal, but they have trouble keeping up. Since 2008, drugs with names like 2NE1, after a Korean girl band, and SS-135, which was NASA's final space shuttle mission, have been appearing at a rate of one a week, according to the United Nations–affiliated International Narcotics Control Board. In July 2012, the US Congress voted to list 26 new chemicals under the Controlled Substances Act. The drugs, however, are sold over the Internet from countries where it is legal to countries where it is illegal. The profits can be enormous. Synthetic marijuana, often labeled "plant food" to confuse police, can earn retail profits of $90,000 to $136,000 a pound, compared to $1000 to $5000 for the real stuff. In March 2013, the Narcotics Control Board labeled new psychoactive substances the fastest growing category of drugs in the world and identified more than 1000 compounds that have entered the market since 2008. According to the US Drug Abuse Warning Network, some 28,000 emergency room visits in 2011 were caused by known marijuana synthetics—more than double the 2010 number. Legal systems for banning drugs are not set up to handle a market in which a new drug emerges weekly. Chinese manufacturers are the main suppliers of the chemical compounds used in synthetics. Most of the suspect ingredients are legal there. After 4 years of meeting with the Chinese, US officials can point to a single success: pushing China to prohibit mephedrone, a cocaine synthetic that is marketed in the US as "bath salts," a rapidly increasing problem.

HEROIN IS BACK

Donna Leinwand Leger (7) in the *USA Today* indicates that heroin is back. In Charlotte, North Carolina, it has become so easy to get that dealers deliver to the suburbs and run specials to attract their young professional, upper-income customers. These lawyers, nurses, policemen, and ministers are showing up in the detox wards at Charlotte hospitals desperate to kick an opiate addiction that often starts with powerful prescription painkillers, such as OxyContin and Vicodin. The Carolinas Medical Center analyzed the patients' zip codes to see where heroin had taken root and discovered that its heroin patients were coming from the five best neighborhoods in Charlotte. They believe they are witnessing a growing and more dangerous wave of drug addiction sweeping the country, ensnaring several hundred thousand Americans into the heroin trap and importing crime to America's suburbs. Prescription painkiller addicts are finding their drug of choice in short supply, so heroin becomes their drug of last resort. As adults move from legitimate prescriptions to the black market of pure precisely measured narcotic pain pills to the dirty world of dealers, needles, and kitchen table chemists, health officials and police are noting sharp increases in overdoses, crime, and other public health problems. One expert indicated that "when you switch to heroin, you don't know what is in there from batch to batch."

The number of people who say they regularly abuse painkillers dropped from 5,093,000 in 2010 to 4,471,000 in 2011, according to the National Survey on Drug Use and Health. Young adults who said they regularly abused painkillers dropped from a high of 1.62 million in 2006 to 1.22 million in 2011. The survey estimated that 281,000 people aged 12 and older regularly used heroin in 2011, up from a decade low of 119,000 in 2003. The number of people seeking treatment for heroin found increases in 30 of 39 states reporting data in 2011 to the Substance Abuse and Mental Health Services Administration. In 2011, 238,184 sought treatment for heroin addiction. The 2013 National Drug Control Strategy released on April 24, 2013, confirms that heroin use appears to be increasing particularly among younger people living in suburban and rural areas. To counter the escalating overdose problem, the strategy includes a plan to make Naloxone—a medicine that can reverse heroin or opiate overdose—more accessible.

OxyContin, a narcotic painkiller in the opiate family, came on the market in 1996. By 2001, it became the nation's bestselling brand-name narcotic pain reliever. Although it's a highly effective drug for people suffering from chronic pain from diseases such as cancer, the Drug Enforcement Administration noted high levels of abuse particularly in West Virginia and Kentucky, where it became known as "hillbilly heroin." To stem abuses of pain pills, authorities over the past decade began cracking down on clinics, and drug companies began creating pill formulations that made them harder to crush and snort for a quick high. As bad as OxyContin is, heroin is worse, and the users of heroin are getting younger and younger. Heroin given intravenously is particularly dangerous because addicts may share needles, exposing themselves to bloodborne disease such as HIV and hepatitis, and can easily overdose when injecting heroin directly into their bloodstreams.

In Charlotte many of the opiate addicts in the Carolinas Clinic started with powerful painkillers prescribed after surgery or a broken bone. As doctors cut off their prescriptions and the black market supply withered, they turned to cheaper, easier-to-find heroin. The going rate for a tiny balloon filled with a dose of heroin is $9. A heavy user may take up to 10 doses a day. In contrast, prescription pain pills containing OxyContin sell for up to $1/mg—$80 for an 80 mg pill.

Thus, once considered an urban drug, heroin has found an unwelcomed home in small towns and suburbs. With the introduction of street drugs came the crime wave. The addicts will do almost anything for a quick dollar, stealing from parents and committing burglaries.

LEARNING TERRORIST PREVENTATIVE TACTICS FROM ISRAEL

Israel is perhaps one of the most targeted nations for terrorists, and per capita it has lost more citizens to terrorist attacks than any other nation (8). As a result, it has spent years developing ways to prevent terrorist plots before they occur. One method is to instill in Israelis a keen awareness of their surroundings. In the 1970s, schoolchildren were taught in the classroom to avoid loaves of bread and cigarette packages on the ground because they could be booby trapped with bombs. People call the police whenever they see an unattended package, especially in airports, bus stations, and train stations, and the sight of a bomb robot is common now in the streets of Tel Aviv and Jerusalem.

In Israel things changed after the 1967 war in which they conquered East Jerusalem and tens of thousands more Arabs became residents of Israel. Jews and Arabs in the new territory mingled in ways they had not before, and Israelis sometimes had difficulty determining friend from foe. Some Jews of Arab or North African descent would wear the six-pointed Star of David as a talisman around their necks to signal that they were no threat. The mingling led to profiling in which Israeli security experts disseminate the characteristics of people who are far likelier threats of terrorist attacks than others. In Israel they won't check an old blond American woman but they will check a dark-skinned young guy who might be of North African descent. They compromise social values to be more efficient.

During the Palestinian uprising called the Second Intifada, suicide bombings killed hundreds of Israelis in cafes and restaurants from 2000 to 2005. In March 2002 alone, 139 Israelis were slain in such attacks. Another way Israel halted such bombings was by stopping them at their source: the Palestinian territory of the West Bank. Israel erected a fence between the West Bank and Israel that has effectively ended most unauthorized travel between the two sides. The state's most important tool for stopping terrorist plots is aggressive surveillance and infiltration of Palestinian society to find and stop the planners. In addition to electronic methods, Israel also employs a network of informants and spies who are recruited with cash. Acts of terrorism, like the bombings at the Boston Marathon in April 2013, may alter the behavior of ordinary US citizens in the future.

MORE WEIGHT → HIGHER AIRFARES

Samoa Air, a tiny South Pacific airline, charges passengers based on their weight, namely 42¢ a pound for each flight (9). Samoans are renowned for their weight. According to the World Health Organization, about 55% of the country's population over 20 years of age is considered obese. Only Nauru and Tonga have a higher percentage, namely 71% and 60%, respectively. The US ranks fourth, 32%, followed by Australia and United Kingdom, each 25%. In contrast, China is 6%. These are 2008 figures.

OCEAN ACIDIFICATION

According to Dan Vergano (10), the ocean's water is shifting toward the acidic side driven by climate change, which has brought increasingly corrosive seawater to the surface along the West Coast of the USA. Normally, plankton in the ocean suck up carbon dioxide via photosynthesis, and the more carbon dioxide they ingest, the less warming of the atmosphere. When those sea plants die, they fall to the depths and some of the consumed carbon ends up dissolved in deep ocean waters. The ocean water in the depths is 3 times more acidic than that near the surface. In addition, the ocean absorbs 23% of all human-made carbon dioxide emitted into the air by burning coal, oil, and other fossil fuels, according to a 2012 *Earth System Science Data* report—more than 8 billion tons of the stuff every year. When conditions are right, strong winds blowing over ocean water along steep coasts, such as along the West Coast of North America, generate "upwelling" of the deep waters.

The more acidic the ocean, the fewer shellfish develop. In recent times, baby oysters grown in some Pacific Coast hatcheries were dying en masse. The entire West Coast oyster business faced collapse without the larvae that seeds the shellfish. The shellfish farmers in 2008 began figuring out that the deep ocean water being more acidic was coming to the surface and was likely dissolving the fragile young oysters. Without industrial emissions of greenhouse gases, however, the upwelling would not be a problem because really corrosive water would not get high enough to reach the surface. It is the extra kick from human-made carbon that is pushing the saturation point higher. Shellfish rely on calcium to build their shells, and more corrosive water makes that harder for them to the point of becoming impossible. Some seawater scientists in 2012 definitively showed that those deep waters do dissolve baby oysters only a few days old, ones which rely on a very soft form of calcium for their initial growth spurt. More carbon in the air means more carbon in the ocean.

Deep water upwelling is not a problem so far on the US's East Coast, but warmer waters there have shifted crab and fish populations, while acidic mud on the main seafloor has hurt clamming. The acidification taking place in the waters along the US West Coast guarantees the same for the rest of the world's oceans in the years ahead.

US UNEMPLOYMENT

As John Cassidy emphasized (11), 12 million Americans are out of work, 8 million are working part-time for economic reasons, and 2.5 million say they want a job but have given up looking. At the start of 2008, when the recession began, the civilian population of the US aged 16 and up (and excluding prisoners and members of the armed forces) was 232.6 million, of whom 154.1 million were in the labor force, that is, they were working or looking for work. Over the past 5 years the working-age population has grown steadily. In February 2013, it was 244.8 million, an increase of 12.2 million since 2008. But the labor force has hardly grown at all. In March 2008, it stood at 155.5 million, a rise of just 1.4 million in 5 years. The proportion of the population in the labor force has fallen

from 66.2% in January 2008 to 63.5% in February 2013. That fall off may not sound very dramatic. If the participation rate, however, were still at its level of 5 years ago, there would be 162.1 million people in the labor force instead of 155.5 million. Thus, as many as 6.6 million workers have vanished from the economy, robbing it of their efforts, skills, and creativity. The result is more personal hardship, a weaker gross domestic growth, lower spending, and less wealth creation.

MOBILE PHONE AT FORTY

It was 1973 when inventor Martin Cooper made the first call on a mobile phone using a prototype Motorola DynaTac (12). The original DynaTac was 10 inches long and weighed 2.5 pounds. The world now has 6 billion cell phone subscribers, and more and more of them are moving into the realm of smartphones. Most modern smartphones weigh between 4 and 6 ounces. Smartphones have changed the world.

E = MC^2: EINSTEIN'S BIG IDEA

A 90-minute *Nova* video has traced the development of the theory establishing the connection between energy, matter, and light (13). The "squared" portion of the theory of *Albert Einstein* (1879–1955) was presaged by *Émilie du Châtelet* (1706–1749), a brilliant and rebellious daughter of Louis XIV's secretary. She discovered advanced math at the age of 23, fell in love with Voltaire, and began an institution to rival the Royal Academy. She dared to challenge Isaac Newton's gravity thesis as "flawed." An experiment of the Dutch scientist *Willem 's Gravesande* convinced du Châtelet that the energy of an object is a function of the square of its speed. In 19th-century London, the very notion of "energy" had not yet crystallized. Energy was thought of in terms of disconnected powers or forces, unique to various materials and activities. *Michael Faraday*, a blacksmith's son, became a lab assistant to *Sir Humphry Davy*, the great physicist of that era. He dumbfounded his mentor by articulating the theory that electrical current "emanated outwards" from wires, rather than flowing through them like water through a pipe. The result was the invention of a primitive electric motor—and new physics.

Einstein grew up in the world of electricity at a time when scientists thought that all forms of energy had been discovered. Far from a model student, he was "obsessed" with the nature of light. The speed of light was computed before the 19th century, but no one knew what light actually was. Einstein, who suffered from poverty and was unable to secure promotion in his job, published five major articles in 1905 establishing the speed of light as a cosmic speed limit and postulating that energy becomes mass at a speed of light. The formula E = mc^2 expresses the unity of matter, energy, and light.

Theoretical physicist *Max Planck* (1858–1947), who originated the quantum theory, encouraged the world's leading physicists to take Einstein seriously. In short order, E = mc^2 became the Holy Grail of scientific research, and Einstein won the Nobel Prize in physics in 1921.

Einstein thought it would take 400 more years of research to develop applications of his theory, but he had not banked on a young Jewish woman in Hitler's Germany, *Lisa Meitner*. She and her collaborator, *Otto Hahn*, studied the atom, about which little was known. As a result of her work, she became the first German woman ever to achieve the title of professor. On the brink of major discoveries she was forced to flee the Nazis, but she continued her collaboration with Hahn by letter. They felt that if they could add neutrons to the 238 in the nucleus of uranium, they could make a heavier element. Hahn's experiments kept producing lighter ones. Eventually, Meitner realized that the uranium atom had become so large it had split. She and her nephew, *Otto Frisch*, published the first article on nuclear fission, but Hahn was given all the credit and the Nobel Prize.

Einstein's theory not only led to the development of the atomic bomb, but also explained the birth of the universe—pure energy becoming matter in the Big Bang—and the process by which stars burn, giving off energy, eventually leading to the emergence of life.

EDITORS, JOURNALISTS, AND PUBLISHERS

I have been a newspaper junkie for decades. I subscribe to *The Dallas Morning News, The Wall Street Journal, USA Today, Barron's,* and several magazines. Additionally, I have collected a number of books on famous newspaper editors/publishers/writers, including Joseph Pulitzer, William Randolph Hearst, Eugene Meyer *(Washington Post),* James A. Wechsler *(New York Post),* Richard H. Meeker, Vermont Royster *(The Wall Street Journal),* Eric Sevareid, Ralph McGill *(Atlanta Journal Constitution),* Hedley Donovan *(Time),* and James Reston. Studying some of their comments, I believe, has helped me in my own editing endeavors.

One of my favorites through the years has been Al Neuharth (Allen Herald Neuharth), who started *USA Today* in 1982 (14). He was born on March 22, 1924, in a German-speaking household in South Dakota, growing up in Eureka and Alpena. His father died when Al was 2, and his mother raised him and his brother by washing dishes and taking in laundry. He was a sergeant in the infantry in World War II and then went to college at the University of South Dakota in Vermillion, where he worked on the college newspaper. After graduation he was hired as a reporter for the Associated Press, but he decided to start his own newspaper by launching a weekly called *SoDak Sports* to cover South Dakota sports in unprecedented detail. In 1954, he moved to Florida to work at the *Miami Herald.* In 1963, he joined Gannett, becoming president in 1970 and chief executive officer in 1973. In the years that followed, Gannett became the most profitable newspaper company in history. In 1982, he started *USA Today,* which in actuality reinvented the American newspaper and set the stage for digital storytelling.

He emphasized that a newspaper must reflect all its readers. He had seen his own mother work for less pay than what men got. Gannett, accordingly, put unprecedented numbers of women and minorities in important jobs. Neuharth tried to shatter those barriers not only inside the newsroom but in the pages of the newspaper itself, where diversity in images and content was stressed from the top.

Selling *USA Today* to Gannett's board of directors was not easy in the shaky economy of the early 1980s. Neuharth chose the name, picked the editors, and approved the newspaper box, designed to look like a television set. Just 2 years after *USA Today* was launched, it was losing $340,000 a day. To raise *USA Today's* profile, Neuharth toured 50 states during "BusCapades" in 1987; the next year he visited 32 countries on a "JetCapade" to meet world leaders. In 1989, he retired as Gannett chairman but started a column that appeared every Friday; since 1989, he wrote over 1000 of them. One Friday in April 2013, I searched for Al's column and it was not there. The next day I learned that he had died.

Al Neuharth was a colorful and controversial figure, but his *USA Today* became the most read newspaper in the country after several years. It surpassed for a time *The Wall Street Journal,* which has subsequently recouped that position. Nevertheless, the fantastic graphics and color of *USA Today* forced most newspapers around the country to change the appearances of their papers. He taught me that most medical publications do not need to be as long as they are. *The American Journal of Cardiology* (AJC) publishes, for example, more articles each year than any other cardiovascular journal in the world, including publishing the most tables and figures. It is the text that is primarily shortened. (I became editor of the AJC the same year that *USA Today* was launched.) I will miss you, Al.

BROTHERS

My brother and I are quite different and almost from the beginning went our separate ways. It was a bit hard for me to understand how two boys growing up with the same parents and raised by the same mother could be so different. Thus, I was elated to see the recent book entitled *Brothers* by George Howe Colt, who demonstrated that differences among siblings are not nearly as rare as I had thought. He gives numerous examples of major differences: the *Robespierres* (Maximilien became the rigid, merciless overlord of the Reign of Terror, known to supporters as the "Incorruptible"; his younger brother, Augustine, became a self-indulgent lover of luxury known to friends as "BonBon"); the *Melvilles* (Gansevoort became a dutiful, responsible lawyer; his younger brother, Herman, became a world traveler and iconoclastic writer known to the family as "The Runaway Brother"); the *Carters* (sober and pious Jimmy became president; his younger brother, Billy, played the court jester and drunken buffoon); the *Browns* (John was the cynical hard-drinking Rhode Island slave trader, and his idealistic abstentious younger brother, Moses, became a leading Quaker abolitionist); the *Capones* (Al became the most powerful gangster in Prohibition-era Chicago, and his eldest brother, Vincenzo, was town marshal and Boy Scout commissioner in a small town in Nebraska and a prohibition enforcement agent responsible for busting up illegal stills).

Colt asked, "How can siblings, who share so much genetically and environmentally, be so different?" Studies in the past 3 decades of intelligence, personality, interests, attitudes, and psychopathology have concluded that siblings raised in the same family are, in fact, almost as different from each other as unrelated people raised in separate families. Paradoxically, Colt indicates that the longer they live with each other, the more different siblings become.

Colt shows that biological siblings share, on average, half their genes; if personality traits were entirely genetic, siblings would be 50% similar and 50% different—even before factoring in the effects of being raised in the same family by the same parents. But biological siblings have personality correlations, according to Colt, of about 15%! (Even identical twins have only about a 50% overlap.) Although siblings share about half of each other's genes, not only is the genetic contribution of each parent halved, but the sequence of those shared genes is re-arranged through a process called *recombination*. The behavioral geneticist *David Lykken* observed that siblings are like people who receive telephone numbers with the same digits arranged in a different sequence. Just as those telephone numbers, when dialed, result in entirely different connections, genes that have been scrambled will express themselves in widely different personalities.

According to Colt, there is a growing amount of research suggesting that siblings may be influenced most strongly by the things they do not share: birth order, age, friends, teachers, and the vagaries of chance. And they do not even really share the things that they appear to have in common—if not identical genes, then seemingly identical parents, homes, and often schools—because each of them perceives these things differently. Psychologists have indicated that the experience of each child within a family is so distinct that each grows up in his own unique "micro-environment"; in effect, each sibling grows up in a different family.

Colt's *Brothers* is a terrific book—brilliantly conceived, daringly organized, endlessly fascinating. Colt, nearly 60, is second in a line of four brothers. They have no sisters. The book is part family memoir, part celebrity biography, and part recapitulation of research about sibling dynasties. The celebrities include not only Edwin and John Wilkes Booth and John and Will Kellogg, but also Vincent and Theo van Gogh, John and Henry David Thoreau, and the Marks brothers, with brief mentions of the Kennedys (four brothers) and the Eisenhowers (six brothers), among others.

Edwin and John Wilkes Booth. Edwin and John Wilkes Booth, <5 years apart, are described in detail. Their father, Junius Brutus Booth, lived two different lives. On the stage he was the greatest American actor of his day, a man of prodigious talent. He also was a drunkard, was intermittently insane, and tried to kill himself at least twice. His other life was a relatively sane one in a four-room log cabin in rural Maryland 3 miles from his nearest neighbor and 25 miles from the nearest theater. Here Booth created a 150-acre sanctuary with dairy, stables, vineyard, orchard, vegetable garden, and swimming pond, to which he could retreat between professional engagements. Here he was known as "Farmer Booth." Here he was a devoted family man to Maryann and their 10 children, six of whom would survive childhood. Booth, unlike most Marylanders, refused to own slaves. He believed that men's souls were reborn into animals' bodies and thus forbade the eating of meat or fish or

the felling of trees or the picking of flowers. The Booth children were not permitted to see doctors. Their illnesses were treated by home remedies. The boy who grew up to commit the most infamous murder in American history was raised as a vegetarian, forbidden to kill even a mouse or to brand a cow for the pain it would cause the animal.

Edwin Booth, the older son, grew up on the road with his father, forced to fend for himself from early on. When his older brother, June, outgrew the task, Edwin was taken from school at the age of 13 to storm the country as his father's dresser and to keep his father sober for the show, sometimes locking him in his hotel room on the day of a performance and after the final curtain tailing him down to waterfront bars and waiting outside before helping his father back to the hotel. When his father was overtaken by madness, Edwin was expected to lure him back to sanity. Edwin listened to the play night after night through the keyhole of the dressing room in which he had been left with his schoolbooks. Edwin made his first professional on-stage appearance at 15. After caring for his father for 5 years on the road, Edwin started his own career and by the time Lincoln had been elected president, Edwin was the nation's most respected and admired actor.

Edwin never had a childhood, unlike John Wilkes, called "Johnny" by his family, who enjoyed a perpetual adolescence right up to his death at the age of 26. While Edwin was babysitting his father in cities and towns across the country, Johnny was being spoiled by his mother on the farm. While Edwin grew up in the company of men traveling by stagecoach on muddy roads, eating and sleeping in flea-ridden beds at theatrical boarding houses, Johnny spent most of his time with his older sister, Asia, who later would devote much of her adult life to writing about her father and brothers in an effort to restore the family name.

If Junius Brutus Booth had been born 150 years later, he would likely have been diagnosed as bipolar. It seemed, according to Colt, as if Edwin and John had inherited a different pole. Edwin was shy, somber, introspective, and frequently depressed. He rarely smiled. His laugh was soundless. John Wilkes (Johnny) reflected his father's maniac side. From childhood he was gregarious, headstrong, and unpredictable. He told his sister, "Don't let us be sad. Life is so short and the world is so beautiful. Just to breathe is delicious." While Edwin liked being alone, Johnny preferred a crowd. He made friends easily and at school became the magnetic center of a circle of boys. Edwin Booth had a profound melancholy; Johnny had an "exaggeration of spirit, almost a wildness." But Johnny seemed the sanest of the Booth children. Edwin grew up expecting *doom*; Johnny grew up expecting *glory*, believing he was destined for fame.

There was another factor that made it seem as if Edwin and John had been born into different families: John Wilkes was his parent's favorite child. Johnny was easy to love: cheerful, charismatic, exuberant, and handsome to the point of beauty. Johnny most resembled, of all the children, his high-spirited father in looks and manner, a fact that surely contributed to his "favorite" status. As an adolescent, Johnny spent his time playing cards, getting drunk, starting fights, skipping school, and pulling pranks. (According to Freud a person who has been the indisputable favorite of his mother keeps for life the feeling of a conqueror, that confidence of success that often induces real success.)

John Wilkes Booth was 9 when Edwin Booth first left home to tour with his father. Johnny was 18 when Edwin returned. Although John admired Edwin, and Edwin, like almost everyone who met John, couldn't help liking his younger brother, they hardly knew each other. Edwin began helping John, casting his brother in several Shakespeare plays. At first, John's acting was crude and lacked confidence; he stuttered and forgot his lines. But Edwin stuck with him and at every opportunity covered up his mistakes, arranging the staging so John was never out of range of the footlights, and gave him more prominent billing than his experience warranted. It was on Edwin's recommendation that John, after only 3 years, was hired for the first time as a leading man.

Several biographers have explained Lincoln's assassination as an extreme case of sibling rivalry, suggesting that John was a second-rate thespian who, realizing he would never eclipse his older brother Edwin and inherit the paternal mantel, was driven to seek fame on another stage. A proud man accustomed to getting his way, he may have resented being given direction by Edwin in their early joint appearances. John was realistic about his own acting, apparently, and in awe of Edwin's. If there was a theatrical sibling rivalry, John had no doubt who was the winner. Although John Wilkes Booth is now remembered only as Lincoln's assassin, at the time of his death he was one of the most popular actors in the USA, with reviews as glowing as those of any other performer excepting perhaps his brother Edwin. John T. Ford, owner of the theater in which Lincoln was killed, observed, "Doubtless he [John Wilkes] would have been the greatest actor of his time if he had lived."

John was all raw instinct and undisciplined bravado. If the brothers' acting style differed, so too did their motivations. Edwin sought excellence; John wanted renown. Edwin was a student of the theater and worked exceedingly hard; John had little patience for hard work and was easily bored. If Edwin was most comfortable alone in his study, John was most at home at the center of a party, telling stories, playing practical jokes, chatting expansively about politics, literature, war, nature, and the theater. He was a familiar sight in Washington's bars, billiard rooms, 10-pin alleys, shooting galleries, and brothels. John was often described as "the most handsome man in America." Like Edwin, John had wavy black hair, fair skin, an aquiline nose, and unnaturally long eyelashes, and he was an inch taller than Edwin and far more muscular (he exercised regularly) and sported a thick mustache. John was besieged by adoring female fans at stage doors, received 100 love letters a week from women he had never met, and was propositioned by women of every social station. His first biographer described him as "one of the world's most successful lovers." The treasurer at the Ford Theater where Lincoln was shot described John Wilkes as one of the simplest, sweetest-disposition, and most lovable men he ever knew.

Even as John's theatrical fame grew, he longed for a more tangible form of glory. Edwin's heroes were the great actors of the past. John Wilkes admired the abolitionist John Brown for his daring. The brothers surprisingly shared a deep fraternal devotion. If John was in awe of Edwin's discipline and talent, Edwin would have liked to possess some of John's easy charm.

In the Civil War, the two brothers took different sides. Edwin, who had spent much of his life in the West and Northeast and whose friends were Northerners, naturally sided with the Union. John had grown up in Maryland, where slavery seemed to be the status quo everywhere except on the Booth farm. During his 2 years in military school, he was friends with the sons of some of the South's most prominent slave-owning families—in a region where, in the 1860 election, only 1 in every 40 votes was cast for Lincoln. John was passionately, virulently for the South. The restrained, circumspect elder brother Edwin was a Northerner, and the impetuous feather-ruffling rebellion-loving younger brother a Southerner. John had a Southern gentlemen's patrician sense of social order, reinforced by the sense of entitlement he enjoyed as the family favorite.

It is not clear when John Wilkes decided to assassinate Lincoln. His sister, Asia, thinks when Richmond fell on April 3, something in her brother snapped. Ten days later, on the night of April 14, while Edwin was on stage in the Boston theater, John entered Lincoln's box at Ford's Theater, held his single-shot Philadelphia derringer pistol 2½ feet from the back of the president's head, and pulled the trigger.

While on the run through the forest and swamps of Maryland and Northern Virginia after killing Lincoln—cold, wet, hungry, and feverish, with a broken leg—John still believed that his act would win him a place among the pantheon of heroes. He was devastated to learn that his act was reviled throughout the USA. Although many people refused to believe that the charismatic John Wilkes Booth could be the assassin, the moment Edwin Booth heard of the president's death and read in the newspaper of the brandished dagger, the cry "*sic semper tyrannis!*" and the leap to the stage, he recognized his brother's histrionic touch. Just as John early in his career had resented being known as Edwin's brother, now Edwin resented being John's brother. Seeking fame for himself, John had inadvertently made Edwin even more famous. In 1889, Edwin founded the Players Club, a gathering place for actors on Gramercy Park South, where he lived in two rooms upstairs. Four years later when he suffered a massive stroke and died at the age of 59, there was a portrait of John on his bedside table.

John and Will Kellogg. In the Calhoun County Courthouse in Southern Michigan in 1917, the plaintiff and defendant in *Kellogg vs. Kellogg* were brothers. The plaintiff, John Harvey Kellogg, the man everyone called "the Doctor," was the flamboyant founder and director of the Battle Creek Sanitarium, a combination spa, hospital, Chautauqua where the well-heeled came to see and be seen as they followed a customized regimen of rest, exercise, and diet. A short (62 inches), plump, 65-year-old Banty rooster of a man, the "Doctor" dressed all in white "to allow more of the health-giving rays of the sun to reach his body." The only person in the courtroom the ebullient doctor didn't try to charm was the defendant, 57-year-old Will Kellogg, known as "W.K.," the founder and president of the Toasted

Corn Flake Company, the rapidly growing business that would one day be known as Kellogg's. The "Corn Flake King," as he was dubbed by the press, was a bald, short (67 inches), beady-eyed, moon-faced man who wore a rumpled suit, Coke-bottle glasses, and a dour expression. Only a few incisive words escaped his pursed lips. During a recess after W.K. had testified, one of the Doctor's lawyers was heard to say, "Don't ask him anything else. He is too smart." In the courtroom the brothers ignored each other. Indeed, for most of the previous decade, the Doctor and W.K. had communicated almost entirely in lawsuits. The case boiled down to one simple question: "which brother had the right to the family name." As in any sibling rivalry, the roots of the conflict went deep.

Growing up in Battle Creek, Michigan, not long after the Civil War, John and Will Kellogg seemed unlikely rivals. Of the 14 children born to John Preston Kellogg, a devout Seventh-Day Adventist who owned a small broom factory, John Harvey, the tenth child, was the most promising. John, the runt of a large litter, made up for his frailty with Napoleonic assertiveness. He was outgoing, headstrong, and ambitious. While his brothers were playing outside, John played the piano and violin, wrote poetry, and made up stories where he cast himself as the hero. He considered games a waste of time. He attended school for only 2 years to work 10-hour shifts in his father's factory, sorting broom corn for $2 a day. John educated himself. He soon exhausted his parents' meager collection of books and began borrowing from neighbors. Words fascinated him. (As an adult he carried a vest-pocket dictionary to peruse in his spare moments.)

The twelfth Kellogg child, Will was uncompromising, cautious, deliberate, and taciturn. A teacher at the Adventist school he attended through the fifth grade assumed he was "dim-witted" because he couldn't read the words on the blackboard. Finally, at 20 he got glasses. Will wasn't much to look at either. But he was a plugger. At the age of 7 he was working as a stock boy at his father's factory after school and on Sundays. On summer mornings, he uprooted, bunched, and washed vegetables for the local market. The summer he was 9, he pulled and topped 350 bushels of Bermuda onions. He was paying for his own clothing at age 10 and supporting himself at 14. There was little time for fun. Later in life he said "I never learned to play." He felt especially self-conscious and inadequate next to his cocksure older brother who rarely let Will forget the 8 years that lay between them. John made Will shine his shoes. He made Will mind his manners. If Will complained, John gave him a whipping.

The Kelloggs weren't the only ones who considered John promising. The family shared a pew at the Battle Creek Tabernacle with elder James White and his wife, Ellen. Impressed by 12-year-old John Kellogg, the Whites invited him to learn the printer's trade at the Adventist publishing plant, where John advanced rapidly from errand boy to apprentice typesetter to proofreader. At 16, he was editing the *Advent Review and Sabbath Herald*. As he worked on various Adventist publications, John was intrigued by the church's minimalistic approach to nutrition. He decided to become a vegetarian. John became the Whites' protégé, living with them for months at a time, helping Pastor White with his writing.

In 1866, the Whites opened a small medical boardinghouse where ailing guests convalesced on a regime of rest, exercise, and hydrotherapy along with a diet of fruits, vegetables, graham bread, and water. But the Western Health Reform Institute, as it was called, didn't attract many customers, and the Whites decided they needed a first-rate physician to distinguish it from the other spas and water cure establishments that were springing up across the country. The Whites sent John to Belleview Hospital Medical College, and he graduated in 1875. The following year they made him physician-in-chief of the faltering institute. John, only 24 years old, changed the name to Battle Creek Sanitarium and added a barrage of new treatments, including massage, calisthenics, electrical stimulation, deep-breathing exercises, and surgery. He led sing-a-longs and played his violin. He wrote pamphlets and magazine articles describing the work. Within 2 years, business at "The San," as people called it, was so good that John tore down the old farmhouse and built a 5-story Victorian building enough for 200 patients—the largest building in Battle Creek.

Will was also singled out by the Whites but for a less exalted position. While John was dissecting cadavers in New York City, 14-year-old Will was driving a horse and cart across Southern Michigan peddling his father's brooms. Though painfully shy, Will was a determined salesman who rarely took no for an answer. When Will's father broke his hip, he put Will in charge of the family business. He did so well that 2 years later when the Whites needed someone to manage a struggling Adventist broom factory, they sent Will. Supervising 60 men 1000 miles from home was a challenge for a shy 19-year-old, but Will turned the company around within a year. Back in Battle Creek, he took a course in bookkeeping at the local business college and prepared to marry his long-time girlfriend, a grocer's daughter he called "Puss." In April 1880, John Harvey Kellogg asked his younger brother to come work for him at the San.

By 1900, the Battle Creek Sanitarium was the largest and most popular spa in the country with 400 guestrooms, two indoor swimming pools, a surgical hospital, a 1000-seat chapel, 20 cottages, a lakeside resort, and 400 acres of farmland. Here some 3000 patients a year pursued what John Harvey Kellogg called "biologic living," described in one San brochure as "daily cold water and air baths, swimming, work in the gymnasium, wearing of light and porous clothing and frequent changes of underwear." The Doctor believed that the key to happiness lay in a healthy diet—defined at the San largely by what people couldn't eat: meat ("only proper food for hyenas and turkey buzzards," said the Doctor), tobacco ("destroys the sex glands"), coffee ("cripples the liver"), ice cream ("unnatural"), vinegar ("a poison, not a food"), oysters ("swarming with bacteria"), bouillon, tea, sugar, cheese, chocolate, alcohol, and spices, to name a few. San cuisine consisted largely of nuts and grains. The San offered 26 basic tithes, but each guest had his or her own customized plan. Ever since the Doctor had visited a colony of orangutans in Algeria and noticed that our primate cousins defecate almost continuously, he had maintained that frequent bowel movements were the key to what he called "getting the stomach right." Not all patients had the fortitude for the recommended five enemas a day, a regiment made possible with the help of a high-speed machine capable, according to the proud Doctor, of forcing 15 gallons of water through the intestines in a matter of minutes. Between meals—and enemas—patients submitted to massages, exercises, hydrotherapies, electric light baths, salt scrubs, etc. At the end of each day, patients gathered on the roof where the Doctor led them in a series of elaborate marching patterns and the official San song, "The Battle Creek Sanitarium March." Although the "biologic living" sounded a bit joyless, there were gym classes, cooking classes, folk dancing classes, greenhouse tours, Indian club demonstrations, picnics, bird walks, sledding and sleigh rides, and nonsectarian weekly church services.

The Doctor was the wizard behind the vegetarian Oz. His goal was to change the way Americans ate, breathed, dressed, exercised, and defecated. To that end, he churned out nearly 50 books, more than 200 medical papers, and so many pamphlets for the lay reader that even the publicity-conscious Doctor couldn't keep count. He founded a nursing school, a school of hygiene, a liberal arts college, and a medical school, which provided the San with a steady stream of low-paid employees. He helped establish more than 30 San franchises across the country. He gave more than 5000 lectures. He made frequent trips abroad to examine the latest exercise equipment or to study advanced surgical techniques or to learn about new bowel cleaning methods. He invented a heated operating table, a vibrating chair that increased blood circulation, an electric belt that massaged the hips, a mechanical exercise horse, a machine that kneaded the abdomen to relieve constipation, and a canvas sleeve that brought fresh air into a patient's bedroom at night without chilling the entire room. An ostentatiously prodigious worker, the Doctor rose at 4:00 AM for an enema, a cold bath, and calisthenics before launching into a 24-hour workday. He bragged of composing between 25 and 50 letters a day, of dictating 18 hours at a stretch, of working 40 hours straight without nourishment, and of performing as many as 25 operations in a day. (He was an accomplished gastrointestinal surgeon, and his precise stitching moved the director of The Johns Hopkins Hospital to remark, "I have never seen such beautiful human needlework.") The Doctor was a skilled multitasker. While taking his morning bath, he listened to staff reports; while dictating, he polished off a few medical journals.

The Doctor percolated with ideas but he depended on Will to carry them out. The Doctor was the San's artistic director, Will its stage manager. The Doctor had hired his brother because he needed a hard worker who was not only good with numbers but willing to do what he was told. Will did everything at the San and was paid poorly by his brother. To support Puss and their three children, Will also took care of a neighbor's house for an additional $3 a week to supplement his $6 a week salary from his brother. Even so, Will went into debt. Will's duties rapidly expanded. By 1900, not only was he responsible for billing, pricing, and purchasing, but he managed Modern Medicine Publishing and a half dozen other companies his brother had

set up to sell his health foods, surgical devices, and exercise machines. He answered the San mail—some 60 to 100 letters a day. He was the unofficial credit manager, a member of the labor committee, a volunteer security guard, and, on occasion, a hospital orderly. Each afternoon he was besieged by wealthy patients requesting extra services; disgruntled employees airing complaints; financially strapped patients seeking discounts on their bills. The Doctor had strict admission standards: no one contagious, no one on a stretcher, no one who looked sick. His ideal patients were overweight or neurasthenic women and overworked and dyspeptic men.

Will might not have minded serving his brother had his contributions been acknowledged. The Doctor never named him business manager, never gave him a title or a job description during his 25 years at the San. It rankled him that he worked there 10 years before his brother allowed him an office, and he worked for 14 years before his brother paid him enough to enable him to get out of debt. It rankled him that, like the 1000 other employees, he was expected to call his brother "Dr. Kellogg." Dr. Kellogg didn't seem to notice that he was humiliating Will. Will worked for 7 years before the Doctor allowed him a vacation. But, the Doctor treated most people that way. The Doctor found it nearly impossible to apologize, admit a mistake, or delegate. He was a czar and a law unto himself, ignoring his associates and subordinates, recalled Will. John was envious of Will for being 5 inches taller; Will envied John for being a doctor. Family members said that Will dreamed of becoming a physician himself but was so busy supporting his family on the meager salary his brother paid him that he never had the opportunity.

The brothers' antipathy was intensified by their differences: the Doctor in fancy white and Will in drab, baggy, inexpensive suits; the Doctor escorted by a convoy of nurses and Will working behind the scenes, a quiet, almost furtive presence; the Doctor expressing himself in hyperbolic verbal torrents and Will speaking slowly and carefully when he spoke at all. The brothers who lived only a few blocks from each other rarely socialized. The Doctor, something of an intellectual snob, spent his spare time hobnobbing with the celebrities who frequented the San. Will, embarrassed at never having gotten beyond sixth grade, spent his with Puss and their children. The Doctor treated his wife, Ella Eaton, more like a business associate than a wife. They spent their honeymoon revising the Doctor's new books. The Doctor believed that sex bred disease and bragged that he and Ella never consummated their marriage and never intended to. Fearful of germs, he tended to shy away from physical contact of any kind. Over the years, however, the Doctor and his wife took in 42 abandoned or needy children, at least nine of whom they formally adopted. Convinced that a healthy diet and proper upbringing could trump any hereditary deficits, the Doctor treated his "waifs," as he called them, more like research subjects than loved sons and daughters. Housed in dormitories on the far side of "The Residence," the Doctor's 20-room Queen Ann mansion, they were raised and homeschooled by Ella and a cadre of San staffers on a modified biologic living schedule of vegetarian meals, chores, and calisthenics. (In the late 1880s,

Ella, who served as San dietician in addition to overseeing the Doctor's adoptees, had a nervous breakdown and lived as a semi-invalid until her death in 1920.)

Whenever the Doctor patronized him or overturned one of his orders to the staff, Will fumed. Will, however, had grown accustomed to living in the shadow of his genius brother. In 1883, a few years after Will came to work for his brother, the Doctor established an experimental kitchen in the basement of the San, where the brothers tried to create palatable recipes from the nuts and grains that dominated the San diet. Over the next 20 years, more than 80 different culinary confections would emerge from the kitchen. The brothers followed their customary modus operandi: the Doctor jotted down his ideas and passed them along to Will, who, after his 15-hour workday, experimented into the night. At one point, Will developed yet another nut and grain concoction and took it to his brother for approval. In 1897, the Sanitarium Food Company, with Will as manager, offered 42 different kinds of biscuits, breads, crackers, and ersatz coffee, available by mail order for those who wished to practice biologic living at home.

In 1895, the brothers began manufacturing Granose Flakes in a barn behind the San. That first year, despite minimal promotion (the Doctor permitted Will to advertise only in San publications), they sold almost 57 tons. Will knew they could sell much more. The Doctor refused to let Will advertise nationally. In 1900, while the Doctor was away, Will visited several members of the San board of directors and told them that, given the opportunity, the San food business would someday be so large that the sanitarium itself would be a mere "side show." The board members agreed to let him build a small factory behind the sanitarium bakery to house the granose operation. When the Doctor returned from his trip and heard that the factory cost $50,000, he was furious. Saying he had not authorized the project, he insisted that his brother pay for it. Will, who had to beg friends and relatives for the money, eventually paid off the debt. But he never forgave his brother. And when a few months later the Doctor pressed ahead on moving the San business office, Will exploded. During the argument that followed, he quit. After 21 years at the San, Will would not find it easy to cut ties to his brother.

On February 18, 1902, 6 months after he left, the San burned to the ground. Having spent more than half of his life there, Will felt a responsibility to help rebuild the place in which he had invested so much. He offered to work without pay for "as long as my services were needed." The Doctor put him in charge of financing the new building. Fifteen months after the fire, during which Will had worked 18- to 24-hour days, a new San rose: a 6-story, 560-foot-long, 1220-bed Italian Renaissance edifice with mosaic marble floors, a solarium, a roof garden, a gymnasium, and a glass-domed courtyard filled with orchids, orange trees, and 20-foot banana palms.

Will might never had broken permanently with his brother had it not been for C.W. Post, a 36-year-old inventor, real estate broker, and blanket manufacturer from Fort Worth, who had arrived at the San in 1891 with a 10-gallon Stetson, an emaciated frame, and an empty bank account. Though he stayed at the San for 9 months and gained almost 50 pounds, Post pronounced his treatment a failure. In 1892, he opened a scaled-down cut-rate meat-serving version of the San across town. A few years later, Post—who had spent much of his time at the San sniffing around its experimental kitchen and peppering the staff with technical questions—began to market *Postum*, a bran and molasses coffee substitute that bore more than a passing resemblance to the Doctor's caramel cereal. By 1898, Postum sales totaled $840,000, and by 1903, they had risen to $10 million. Will was envious. Post was doing exactly what Will had urged the Doctor to do: pouring money into advertising and promotion. It galled Will to slave 16 hours a day for meager pay while others made fortunes pirating the San work. He begged his brother to let him take on the competition. The Doctor refused. Not only was he parsimonious by nature, he worried that associating his name with commercial advertising would jeopardize his reputation in the medical community. Will grew frustrated with his brother. At times they quarreled fiercely; at times they stopped speaking to each other.

Hoping at least to distinguish the San cereals from their imitators, Will suggested that they use *his* name on the packaging, making it clear that Will, not the Doctor, was endorsing the product and thereby protecting the Doctor from accusations of venality. The Doctor gave in. In 1903, these red-inked words began appearing on a few San products: "Beware of imitations—none genuine without the signature—W.K. Kellogg." It was the first step not only in differentiating San products from those of its competitors but in differentiating Will (or W.K. as he would soon be known to the world) from his brother.

In 1898, the Kellogg brothers had produced a flaked corn cereal, but it lacked flavor. In 1902, they added malt to their flakes, which gave them a richer, nuttier taste. The Doctor, however, discouraged promotion, insisting that their mail order sales were perfectly respectful. Fed up with his brother, galvanized by Post, Will forged ahead without the Doctor's permission. He sent salesmen door to door with free samples. He advertised in newspapers, put up street car signs, and sponsored store window displays. Reasoning that there were more well people in the world than sick, he marketed cornflakes as something tasty rather than something healthy. In 1905, while the Doctor was on a trip to Europe, Will did the unthinkable—he coated the flakes with sugar. When the Doctor returned, he had a fit but sales soared and the sugar stayed.

The end came when insurance executives came from St. Louis and offered to help finance a company devoted solely to cornflakes. Will presented the idea to his brother but the Doctor wasn't interested. Will offered to buy the cornflake rights from his brother; they haggled for 6 months before the Doctor, still in debt from the fire, settled for $35,000 cash and more than half the new company's stock. In February 1906, Will opened the Black Creek Toasted Corn Flake Company. Although Will was president and chief executive, the Doctor, as majority stockholder, retained the controlling interest. Not believing his brother's company would amount to much, the frugal Doctor distributed chunks of his stock to San physicians in lieu of salary increases before traveling to Russia to observe the work of a physiologist named *Ivan Pavlov*. He returned several months later to find that while he had been watching dogs salivate, his younger brother had been tracking down and buying up the stock that the Doctor had so cavalierly given away. Will now had the controlling interest in his own company. On the eve of his 46th birthday, he was no longer his brother's lackey.

Will Kellogg liked to say he was "an old man" when he finally went into business for himself, but he quickly made up for lost time. In his first year, he handed out 4 million free samples, convinced that once people tried his cornflakes, they would continue to buy them. He spent $30,000—one third of the company's initial working capital—on a single full-page ad in *Ladies Home Journal*. By the end of 1906, Will was indeed selling cornflakes by the carload. Although his plant burned down the following year, Will had a Chicago architect on site within 12 hours and a new fireproof plant in full production within 6 months. In 1907, while the Doctor was abroad, Will changed the name of his product to Kellogg's Toasted Corn Flakes. The Doctor was infuriated by his brother's success. Will wrote his brother, "For 22½ years I had absolutely lost all my individuality to you. I tried to see things with your eyes and do things as you would do them. You know in your heart whether or not I am a rascal. You also know whether or not I would defraud anyone, under any circumstances."

The war began in 1908 when the Doctor, claiming he had never liked the name, changed the Sanitas Nut Food Company to Kellogg Food Company. Will was outraged. The Doctor had never shown the slightest interest in using the Kellogg name on his products—indeed, he had insisted on not using it—until his brother began printing it on his cornflake boxes. This suit was settled the following year with an out-of-court compromise in which the Doctor agreed not to use the word Kellogg on any flake cereal food or display it conspicuously on any packaging. The truce lasted, however, only a few months. Their suits continued for a number of years. Even as they battled in court, the Kelloggs goaded each other to greater achievements. The San prospered in that magnificent new building Will's work had made possible. Its 1390 beds filled with movers and shakers, including Upton Sinclair, Henry Ford, Amelia Earhart, Johnny Weissmuller, Charles Edgar Welch, President William Howard Taft, and William Jennings Bryan.

The brothers later tried to rival each other in philanthropy. Each tried to give away more money than the other. The Doctor gave away his money as soon as it came in. Will let his money grow and then gave it away. The W.K. Kellogg Foundation became one of the largest charitable organizations in the US. The man who had never learned to play was determined that others might have the opportunity: he built schools, libraries, parks, playgrounds, swimming pools, gymnasiums, auditoriums, Boy Scout camps, hospitals, bird sanctuaries, and farms. Kellogg's was one of the first companies to institute 8-hour shifts and 5-day weeks and provide insurance, a health plan, and day care.

In all nonfraternal matters, Will preferred anonymity. Though he was now at least as famous as his brother, Will shunned publicity. He declined honorary degrees, refused to be listed in *Who's Who*, and rarely appeared at public gatherings,

especially those designed to honor him. If he couldn't avoid being present, he sat in the back row. He often traveled under a pseudonym to avoid being recognized. Asked to prepare a short autobiography, Will came up with a mere 16 sentences, dismissing his quarter century at the San in a single phrase: "Took a job in April 1880, continued same for 25 years."

Despite Will's success, he was an insomniac. Like the Doctor, Will rarely handed out compliments and didn't tolerate failure. He was a strict moralist who always interfered in his children's personal lives. Although he went out of his way to help his employees enjoy themselves, he didn't know how to do so himself. He replaced his modest stucco home with a 30-room Tudor mansion, complete with a seven-car garage, tennis court, croquet pitch, greenhouse, and 800-acre Arabian horse ranch in Southern California, a home in Palm Springs, an Italian style villa on the Gulf Coast of Florida, and an apartment building across the street from the San, from which he could keep an eye on his brother's operation. He began traveling and feasted on his forbidden favorites—lobster, chocolate, and oysters—despite suffering from gout. Despite his wealth, Will was no less shy than he had been as a boy. He appeared to always feel inadequate next to his charismatic brother. Will was always formal and self-conscious with his children, hugging them only when he knew no one was watching. He did not approve of strong feelings of any kind unless pets were concerned. He was considered by his friends to be a lonely, isolated individual.

For all his ebullience, the Doctor too was lonely. He had thousands of acquaintances around the world, many of them famous, but few close friends. After his wife died, he never re-married. He remained proudly and publicly celibate. He seemed hardly able to keep track of his adopted children.

As the brothers aged and their lawsuits faded into the past, their relationship seemed at times almost guardedly cordial. Pride, however, kept both brothers from reaching out far enough to forgive each other. Although rivalry usually mellows with age, this was not so with the Kellogg brothers. On October 3, 1942, Will called on his brother. At 90, the Doctor had difficulty hearing and, even with an eyepiece, could barely recognize himself in the photos he autographed for San guests. Eighty-two-year-old Will had been diagnosed with glaucoma 5 years earlier and was completely blind. He got around with the help of a white cane and a German shepherd. The conversation, which lasted more than 5 hours, did not go well. Will tried to convince his brother that he was too old to control the San. If he wasn't willing to relinquish control, then he should at least let an old Adventist colleague help him. The Doctor rejected his brother's advice. After 66 years running the place, he wasn't about to give up the San. The Doctor died at 91, and 3 years later at 85 years old, Will Kellogg resigned from the Kellogg board of directors, although he continued to keep track of each new advertisement, salary increase, and sales report. Although his children and grandchildren would have liked to visit more often, they were afraid to show up at his house without an invitation, and Will wasn't the inviting kind. He spent several Christmases alone with his household staff. He was, perhaps, closest to his nurse, who read aloud to him and listened to him talk about the vicissitudes of his life. Will expressed regrets several times that he and John Harvey never reconciled. At 91, on October 6, 1951, Will Kellogg died. Although he had outlived his brother by 8 years, he was 3 months younger than the Doctor when he had died. Will was buried next to his brother. In happier times, Will and the Doctor had put up matching twin monuments on their plots. At some point during their estrangement, however, Will had ordered his monument torn down and replaced by another: a bronzed sundial on which a robin tugged a worm out of the earth. Will, it seemed to say, was the proverbial early bird who got the worm—or at least before his brother got it.

In contrast to the Kellogg brothers, some famous brothers worked together beautifully: the *Wright* brothers ("Whatever it was they would do it together"); the *Mayo* brothers (Will and Charlie always remained as close as they had been in childhood, sharing a bank account and for a long time living next door to each other); and the *White* brothers (Sam, a physician, and Byron, a Supreme Court justice—Byron was asked once who he admired most: "My brother Sam" was his response) (16).

William C Roberts

WILLIAM CLIFFORD ROBERTS, MD
6 May 2013

1. Siegel A, Etzkorn I. *Simple: Conquering the Crisis of Complexity*. New York: Twelve, 2013 (237 pp.).
2. Vaillant GE. *Triumphs of Experience: The Men of the Harvard Grant Study*. Cambridge, MA: Belknap Press of Harvard University Press, 2012 (457 pp.).
3. Angell M. What is a good life? *New York Review*, May 9, 2013.
4. Burns S. Test your wealth with 4 questions. *Dallas Morning News*, March 31, 2013.
5. Reddy S. When email is part of the doctor's treatment. *Wall Street Journal*, March 26, 2013.
6. Dwaskin E. A global effort to stop designer drugs. *Bloomberg Businessweek*, April 18–21, 2013.
7. Leinwand Leger D. Heroin is back: your neighborhood could be next. *USA Today*, April 25, 2013.
8. Dorell O. In Israel, keeping your eyes open has become a way of life. *USA Today*, April 17, 2013.
9. Craymer L. Weigh more, pay more: Samoa Air pegs ticket prices to passenger pounds. *Wall Street Journal*, April 4, 2013.
10. Vergano D. How climate change threatens the seas—and yes, seafood. *USA Today*, March 28, 2013.
11. Cassidy J. Meet the 'missing millions' who've vanished from the economy. *Fortune*, April 8, 2013.
12. Molina B. Mobile phone at 40: one long shrinkage spurt. *USA Today*, April 4, 2013.
13. James S. Einstein's big idea: the story behind the world's most famous equation, E = mc². *Nova*, October 11, 2005. Available at http://www.youtube.com/watch?v=jqiRoKy0Gyo.
14. Colton D, Hampson R. *USA Today* just one Neuharth legacy. *USA Today*, April 22, 2013.
15. Colt GH. *Brothers. On His Brothers and Brothers in History*. New York: Scribner, 2012 (465 pp.).
16. Hutchinson DJ. *The Man Who Once Was Whizzer White. A Portrait of Justice Byron R. White*. New York: Free Press, 1998 (577 pp.).

Chapter 12

October 2013

ALTERNATIVE MEDICINE

That includes everything from herbal supplements to crystal healing and acupuncture. About 50% of Americans use alternative medicine and 10% use it on their children, according to Paul Offit, the author of *Do You Believe in Magic? The Sense and Nonsense of Alternative Medicine* (1). Consumers of alternative medicine range from healthy people who pop the occasional supplement, hoping to ward off a cold, for example, to the seriously ill, who turn over their life savings to gurus promising miracles. Offit indicates that alternative medicine is a $34 billion a year industry whose key players are adept at using lawsuits, lobbyists, and legislation to protect their market. More than 54,000 varieties of supplements are on the market. There is a Congressional Dietary Supplement Caucus of legislatures who look favorably on the industry. One congressman indicated that the alternative medicine industry is as tough as any industry lobbying in Washington. They want as little legislation as possible.

Alternative medicine proponents say it is popular because people want more control over their health. While some supplements are just high-priced placebos, others carry serious risks. Dietary supplements can be prescription medications in disguise. The most common offenders tend to be the "natural" supplements claiming to melt fat, build muscles, or boost sexual performance. The Food and Drug Administration (FDA) has found that hundreds of brands actually contain real drugs, including anabolic steroids and the active ingredient in Viagra. In April 2013, the FDA indicated that it had received 86 reports of illness and death due to body-building supplements that illegally contained a stimulant called DMAA, which is especially risky when combined with caffeine because it can raise the blood pressure with its consequences. The FDA in 2012 estimated that supplements cause 50,000 adverse reactions a year.

Some patients with serious illnesses delay proper therapy as they opt for alternative medicine. Apple founder Steve Jobs' faith in alternative medicine may have cost him his life. Jobs was diagnosed with pancreatic cancer in 2003, and although revered for his brilliant mind, chose to delay surgery for 9 months in favor of acupuncture, herbs, and special diets. Jobs eventually had surgery and, later, a liver transplant, but it was too late. He died in 2011, 8 years after diagnosis. According to his physician he had the only kind of pancreatic cancer that is treatable and curable.

According to Offit, consumers are often taken in by the outrageous claims of the supplement producers or because they fall victim to hucksters' charismatic personalities.

Many Americans also are unaware that supplements, unlike drugs, do not need to be approved by the FDA or tested for safety before going on the market! During all these years the FDA has banned only one supplement, namely Ephedra, which was taken off the market in 2004 after it was found to increase the risk of heart problems and death. The FDA's authority with supplements is mostly "reactive." The agency must wait for people to get hurt or die before it can remove an unsafe supplement from the market.

Beware of supplements!

MEDICAL SPAS

A piece by Melinda Beck indicates that states are tightening regulations on medical spas and wading into some disputes over where beauty treatments stop and the practice of medicine starts (2). Medical spas are fast-growing hybrids between day spas and doctors' offices. They typically offer Botox injections, facial peels, laser skin treatments, and other minimally invasive cosmetic procedures. Some even add breast implants, tummy tucks, and chin, face, brow, and eyelid lifts. The International Spa Association now counts 1750 medical spas across the US, up from 471 in 2003. Some of the growth comes from dermatologists and plastic surgeons adding such services and amenities to their practices. But physicians trained in unrelated specialties, such as obstetrics or orthopedics, also are supplementing their incomes with the lucrative procedures that rarely are covered by insurance. Most of the services are performed by nonphysicians.

State regulations vary widely. Only a few require medical spas to be licensed. In some states, procedures from laser hair removal to liposuction can be performed by nonphysicians. Most require physician oversight, though the physician does not necessarily have to be on site or even in the same state.

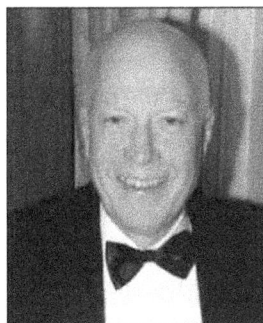

William C. Roberts, MD.

Some serious injuries have prompted crackdowns. Florida now requires that liposuctions removing >2 pounds of fat be performed in a state-licensed surgical center with emergency equipment on hand. A new state law in Maryland requires the state health department to oversee cosmetic surgery facilities. Pennsylvania is presently weighing tighter rules on who can provide laser treatments. Some of the push for more regulation is being driven by dermatologists who say allowing nonphysicians to perform cosmetic procedures puts physicians at risk. Only a few states require medical spas to report injuries.

Laws requiring physicians to perform procedures do not guarantee confidence either. Several groups have sprung up to teach cosmetic procedures to physicians from other fields. The National Society of Cosmetic Physicians, for example, advertises 2-day workshops on laser liposuction, breast augmentation, and tummy tucks. The proposed medical spa law in New York would require physicians advertising themselves as "board certified" to specify which board. This kind of medical business is obviously quite profitable to those who do it.

THE REAL CHOLESTEROL-LOWERING MAGIC BULLET

My friend, cardiologist Robert L. Rosenthal, sent me a *New York Times* piece entitled "Rare mutation ignites race for cholesterol drug" (3). The article by Gina Kolata describes the development and early testing of a monoclonal antibody, made in living cells, with the ability to lower the low-density lipoprotein (LDL) cholesterol (the bad one) to levels lower than they were at birth, to as low as 12 mg/dL. The story began about a decade ago when some French researchers published a note in *Nature Genetics* describing three generations of a family with extremely high LDL levels—up to 466—and a strong history of coronary heart disease. The researchers found that the family had a mutation in a gene called *PCSK9*, which slowed the body's ability to rid itself of LDL. The mutated gene leads to the soaring cholesterol levels.

The French study gave Jonathan C. Cohen and Helen H. Hobbs of the University of Texas Southwestern Medical Center in Dallas an idea. If a mutation in *PCSK9* could lead to high LDL levels, perhaps there were mutations that did the opposite, namely lead to very low levels of LDL and protect against atherosclerosis. Cohen and Hobbs found in data from a Dallas study that about 2.5% of blacks had a single mutated *PCSK9* gene that no longer functioned, and about 3.2% of whites had a less powerful mutation that hampered the gene but did not destroy it. Because people have two copies of every gene, one inherited from each parent, those with the newly discovered mutation did not have two mutated genes, but instead had one fully functioning *PCSK9* gene and one that was disabled. Blacks with the mutation ended up with LDL levels averaging 100 instead of the usual 138, a 28% reduction; whites with a less powerful mutation had LDL levels averaging 117, about 15% lower than average. The people with one disabled gene had lower than normal LDL levels for their entire lives. Hobbs and Cohen found that blacks aged 45 to 64 with a single mutated gene seemed almost immune to coronary heart disease during a 15-year follow-up, and whites, who had the less powerful

mutation, had a 46% reduction in the incidence of coronary heart disease. These findings led them to search for a mother and father who each carried the single mutated gene. They found one such couple and tested their daughter who had the rare double inheritance. The daughter was a 32-year-old aerobics instructor living in a Dallas suburb with her two young children. She was healthy. Her LDL was 14, a level unheard of in healthy adults. This aerobics instructor was only 1 of 2 people thus far found on planet Earth with the rare gene mutation inherited from both parents; the other person, a young healthy Zimbabwean woman, had an LDL of 15.

The discovery of the mutation and the two women with their extremely low LDL levels has set off one of the greatest medical chases ever among three pharmaceutical companies, Amgen, Pfizer, and Sanofi, to test and win approval for a drug that mimics the effects of the mutation, drives LDL levels to new lows, and prevents coronary heart disease and other forms of atherosclerotic disease. All three companies now have drugs in clinical trials and report that the results so far are exciting. Each company's drug is a biologic. The drugs will be injected, probably twice a month. This is great news on the horizon for our most frequent cardiovascular disease, namely atherosclerosis, and its most frequent form, coronary heart disease (heart attack).

PREVENTING HEART ATTACKS WHEN MOUNTAIN CLIMBING

Novice mountaineers may lower their risk of having a fatal heart attack if they acclimate themselves before a high-altitude recreational hiking or skiing expedition according to a study published in the *American Heart Journal* (4). The risk of dying of a heart attack on the first day of vigorous mountain exercise was more than 5 times as high in individuals who had slept at lower elevations on the previous evening compared with those who had slept at higher elevations. The study from mountainless Dallas analyzed 301 sudden cardiac deaths occurring during weeklong expeditions in the Austrian mountains from 1985 to 1993. Of the 301 victims, 149 died on the first day of climbing and 152, on a subsequent day; 29% of the deaths occurred around noon after 2.5 hours of activity. Sleeping altitude was the only significant predictor of sudden cardiac death on the first day. Those individuals who died on the first day slept at an altitude about 1000 feet lower than those who died on a subsequent day. Deaths in both groups occurred at altitudes of 5354 to 5899 feet. Try to spend the first night at a higher altitude.

EXERCISE AND WEIGHT LOSS

Through the years I have heard many people talk about their desire to lose weight. Many have commented that they needed to exercise more. Dwyer-Lindgren and colleagues (5) in a recent article provide evidence that, although exercise can provide many health benefits, weight loss is usually not one of them. US obesity levels have risen over the past decade despite an increase in physical activity. For every 1% increase in physical activity, obesity rates declined by only one tenth of a percent. The researchers concluded that exercise alone is not enough to lose much weight.

COWS, NUMBERS, DROUGHT, AND PRICES

Wholesale beef prices rose in 2013 (6). The meatpackers have been paying more for cows after droughts the past two summers in Texas, Oklahoma, and other big cattle-ranching states. The dry weather parched pastures and drove up feed costs, forcing many ranchers to cull their herds. The nation's cattle herd shrunk by 2% at the end of 2012 from a year earlier to under 90 million cows, the lowest level since 1952. That means fewer beef carcasses are making it through the industries' supply chain. In 2012, Americans spent $288 per person on beef, a 4.2% rise from $277 a year earlier, as retail prices rose. US beef sales in 2012 reached $91 billion, up from $86 billion in 2011. The sales of beef in the first half of 2013 fell 1.7% from a year earlier. In contrast, pork volumes rose 3% and chicken volumes were flat. As beef prices rise, less beef is consumed. Because most Americans devour bovine muscle, an increase in price may be the only way to really decrease its consumption. The same happened with cigarettes: as the price rose, the number of smokers declined. It continues to be true: we kill the cows and then the cows kill us.

E-CIGARETTES

These are the battery-powered devices that turn heated nicotine-laced liquid into vapor (7). The market for this type of cigarette presently is small but growing rapidly, in part because it is increasingly seen as less harmful than conventional cigarettes. E-cigarettes, unlike traditional smokes, currently are not federally regulated. The FDA warned consumers in 2009 that the new technology could pose its own health risks and stressed the need for more study. The agency has said it is planning regulations that would treat e-cigarettes as tobacco products, but has provided no details thus far. More than a dozen states have banned e-cigarette sales to minors, and others have outlawed their use in enclosed public spaces.

The long-term impact of inhaling e-cigarette vapor, which contains other substances such as propylene glycol, has yet to be determined. But, could e-cigarettes, which currently offer flavors such as chocolate, strawberry, and pina colada, serve as a gateway to traditional cigarettes for young people? What kind of age restrictions and warnings should e-cigarettes carry? What about advertising? E-cigarette sellers are not currently allowed to make health or smoking cessation claims. Nevertheless, the potential market for e-cigarettes is huge. Industry experts say US retail sales of e-cigarettes could reach $1 billion in 2013, just 1% of the country's cigarette market but twice that of 2012. It's better not to use a-, b-, c-, d-, or e-cigarettes!

CARE GIVING FOR THE ELDERLY

Kelly Greene (8) discussed the problem of overseeing home health care for elderly patients. In 2011 alone, the most recent data available, so-called informal caregivers provided at least 11.2 billion hours of unpaid care to family members and friends. That commitment is expected to escalate. In 2010, about 4% of adults under age 65 were providing unpaid care to relatives or friends who were 65 and older. By 2050, demand for informal caregivers could double to 8% as the younger population shrinks relative to the elderly population. Elderly people and their families also spent at least $3 billion on their own in 2011 on long-term care in the community, mainly at home, in addition to $36 billion on nursing homes and other long-term care facilities. And those figures do not necessarily include drugs not covered by Medicare and other unreimbursed expenses, such as food for special diets, increased utility costs, home renovations, and special supplies. One third of adults 65 or older and two thirds of those who have reached their mid 80s have functional limitations, needing help with tasks ranging from eating and bathing to preparing meals or paying bills. Four out of five older adults who fit that description still are living in the community rather than in a nursing home.

Greene provided suggestions for helping families cope with paying for more care at the same time they are stretched by the unpaid time they are spending providing it themselves:

1. *Hire your own homecare professional or become one yourself.*
2. *Take the tax breaks.* Many elder-care expenses qualify for a medical expense deduction from federal income taxes. It is still 7.5% for people 65 and older. If you hire paid caregivers on your own, rather than working through an agency, the parent has to report the caregivers' income, either on a W-2 or 1099 form, to be able to deduct the expense. The adult child can take deductions only if the parent is a dependent and the child pays. Home improvements made with a physician's prescription are tax deductible also. Such remodeling could include adding an elevator, swimming pool, central air conditioning, or ramps. The key is getting the physician's note and deducting only the amount "over and above the amount it increases the home's value." One other possible medical expense deduction is entrance fees to a continuing-care retirement community, which provides care ranging from independent living to skilled nursing. The fees can run to >$100,000.
3. *Designate a bookkeeper.* People planning for later life should decide who should handle their finances in a health crisis, including designating who in the family should take control of the parents' finances when needed, taking inventory of the parents' resources, making sure the parents' will and power of attorney are current, and pinpointing resources to pay for care costs.
4. *Remember the veterans.* The "aid and attendance" benefit of wartime veterans pays up to $2054 a month to married veterans who qualify. Single veterans and surviving spouses can qualify for smaller amounts. To qualify, veterans generally must have served at least 90 days of active military service, including at least one day during a war. The income limits are met after deducting unreimbursed medical expenses, including any long-term care expenses.
5. *Embrace respite care.* Respite care is short-term care designed to give the regular caregiver a break. One person who cared for her mother sometimes would take her mother to a hospital facility for a week for what was called respite care. These respite programs are available nationwide through

social service agencies, nonprofit groups, and long-term care providers (eldercare.gov).

6. *Know when to consider a permanent facility.* Home care works best if you need a visiting nurse 3 or 4 times a week. But dementia requires round-the-clock care, and in these circumstances a nursing home or assisted living facility can be considerably less expensive.

As George Burns said, "Getting old is not for sissies."

HOSPITAL CACOPHONY

Hospital noise is constant: the beeping of a heart monitor; the opening of doors by a nurse to take vital signs; changing shift conversations; overhead pagers; a visitor's cell phone conversation; television; rattling dishes in a moving cart; an alarm going off when an intravenous medication is finished (9). Noise reduction efforts began gaining momentum in 2012 when Medicare began basing a portion of hospital reimbursement on quality measurements, including patient ratings of the quality of care. (Noise consistently gets the worst marks on patient surveys!) The latest data from the federal program for the year ending June 2012 showed that only 60% of patients said the area outside their room was quiet at night, the lowest satisfaction score among 27 questions about the hospital experience.

Several hospital administrators have cited changing behavior and culture as the biggest challenge to reducing hospital noise. Many hospitals now have only private rooms. Noise remains harder to control in shared rooms. A complicating factor is hospitals' increasing openness, including more liberal visiting hours and policies that permit cell phones and other devices. Some hospitals have formed "quiet teams" to identify ways to reduce noise. Some are reducing the frequency and intensity of medical alarms, dimming lights in the evenings, and replacing nurses' pagers and walkie-talkies with mobile headsets. Patients are getting Quiet Kits, white-noise machines and headsets for TVs and iPads. Some hospitals have hired consultants offering "sound scrapping" solutions, including architectural changes and the use of ambient sound.

Some consultants apparently suggest that hospitals "stop chasing silence" and increase the ratio of good sounds to bad sounds. Complete silence can actually be worrisome and isolating. The sickest patients may want quality sleep, but they also want to feel connected to their caregivers and know that they are not far away in case of an emergency. Some hospitals are asking staffers to use "library" voices because quiet murmurs can be more comforting than normal speaking tones. A recent study at Baylor Health Care System's Heart Hospital in Plano found that white-noise machines made no difference in patients' perception of noises in rooms. Terri Nuss has indicated that smooth hard surfaces enhance noise but they are easy to clean and help fight infection. Ms. Nuss indicates that Baylor University Medical Center at Dallas is trying to figure out what is an acceptable sound level. We can all be a little quieter.

END-OF-LIFE PREFERENCES

Ellen Goodman, a favorite of mine, retired as a widely syndicated columnist about a year ago and founded the Conversation Project (theconversationproject.org), a national campaign to encourage conversations about our wishes for end-of-life care (10). Dying is not easy today. Too often, of course, feeding tubes and life support abound. A fractious family may play out its contentious relationships. Every day in this country, Ellen Goodman opines, thousands of families face these crises without being able to call on the voice of the person they love. It is a familiar drama in an era when death is no longer likely to be natural. How do we know when medical technology extends life and when it prolongs suffering? Goodman indicates that the thousands of people who have used the Conversation Starter Kit on the website state that with help these talks can be far more intimate than intimidating. Goodman indicates that since she launched the project it seems as if everyone has a story to tell of a good death or a hard death. The difference often hinged on whether people they loved had expressed their wishes and, in turn, had those wishes respected. It is clear that too many people are dying in a way they would not choose. Surveys indicate that 70% of Americans want to die at home, yet 70% end up dying in hospitals and institutions. At home, one is at least surrounded by loved ones in comfort and in peace. Too many survivors are left not just mourning but feeling guilty, depressed, and uncertain of whether they have done the right thing—done what their mother, father, husband, friend would have wanted, if he or she had said. Have you had the conversation?

GUIDELINES ON FOOD IMPORTED TO THE US

In July 2013, the FDA proposed new steps to ensure that fresh produce, cheeses, and other foods imported to the US are safe (11). The proposed rules, required by a sweeping Food Safety Law passed by Congress 2 years ago, are meant to establish better checks on what has long been a scattershot effort to guard against unsafe food imported from >150 countries. Only around 2% of that food is inspected by the US government at ports and borders. About 15% of the food Americans eat is imported, including about 50% of fruits and 20% of vegetables. An estimated 3000 people die from food-related illnesses in the US every year.

The proposed guidelines require US food importers to verify that the foreign companies they are importing from are achieving the same levels of food safety required in the USA. The rules, which would also improve audits of food facilities abroad, could cost the food industry up to $470 million annually.

Since Congress passed the Food Safety Law in December 2010, several outbreaks have been caused by imported foods, including an occurrence of Listeria in imported Italian cheese in 2012 that killed 4 people. Other illnesses were linked to tainted papayas, mangoes, and nuts and spices used as ingredients. Like rules for domestic farmers and food companies released in early 2013, the idea of the new guidelines is to make businesses more responsible for the food they sell or import by proving that they are using good food safety practices. Currently, the government does little to ensure that companies are trying to prevent food safety problems rather than waiting and responding to outbreaks after they happen. Requiring better prevention was the intent when Congress passed the bill. Since then, however, the law has run into several obstacles, including FDA delays in issuing the guidelines, a lack of congressional funding, and increasing opposition from some rural members of Congress who represent worried farmers. FDA regulators say the new rules are necessary as the food system becomes more complex and more global. Food often stops in several locations and passes through several different hands in a matter of days before it hits grocery shelves. A lack of funding also has given the FDA little oversight over what is produced. The agency inspects most food companies in the US only once every 5 to 10 years, and it does even fewer inspections abroad. The Food Safety Law requires the agency to step up those inspections. In 2012, the FDA inspected about 1300 facilities in foreign countries, up from 300 in 2010. That is still just a fraction of the companies that import to the USA. Sounds reasonable.

DESTROYING CHINA'S EARTH

Josh Chin and Brian Spegele (12) recently described some experiences of farmers in central China's Hunan province. They highlight an emerging and critical front in China's intensifying battle with pollution. For years, the focus was on the choking air and contaminated water that plagued China's ever-expanding cities. A series of recent events, however, has highlighted the spread of pollution outside of urban areas, now encompassing vast swaths of countryside, including the agricultural heartland. Estimates from state-affiliated researchers indicate that anywhere from 10% to 20% of arable land, some 25 to 60 million acres, may be contaminated with heavy metals. A loss of even 5% could be disastrous, taking China below the "red line" of 296 million acres of arable land currently needed, according to its government, to feed the country's 1.35 billion people.

Rural China's toxic turn is largely a consequence of two trends: the expansion of polluting industries into remote areas a safe distance from population centers and heavy use of chemical fertilizers to meet the country's mounting food needs. Both changes have been driven by the rapid pace of urbanization in a country that in 2012 for the first time had more people living in cities than outside of them. Yet, the effort to keep urbanites comfortable and well fed has also led to the poisoning of parts of the food chain, and some of that pollution is traveling back to the cities in a different guise. Judith Shapiro, the US-based author of the recent book *China's Environmental Challenges*, indicates that pollution can be displaced only to an extent and that it cannot be walled off. She among others has warned that pollution poses an existential threat to the current regime. Shapiro says that the single most significant determinant of whether the Communist Party will maintain its legitimacy in coming years will be its ability to control that pollution.

China has sought to industrialize its countryside for the last 50 years when it began urging peasants to set up backyard steel furnaces at the expense of agricultural output. The cumulative impact of decades of building up rural industry is now taking an environmental toll, particularly as industrial growth surges forward in China's breadbasket. In some cases, factories are moving to the countryside to take advantage of cheaper land, often made available with the help of local officials who want to boost

growth. In other cases, urban leaders want factories to move out of crowded cities. The ensuing problems of rural pollution are exacerbated by the fact that many small-town governments have less capacity to properly regulate complex industrial activities than their counterparts in big cities. The consequences of this shift catapulted to national attention in February 2013 when China's Ministry of Environmental Protection refused to release the results of a multiyear nationwide soil-pollution survey, calling the data a "state secret." The decision sparked an outcry. Many farmers who farmed lands adjacent to various factories now cannot eat what they grow but by still farming the land they receive payments from the factory owners to compensate for polluting the ground. Bad deal!

US MEDICAL COSTS

As nearly everyone knows, Americans pay more for almost every interaction with the medical system than do people residing in other developed nations (13). They are typically prescribed more expensive procedures and tests than people in other countries, regardless of whether those nations operate a private or national health system. A list of drug, scan, and procedure prices compiled by the International Federation of Health Plans, a global network of health insurers, found that the US came out the most costly in all 21 categories and often by a huge margin. Americans pay, on average, about 4 times as much for a hip replacement as patients in Switzerland or France and >3 times as much for a Cesarean section as those in New Zealand or the UK. The costs of hospital stays in the US are about triple those in other developed countries, even though they last no longer. While the US medical system is famous for use of drugs costing hundreds of thousands of dollars and heroic care at the end of life, a much more significant factor in the nation's $2.7 trillion annual health care bill is not the use of extraordinary services but the high price tag of ordinary ones. The US pays providers of health care much more for everything. Colonoscopies are the most expensive screening test that healthy Americans routinely undergo. They often cost more than childbirth or appendectomy in most other developed countries. Their numbers have increased many fold over the last 15 years, and data from the Centers for Disease Control and Prevention suggest that more than 10 million people get them each year, adding up to more than $10 billion in annual costs. Largely an office procedure when widespread screening was first recommended, colonoscopies have moved into surgery centers where they are billed like a quasi-operation.

As Elisabeth Rosenthal writes, "Hospitals, drug companies, device makers, physicians, and other providers can benefit by charging inflated prices, favoring the most costly treatment options, and curbing competition that could give patients more and cheaper choices. And almost every interaction can be an opportunity to send multiple, often opaque bills with long lists of charges."

The United States spends about 18% of its gross domestic product (GDP) on health care—nearly twice as much as most other developed countries. While the rise in health care spending in the US has slowed in the past 4 years—to about 4%

annually from about 8%—it is still expected to rise faster than the GDP. Aging baby boomers and tens of millions of patients newly insured under the Affordable Care Act are likely to add to the burden.

Consumers of medical care, the patients, do not see prices until after a service is provided, if they see them at all. Patients with insurance pay a tiny fraction of the bill, providing scant disincentive for spending. Physicians often do not know the cost of the tests and procedures they order. Without posted prices, how can one make an intelligent decision? This situation is unique to medicine, where payments are often determined in countless negotiations between a physician, hospital or pharmacy, and an insurer, with the result often depending on their relative negotiating power. Insurers have limited incentive to bargain forcefully since they can raise premiums to cover costs. How medicine got into this situation is a bit unclear to me, and determining a reasonable solution will be a challenge for all.

TEXAS DEBT

According to Steven Malanga (14), Texas' combined state and local debt as of 2011 is just over $233 billion! While state government debt stands at $40 billion, or $1577 per resident, local government debt is >4 times as high: $192 billion, or $7505 per person, the second highest sum in the nation behind only New York's municipalities and far ahead of third place California. During the last 10 years local debt in Texas has increased 144%, much faster than the rate of population increase plus inflation.

Where is all this debt coming from? One place is the huge expenditures by local school districts on athletic facilities. Allen, for example, just spent $60 million on its new high school stadium, and its population is only 83,000. The 18,000-seat facility, which boasts a massive high-definition TV screen, was built from funds generated by a $119 million bond offering. More than 100 new high school stadiums have opened in Texas during the last 5 years, and that does not include pricey upgrades in several.

Debt owed by public school districts constitutes the biggest chunk of the state's soaring local obligations. Over the last decade, it has increased 155%, even as the state's student population has grown just 21%. Interest payments on these school debts now constitute 10% of school spending ($5.5 billion).

Debt is also growing rapidly among the state's 81 retirement systems for local government workers. These systems are underfunded. A result of this underfunding means that the contributions to pension systems that municipalities must make each year are rising, eating up large portions of local budgets. Additionally, employee costs are rising locally, going from 15% of city budgets to 30%. Those cost increases are partly to blame for sharp increases in property taxes: 38% in the last decade. I thought California, New York, and Illinois were the big debt states, but that seems not to be the entire story.

HIGHEST-PAID STATE EMPLOYEES

My friend, Robert Doroghazi of Columbia, Missouri, a retired cardiologist who writes a wonderful biweekly investor newsletter, *The Physician Investor Newsletter* (www.thephysicianinvestor.com/

members), to which I have subscribed for several years, recently had a piece on the highest-paid state employees in the USA (15). They were as follows: football coach, 27; basketball coach, 11; football/basketball coach, 1; hockey coach, 1; college president, 4; medical school dean/administrator, 5; and law school dean, 1. Thus, our society, as Doroghazi comments, rewards sport coaches more than university presidents and medical school deans. Our society also rewards the average Major League Baseball players 5 times more than the average physician ($1.3 million vs. $241,000) (16).

TOP CITIES FOR JOBS

Between 2009 and the end of 2011, Texas added 428,000 jobs to restore the Lone Star State to its prerecession employment level, which it achieved faster than any other state (17). Of the top 10 US cities for jobs, four are in Texas, including Fort Worth, #4; Houston, #5; Dallas, #6; and Austin, #10. Since 2001, employment in Houston has expanded 20%; in Fort Worth, 16%; in Dallas, 11%; and in Austin, 27%. The oil and gas boom has been a big factor, particularly in Houston, but growth has also been strong in technology, manufacturing, and business services. Good for Texas!

STEM JOBS

They are jobs that require some knowledge of science, technology, engineering, or math. A June 2013 report from the Brookings Institution disclosed that the number of US jobs that now require STEM knowledge is 26 million as of 2011, or 20% of all jobs (18). In Dallas–Fort Worth, STEM jobs also make up 20% of all jobs. Pay and employment rates are higher for all STEM workers compared to non-STEM workers. For all STEM jobs in the Dallas–Fort Worth area, the average pay is $70,000, whereas for non-STEM jobs, it is $40,000. For jobs requiring a bachelor's degree or higher, the average STEM salary is $88,000 and the average non-STEM salary is $68,000. Study hard, young folks, particularly in science, technology, engineering, and math courses.

SMARTPHONE ADDICTION

In-Soo Nam (19) described smartphone addiction in high school students in South Korea. She defined this addiction as spending >7 hours a day using the phone and experiencing symptoms such as anxiety, insomnia, and depression when cut off from the device. She indicated that roughly 1 in 5 students in South Korea are addicted to the smartphone. In July 2013, the South Korean government said it plans to provide nationwide counseling programs for youngsters by the end of the year and train teachers on how to deal with students with addiction. Taxpayer-funded counseling treatments already exist in South Korea for adults addicted to smartphones.

South Korea, home of the world's biggest smartphone maker, Samsung Electronics, prides itself on being the global leader in high-speed Internet and advanced mobile technology. Koreans are some of the first adopters of new digital devices. Their mobile phone penetration rate is more than 100%, meaning that some individuals carry more than one handset, and smartphones are nearly two thirds of those devices. In contrast, the smartphone penetration rate in the US was 50% as of June 2013. (Korea also has had problems with online game addiction among teenagers for years thanks to widespread availability of high-speed Internet services.) The smartphone penetration rate in children aged 6 to 19 tripled to 65% in 2012 from a year earlier. The smartphone addiction rate among teens was 18%, double the addiction rate of 9% for adults. In the US in 2012, 37% of teens had smartphones.

The same problem appears to be surfacing also in other tech-savvy places such as Japan and Taiwan. According to experts, in addition to distracting students from their studies, smartphones are damaging their interpersonal skills. Students today, for example, are poor at reading facial expressions. One professor commented, "When you spend more time texting people instead of talking to them, you don't learn how to read nonverbal language." In Taiwan, the phenomenon of constantly checking e-mail or social media has led to the label "heads-down tribes." The number of people in Taiwan accessing the Internet via laptops, tablets, or smartphones in the past 6 months has doubled to a record of 5.35 million from a year earlier.

It is now standard practice in Korean schools for teachers to collect mobile devices from their students during school hours. One teacher there commented that smartphones are often the most important possession for a young person.

POWER-GENERATING WIND TURBINES AND BIRDS

Wind turbines may exceed 400 feet in height, a space extending into bird flight paths (20). The spinning rotors can cover an area >1 acre. Birds scanning the ground for prey flying at night or gliding with the wind may fly directly into the path of a wind turbine, slamming into spinning blades, metal towers, or other structures. The blade tips can travel more than 150 miles per hour. A recent study estimates that approximately 575,000 birds, including species protected by federal law, are killed each year by collisions with power-generating wind turbines. That number could reach 1 million a year by 2030 as utilities install more wind farms. No matter what the power source, be it coal, oil, gas, water, or wind, there is suffering, be it from humans or salmon or birds or other species. There is really no such thing as "clean energy" despite what some of us might like to think.

BASEBALL DOWNTIME

My friend, Baylor surgeon G. Ken Hempel, recently took me and two others to a Texas Rangers baseball game. It was a wonderful evening. Ken picked me up at 5:15 PM, the game started at 7:05, and Ken dropped me back home about 11:00 PM. That nearly 6-hour period produced a great deal of relaxation and a few minutes of excitement. *The Wall Street Journal* recently had a piece on baseball downtime (21). During an average 3-hour Major League Baseball game, the inaction amounts to 2 hours 40 minutes, and the action about 20 minutes. The inaction provided much time to talk. During the game David Murphy hit a home run over the centerfield fence, which stands 425 feet from home plate. The question arose as to the longest home run ever hit. It was by Mickey Mantle, who hit one

634 feet—200 feet longer than David Murphy's big blast and over two football fields in length.

In any given year, roughly 70 million people attend a Major League Baseball game. One thing every one of those fans sees is a bunch of grown men standing in a field doing absolutely nothing "about 90% of the time." Baseball is known for its moments of action, but they are fleeting. Nevertheless, it is clear why this game is known as our "national pastime."

TURNING NIGHT INTO DAY

Darkness was, for all of human existence, a universal obstacle to human happiness. In the late 19th century, the yearning for more light became more urgent. Many forms of work in the new industrial age, both in factories and offices, made more demands on the eyes, requiring greater attention to detail. At the same time, the urban world had grown darker, as tall buildings cast their shade and burning coal belched its smothering pall, blocking sunlight and coating windows with grime.

My father was born into this darkness when he entered the world in 1878; no city in the US was lit at that time. Although Thomas A. Edison had started working on the incandescent bulb in 1877, a year later there was still no reliable bulb. Although Edison made no claim that he had invented the first working light bulb, what he did create was a complete lighting system that linked his powerful and efficient dynamo, through a central main, to feeders and switches to his incandescent bulb of superior design. His system delivered a steady supply of current to hundreds of lights, at varying distances from the source of power, and used parallel circuits to maintain the current even when some of his lights burned out or were turned off. His bulbs used a filament of high resistance, a crucial innovation that saved money by using a relatively small amount of current for each lamp. In the 14-week light exposition in Paris in 1881, Edison showed that electric light not only worked but could be distributed some distance from a central station, a system with the potential to become large and economical enough to challenge the gas companies. Other inventors had shown that they could light a house, but Edison was on his way to lighting an entire city.

Ernest Freeberg recently published *The Age of Edison: Electric Light and the Invention of Modern America,* and what follows comes from his book (22). From the start, all recognized electric light as an agent of creative destruction that would only survive and thrive by stealing away gas customers. The gas companies were among the most heavily capitalized companies in the Western world. Right away, however, people saw that electric light was preferable to gas.

The first American showcase for street lighting (23 arc lamps) was a three-quarter mile stretch of Broadway in New York City installed by Charles Brush in 1880. Leaders in other cities sent delegations to see "the Great White Way" for themselves and to investigate the claims of the various lighting systems. Electric light's first entrance into each new town was always a cause for civic celebration. The market for electric light grew rapidly in part because Americans embraced the idea that their town standing could be measured by its ability to provide residents with the latest technological conveniences. My hometown, Atlanta,

Georgia, was called by Henry Clay, the great editor of the *Atlanta Constitution*, "the poorest lighted city of her size in the country." That changed in 1883, just over 4 years after my father's birth in Oxford, Georgia, a small town 20 miles from Atlanta where Emory University originated, with the arrival of a shipment of light poles. "Let us have light," the newspaper urged.

The dark cities of the Gilded Age were dangerous and lighting companies marketed their product as nothing less than a police force on a pole. After nightfall, urban parks became notorious danger zones, a haven for the cities' dregs and a playground of indecency. Now all that could end by harnessing light's power of exposure. The mayor of Baltimore remarked, "An electric light is a nocturnal joy to an honest man, but a scarecrow to a thief." One British reformer remarked, "Each electric light is as good as a policeman." Gas light was only half as powerful as electric and thus only half as effective in fighting crime. The link between strong light and safe streets became so axiomatic that some worried that a prolonged blackout would produce a crime wave.

While electric light made the urban night less dangerous, it also made it less private, exposing behavior that was not illegal but illicit. Everyone understood that in a world of crowded tenements, city parks provided a place not only for breathing but also for courting. By the middle of the 1880s, most town dwellers in America lived with a new light on a daily basis. Most, however, experienced the new light on the town's main boulevard or park, in a department store, theater, or hotel lobby, and perhaps in the office or factory where they worked. But at the end of the evening, most returned to houses still lit by gas, kerosene, or oil lamps. Gas had not been driven from the field in the first decades of the electric light.

In the months following his 1881 triumph in Paris, Edison worked with his team to introduce improvements and efficiencies in every aspect of his invention, as he prepared to install his first central power station in downtown New York. He won permission to dig up the city streets and had the technical challenge of running 18 miles of copper mains and wires along with the fuses, meters, switches, and fixtures to serve >1000 customers. All of these elements were connected to his six 30-ton dynamos powered by coal housed in a 4-story building on a rundown block centrally located to reach downtown Manhattan customers for half a mile in every direction. By September 1882, Edison fired up thousands of lamps in a square mile of lower Manhattan. After years of painstaking preparation and a half million dollars of invested capital, the system turned on without a hitch. In place of the usual dim flicker of gas, the bamboo filaments of the new lamps provided a steady glare, bright and mellow, which illuminated interiors and showed through windows. The Edison bulb would become so ubiquitous, so mundane, that it would become invisible. Those using the first ones marveled that they were simplicity itself—a glass globe shaped like a dropping tear, enclosing a slender horseshoe of glowing carbon. There was no nauseous smell, no flicker, and little heat. Each light socket contained a key whereby the lamp may be turned on or off at pleasure. Oil lamps and candles in contrast required wick trimming and soot cleaning, while gas burners demanded even more technical skills from customers, who had to adjust meters

and burners in addition to regular cleaning. The electric light required no maintenance while the source of power hummed out of sight, sometimes many city blocks away. The bulb worked for about 600 hours until it either broke or began to blacken and dim. Then an electric company worker could replace the expired bulb in a minute or two. The light bulb was safe enough for a child and simple enough for all to use. The functioning light bulb represented the culmination of decades of scientific insight, inventive genius, and technical skill.

Both Edison and his rival electricians sold standalone systems, single dynamos that fired a string of lamps, enough for a large house, store, or ship. But after the successful test of his Pearl Street station, Edison hoped to move forward with his much grander vision for an electrical grid, installing his central system in the urban core of every major city. Each territory offered a potential market of tens of thousands of lamps for office buildings, theaters, and the private residences of the elite. Edison's company planned to sell its equipment to a local utility which would pay royalties and assume responsibility for finding and serving its customers. Once free from the obligation to oversee the daily operation of his New York power station, Edison devoted his time and resources to improving every aspect of his system. He founded a series of interlocking companies. He supervised their work in developing and manufacturing dynamos, underground conduits, fixtures, and bulbs. Edison set out to apply this strategy not only to the US, but around the world. He arranged similar partnerships with local utility operators in major cities in Europe, Asia, Central and South America, and Australia.

As the popularity of electric lights grew, the electric companies strung numerous high-tension wires along streets already thick with wires for telephones, telegraphs, fire and police alarms, and stock tickers. At dense urban intersections a pole might carry as many as 200 different wires. Those wires were unsightly. Initially, those wires used only a moderate current that posed no danger. All that changed when electric companies added their powerful and fully insulated high pressure arc wires to the mix. These often broke loose and fell across the web of other overhead wires. Traffic stopped and crowds gathered as wires burned and sparked. Once in contact with broken or sagging arc wires, harmless telegraph, fire alarm, and telephone wires delivered awful, even deadly shocks. At other times, they burned and melted, causing numerous fires. The firemen who came to the rescue faced not only the risk of the blaze but also the danger of electrocution.

For late 19th-century city dwellers, the sky overhead became increasingly ominous, thick with wires that might pour down a lightning bolt without warning. One medical journal declared that "the overhead system is a standing menace to life and health." Every week the newspapers ran stories of this very modern form of sudden death. A Memphis man tied his mule to an iron lamp post that had been accidently electrified; the powerful current knocked the screaming mule off its feet and when its owner came to the rescue he leaned against the post himself and was instantly killed. Similar stories multiplied.

Most electric light victims worked for the companies, at a time when the properties of powerful currents were barely understood and safety standards for the industry were just being invented. Many more were struck down while working around the dynamos, accidently completing a circuit that sent the powerful current through their bodies. At a time when prison reformers were exploring the use of electricity to execute prisoners, one editor suggested that death row inmates should simply be apprenticed to work for an electric light company because sooner or later the job would carry them off.

For all of human history, the rhythm of night and day exerted a powerful influence on how people arranged their lives. Nature seemed to intend the daylight hours for toil and the night for rest. This rough rule of thumb made sense in early America's agricultural society but came under challenge during the 19th century's illumination revolution. Although gas light and the new pressures of industrial production had already begun to blur the line between day and night, the more powerful electric light threatened to erase the distinction entirely. The electric light particularly complicated the primordial bifurcation by adding a third option—illuminating evening that mixed elements of brilliance and shadow, looking and feeling like nothing any human had experienced before. These lit hours between sundown and bedtime became a new piece of time. In many industries owners embraced electric lights' economic potential, eager to keep their factories, mills, and shops open and their goods moving. Their workshops had required an enormous outlay of capital for expensive machinery and expanded facilities. To earn the best return on that investment, owners needed to keep those machines running as much as possible. As Henry Ford said some years later, "Expensive tools cannot remain idle. They ought to work 24 hours a day." Thus, electricity would make possible the perpetual workday.

In the early days of the Industrial Revolution, workers relied on sunlight as their primary light source, often setting their benches as close as possible to the factories' tall windows. The introduction of gas offered a stronger light for night work, but gas light was expensive, still caused fires and explosions, and, since it was not portable, proved useless in many work situations. Workers immediately noted the advantages of electric lights. The new light relieved them from the nasty smell and oppressive atmosphere of burning gas or oil lamps. In addition to having clearer heads, they enjoyed clear vision, no longer deceived by the flame's yellow flicker. In some trades the more powerful light proved a useful tool of production, making work not only safer and faster, but also more accurate. Newspapers became early adopters of the new technology and often its greatest fans.

The transportation industry was another early adopter of the electric light, using it to extend the reach and value of the era's powerful new railroads and steam ships, culminating by the early 20th century in a 24-hour per day distribution network. Lighthouses became popular.

Electricity was changing not only the way goods were produced but also how they were sold. Over time, merchants became sophisticated masters of light's power to seduce customers. Stores installing electric lights were believed to have nothing to hide.

Physicians immediately recognized the potential value that the new light might provide to the healing arts, another field profoundly improved by its ability to illuminate a once invisible world. The electric light amplified the power and consistency of the microscope, which in turn helped to confirm the germ theory of disease. The conventional microscope had long revealed minuscule creatures in water and organic matter. The British scientist John Tyndall used a beam of electric light to demonstrate that the air itself carried an organic swarm of spores, bacteria, and other minute solid particles, a startling discovery that unsettled many but added support to Louis Pasteur's germ theory. Electric lights powered to reveal this hidden world proved valuable to health officials as they tried to publicize these radical new ideas about the source and prevention of devastating urban scourges, such as cholera and typhus. Even as 19th-century science asked the public to accept its claims about a world beyond human senses, the new technology gave some of this a tangible reality. A drop of water presented the most extraordinary monsters imaginable, one reported after seeing one of these germ slides.

Surgeons embraced electric light technology almost immediately, another part of the late 19th-century revolutionary improvement in medical practice. Over the centuries, physicians had tried using candles and mirrors to reflect light into the body's darkest corners and performed operations under skylights. Experts had recommended using the "cold north light" whenever possible since it cast less heat on the surgeon and fewer shadows on the patient. Physicians also had rigged devices to concentrate the beam of a candle or oil light, using it to illuminate translucent flesh and reveal the shadows casts by tumors and abscesses. The incandescent bulbs were cooler, flexible, and much brighter, and physicians used them almost immediately to provide the first clear look at the living tissues of the throat, nasal passages, urinary bladder, and other portions of the body. Within a few years, instrument makers had crafted a series of specialized surgical lights, each adapted for the unique challenges posed by the various surgical procedures. Physicians improved their power of diagnosis, sending the focused light of incandescent bulbs into every opening in the body. Dentists benefited as well, finding the light cool enough to use right against the teeth and gums, illuminating defects otherwise hidden beneath the surface. Along with the development of anesthetics and aseptic practices, electric light laid the foundation for modern surgery.

Still others explored the idea that the electric light itself might be good medicine. Patients with nervous diseases and depression were advised to replace their clear glass window panes with blue glass, and a Southern dentist swore by the use of an electric blue light for "the painless extraction of teeth." Dr. John Harvey Kellogg pioneered the medical use of plain white electric light in his "laboratory of hygiene," experimenting with the tonic effects of electric light. If the new urban environment disrupted sleep patterns and frayed nerves, producing a generation of Americans who retreated to sanitariums looking for a cure, then it was fortuitous for Kellogg to discover that the electric light, which had done so much to create these modern maladies, could also be used to cure them. Kellogg thought that electric light was "nothing more nor less than a form of resuscitated sunshine." Kellogg delivered light to thousands of patients, using what he called the "electric light bath." The bather sat in a small cabinet, its interior lined with mirrors and studded with 60 incandescent bulbs. In this way patients dipped themselves into a healing "sea of light." Kellogg claimed, "Shed upon the nude surface of the body the rays will enliven the nerves with renewed force and will dissipate and destroy the enumerable malefic influences which imperil health and life." His electric light cabinet proved a good place to work up a sweat, stimulating the skin, accelerating respiration, and somehow encouraging the internal organs in their eliminative work. Saturating the body in the warm glow of incandescent light, Kellogg claimed, would prevent disease, heal skin conditions, nourish the body, and was the most agreeable means of reducing flesh, especially when the bather followed the electric bath with a brisk rubdown with salt or ice cold mittens.

And now the incandescent bulbs, in wide use since Thomas Edison received a patent for his version in 1880, are being phased out (23). A federal law passed in 2007 will end incandescent manufacturing and importing in the USA by the end of 2014, although stores will be allowed to keep them on the shelves until the inventory is gone. In their place will be the energy-efficient replacements (Halogen, CFL [compact fluorescent lamp], LED [light-emitting diode]), which are more expensive but last longer and require much less energy. Mr. Edison, thank you for the long and good run!

William C Roberts

WILLIAM CLIFFORD ROBERTS, MD
12 August 2013

1. Offit P. *Do You Believe in Magic? The Sense and Nonsense of Alternative Medicine.* New York: Harper Collins, 2013 (336 pp.).
2. Beck M. Medical spas get a checkup. *Wall Street Journal,* June 5, 2013.
3. Kolata G. Rare mutation ignites race for cholesterol drug. *New York Times,* July 10, 2013.
4. Lukits A. Sleep advice for tackling a mountain. *Wall Street Journal,* July 23, 2013.
5. Dwyer-Lindgren L, Freedman G, Engell RE, Fleming TD, Lim SS, Murray CJ, Mokdad AH. Prevalence of physical activity and obesity in US counties, 2001–2011: a road map for action. *Popul Health Metr* 2013 Jul 10;11(1):7 [Epub ahead of print].
6. Gee K, Berry I, Thacker C. Pricey beef puts heat on U.S. grilling season. *Wall Street Journal,* May 25–26, 2013.
7. Esterl M. E-cigarettes fire up investors, regulators. *Wall Street Journal,* June 10, 2013.
8. Greene K. The parent trap. *Wall Street Journal,* July 20–21, 2013.
9. Landro L. Hospitals work on the most frequent complaint: noise. *Wall Street Journal,* June 11, 2013.
10. Goodman E. Another Mandela inspiration. *Dallas Morning News,* July 17, 2013.
11. Hamburg M. FDA urges new guidelines on food imported to U.S. *Dallas Morning News,* July 27, 2013.
12. Chin J, Spegele B. China's bad earth. *Wall Street Journal,* July 27–28, 2013.
13. Rosenthal E. U.S. medical costs are world's highest, by far. *Dallas Morning News,* June 2, 2013.
14. Malanga S. Deep in the debt of Texas. *Dallas Morning News,* May 26, 2013.
15. Doroghazi R. *Physician Investor Newsletter,* July 1, 2013.
16. Boeck S, Nightengale B. Baseball salaries: MLB team breakdown. *USA Today,* April 1, 2013.
17. Kotkin J, Shires M. Top cities for jobs. *Forbes,* June 10, 2013.
18. Jean S, Oxford T. Science, math used in some not-so-obvious fields. *Dallas Morning News,* June 10, 2013.
19. Nam IS. Rising addiction among teens: smartphones. *Wall Street Journal,* July 23, 2013.
20. Cappiello D. Unprotected species. *Dallas Morning News,* May 15, 2013.
21. Moyer S. Play ball … please! *Wall Street Journal,* July 13, 2013.
22. Freeberg E. *The Age of Edison: Electric Light and the Invention of Modern America.* New York: Penguin Group, 2013 (354 pp.).
23. Lights out for old bulbs. *Dallas Morning News,* March 8, 2013.

Chapter 13

Janury 2014

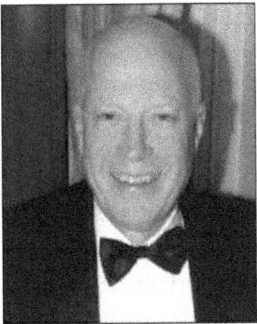

William C. Roberts, MD.

BLACK GOLD

Most physicians, nurses, and administrators are able to get to work every day because of petroleum. Most of us in the USA and indeed in the Western world are at the mercy of petroleum. I became conscious of its importance 40 years ago, as did so many others, when the world experienced its first "oil shock" as Arab exporters declared an embargo on shipments to Western countries on October 17, 1973. The embargo of the Organization of the Petroleum Exporting Countries (OPEC) was prompted by US military support for Israel, which was repelling a coordinated surprise attack by Arab countries that had begun on October 6, the sacred Jewish holiday Yom Kippur. The prices of gasoline quadrupled over the next few months. The crisis challenged the US's position in the world, polarized its politics at home, and shook the country's confidence. I remember reading a number of articles at the time indicating that the world's supply of oil would be depleted within 30 years, which meant of course 2003. But instead, the crisis produced the birth of the modern era of energy.

Although the OPEC embargo seemed to provide proof that the world was running short of oil reserves, the move by Arab exporters did the opposite: it provided massive incentive to develop new oil fields outside the Middle East—what became known as "non-OPEC"—led by drilling in the North Sea and Alaska. Although the Prudhoe Bay oil field was discovered in Alaska 5 years before the crisis, environmentalists had prevented approval for a pipeline to bring the oil down from the North Slope. Only in the immediate aftermath of the embargo did a shaken Congress approve a pipeline that eventually added, at its peak, as much as 2 million barrels a day to the domestic supply.

The push to find alternatives to oil boosted nuclear power and coal as secure domestic sources of electric power. The 1973 crisis spawned the modern wind and solar industries also. The same year Congress passed the first Corporate Average Fuel Economy Standards, which required automakers to double fuel efficiency—from 13.5 miles per gallon to 27 miles per gallon—

ultimately saving 2 million barrels of oil per day. (In 2012 the standards were raised to 54.5 miles per gallon by 2025.)

The crisis also set the stage for the emergence of new importers. In 1973, most oil was consumed in the developed economies of North America, Western Europe, and Japan. These regions consumed two thirds of the oil as recently as 2000, but now oil consumption is flat or falling in those economies and virtually all growth and demand is in developing economies, now better known as "emerging markets." They represent half of world oil consumption today, and their consumption and share will continue to increase. In October 2013, China overtook the US as the world's largest net importer of oil!

The 1970s also were years of natural gas shortages, which turned into a bitter political issue. What has solved the shortages were not more controls but their elimination, which resulted in an oversupply that became known as the "gas bubble." Today, natural gas is the default fuel for new electricity generation.

The oil crisis of 1973 resulted later in major political shifts for the US in political friends. In 1973, Iran was one of the US's strongest allies in the Middle East. Indeed, Tehran did not participate in the embargo and pushed oil into the market. Since the 1979 Islamic Revolution, however, Washington and Tehran have been adversaries. Meanwhile, Saudi Arabia, which was at the center of the 1973 embargo, is now the US's strongest Arab ally.

The real lesson of the shock of 1973, and the second oil shock set off by the overthrow of Iran's shah in 1979, is that they provided incentives and imperatives to develop new resources. Today, total world oil production is 50% greater than in 1973! Exploration in the North Sea and Alaska was only the beginning. In the early 1990s, offshore production expanded into the Gulf of Mexico, opening up deep water as a new oil frontier. In the late 1990s, the Canadian oil sands embarked on an era of growth, and today it is a larger source of oil than Libya before its 2011 civil war.

Most recent is the development of "tight oil," the spinoff from shale gas which has increased US oil output by more than 50% since 2008. This boom in domestic output has increased the energy supply, and combined with shale gas has had a much wider economic impact on jobs, investments, and household income. As these tight oil supplies increase, and as the US auto fleet becomes more efficient, oil imports have declined. Imports reached 60% of domestic consumption in 2005, but they are now down to 35%, the same level as in 1973.

As the US imports less oil, its energy is more secure. There are several million barrels of oil now "missing" from the world oil market, owing to sanctions on Iranian oil, disappointments in Iraqi production, and disruptions to various degrees in Libya, South Sudan, Nigeria, and Yemen. The shortfall is being partly made up by Saudi Arabia, which is producing at its highest level. But the growth in US oil output has been crucial in compensating for the missing barrels. Without it, the world would be looking at higher oil prices, there would be talk of a possible new oil crisis, and no doubt Americans would once again start seeing images of those gas lines and angry motorists from 1973.

Most of the above came from the work of Daniel Yergin, the most influential voice on energy in the world. His book *The Prize*, published in 1991 and containing 908 pages, was the bible for oil history (1). Because of the many changes between 1991 and 2011, Yergin wrote *The Quest*, an 804-page book examining what has happened since 1991, and he provides many suggestions to further decrease our consumption of oil and therefore improve our environment (2). Whether we like it or not, he opines, oil will be our major source for transportation worldwide for at least the next 20 years.

CLIMATE CHANGE

My brother sent me Linda Marsa's recently published book, *Fevered: Why a Hotter Planet Will Hurt Our Health—and How We Can Save Ourselves* (3). Whether we like it or not, the climate is changing and changing for the worse, and the changes will lead to more health problems than ever before. Marsa writes, "While 2012 was the warmest year on record—and the continental United States was gripped by an unprecedented number of droughts, floods, and super storms—what we are seeing is, quite literally, the tip of the iceberg." We are on the threshold of transformative changes in which natural calamities will convulse the globe, possibly leading to unlivable cities, widespread famine, civil unrest, wars over dwindling resources, the extinction of at least half the species on Earth, the death of the oceans from growing acidity, and hundreds of millions of desperate people uprooted by drought, floods, fires, and other weather-induced catastrophes.

Dust storms. Marsa begins with a description of the Black Sunday Dust Storm on Palm Sunday in April 1935. Although there had been almost 50 dust storms in the previous 3 months, the one on that fateful Sunday howled across a parched landscape baked by years of drought and record-breaking heat that often soared into the triple digits; these storms had already blown out 5 million acres of farmland and destroyed most of the wheat crop in Kansas, Nebraska, and Oklahoma. But on that day, a severe storm front had been building 800 miles to the north along the Canadian border, where a warm high-pressure system that had been squatting over the Dakotas collided with a cold front from the Arctic, producing blizzards with gale-force wind, frigid temperatures, and heavy snow in Montana. As the cold front moved southward across the high plains and the Texas Panhandle, the churning winds collected

even greater force, kicking up a black wall of soil >10,000 feet high, containing 300,000 tons of dirt and generating enough static electricity to power New York City. The storm creeping across the Great Plains started as a faint roar in the distance. Birds grew agitated, nervously fluttering and chattering. Cattle tied up in barns bellowed in fear, and rabbits frantically galloped across the prairie. By the time the roar reached its deafening crescendo, whole ranches were buried under a rolling wall of black dust. In many areas, the brutal storm arrived with little warning, leaving many stranded outdoors with no protection. Hundreds of people were buried alive and countless heads of livestock chocked to death. In autopsied carcasses, animals' insides were found to be packed with mud. Trains derailed and cars stalled on the sides of roads, their engines clogged with dirt and their occupants slowly suffocating.

Black Sunday, the occasion of the worst dust storm in US history, provides a grim snapshot of the devastation of the 1930s Dust Bowl and what happens when the weather goes haywire in a landscape that has been drastically altered by human development. Drought and destructive agricultural practices that had eroded the soil set the stage for the worst environmental disaster in American history. Just a few inches underneath the fertile soil that extends over the hundreds of thousands of square miles of the Great Plains is sand. These vast expanses of land were once semiarid grasslands only lightly grazed by buffalo and traveled by the Native Americans who subsided on them for thousands of years. This environmental devastation and its human aftermath were famously captured in John Steinbeck's *The Grapes of Wrath*.

Linda Marsa states that the Midwest and Southern Plains are likely to tip into desert once again as temperatures continue their inexorable climb. The effect of a warming planet on our health is a threat that has been completely neglected, marginalized, and ignored by the global health community and by policy makers, and yet in terms of our well-being, in terms of our survival over the next 100 years, it is absolutely the top public health issue that we should be talking about.

Marsa indicates that the Great Plains actually were unsuited to farming but an unusual stretch of wet weather, new technologies that produce more efficient tractors and combines, and inflated grain prices triggered a land boom that resulted in the plowing of >100 million acres, from a relatively scant 12 million acres a few decades before. When it rained, livestock flourished, crops were abundant, and farmers celebrated record-breaking harvests. Throughout the 1920s the prairie was a beacon of prosperity in an America that would be ravaged by economic calamity by the 1929 stock market crash, which led to the Great Depression. But when drought struck in 1931, no one was prepared. That the very process of cultivating the land would somehow change the climate was not considered. Crop prices crashed as the Great Depression deepened and emaciated cattle died in the fields. Some who chose to hang on in their houses crammed every cranny with wet clothes, sheets, and gunny sacks in futile attempts to keep out the dust. Even on clear days the air was so dry that just breathing would sear the lungs, forcing people to wrap damp bandanas over their mouths and noses and coat their nostrils with petroleum jelly if they dared to venture outside. Many were isolated by the storms, which crippled cars and machines; they were marooned for days on end without food, barely surviving on the ragged edges of poverty. Some were driven mad by the never-ending dust.

By 1935, inhabitants began to abandon the Plains in what became the largest mass migration in US history. By the end of the decade, on the eve of World War II, >2 million people had been uprooted—including 85% of the population of Oklahoma—and 500,000 more were left homeless. Deserted farm houses covered the landscape, and the community schools, churches, banks, and businesses were shuttered, leaving behind ghost towns.

Aside from the profound psychological toll, there also were serious health consequences from living in a dust-choked environment where summer temperatures soared to 120°F and air-conditioning was extremely rare. Simply venturing outdoors could prove fatal. Many suffered from malnutrition and starvation, and many subsisted on pickled tumbleweed, yucca roots, and road kill. Even the dust itself was lethal: the churning winds milled the soil into an extremely fine particulate with a high silica content, which scratched throats and eyes and penetrated deep into the lungs, causing a potentially lethal condition known as dust pneumonia or the brown plague, similar to the black lung that developed in coalminers. Although no definitive public health records were kept during that period, it is estimated that 7000 people suffocated from the dust and thousands more were permanently incapacitated, condemned to a lifetime of hacking coughs and respiratory difficulty.

Will we see the Dust Bowl conditions again? Marsa's answer is "absolutely." She indicates that by the end of this present century we can expect the midsection of the USA to be gripped by extreme droughts and baked by 90°F days for more than half the year. We will no longer call them droughts because the weather patterns will have permanently shifted and the land will simply become desert. The cover of the November 1, 2012, *Bloomberg BusinessWeek* noted after Hurricane Sandy turned much of the northeastern USA into a gigantic disaster zone: "It's global warming, stupid."

Rising temperatures and greenhouse gases. Starting in March 2012, much of the nation sweltered under triple-digit temperatures—3282 daily temperature records were broken in the month of June 2012, and July was the hottest month since recordkeeping began in 1895. A severe wind storm, a type called "Derecho," swept across hundreds of miles, with wind gusts up to nearly 60 miles per hour and lasting >6 hours, and cut off electrical power to nearly 4 million people in Ohio, Pennsylvania, West Virginia, and Virginia for up to a week. The exceptionally dry conditions ignited raging wildfires across the Western USA that incinerated >7 million acres. The heat also contributed to the record-breaking drought, the worst since Dwight Eisenhower was president, that engulfed 80% of the continental US by mid July, affected 165 million Americans, and decimated 65% of cattle production and 75% of the corn crop.

At the end of October 2012 came Hurricane Sandy, which has been described as "historic" and "unprecedented." The sheer energy generated by the storm surge and the destructive potential of the waves in its wake reached 5.8 on the National Oceanic and Atmospheric Administration 0 to 6 scale, the highest ever measured. Exceptionally high ocean temperatures brought this very last season Atlantic hurricane barreling up the East Coast to crash into a cold front that was coming down from Canada. The front's frigid air was fueled by the unprecedented September melting of Arctic ice, which had shriveled to 1.3 million square miles, the smallest ever recorded and less than half the area it had occupied only 40 years earlier. The collision of these two weather systems turbocharged Sandy and transformed it into a "Frankenstorm" that stretched about 850 miles and caused historic destruction and catastrophic flooding in the nation's most populated regions. At least 110 people were killed and thousands lost their homes. Enormous swatches of the electrical grid failed, leaving millions—including much of lower Manhattan—without power for days and some for weeks. New York's entire subway system was shuttered for days; LaGuardia Airport was submerged, and many of New Jersey's iconic beachfront resort towns were turned into piles of kindling. As the weeks wore on, many stranded residents were sickened by serious respiratory infections and developed what came to be known as "Rockaway Cough." As the planet gets hotter, we will live sicker and die quicker!

Indisputably, the planet is heating up. For >100 years, scientists have cautioned that burning fossil fuels like coal and oil would cause global warming because these fuels add enormous amounts of carbon dioxide to the atmosphere. Carbon dioxide is considered a "greenhouse gas" because it creates a hothouse effect by absorbing infrared radiation from the sun, inhibiting the planet's natural cooling mechanisms. While greenhouse gases are normally present in the environment—plants use CO_2 for photosynthesis and we exhale CO_2 every time we breathe—we have released tons more into the atmosphere since coal came into widespread use in the early 19th century at the dawn of the Industrial Revolution. With more carbon-spewing vehicles and factories constantly coming online to accommodate population growth, carbon emissions continue to climb. By 2011, annual global carbon dioxide emissions had reached 31.6 gigatonnes, an increase of 3.2% over the previous year. (A gigatonne is 1 billion tonnes, equivalent to about twice the mass of all 7 billion people on Earth *twice*. This means that 31.6 gigatonnes is more than 60 times the aggregate weight of every single person on planet Earth.) That figure is expected to rise about 3% annually as the population swells and more people around the globe enter the middle class and consume more energy.

According to some scientists, the temperature will rise by about 4°F by the end of this century, which could make the Earth hotter than it has been since the dawn of civilization. The planet today on average is 1.4°F warmer than it was 100 years ago and probably hotter than it's been in at least 1000 years. The sea ice is retreating; permafrost and glaciers are melting; species are migrating northward to find more hospitable climates. Tree-ring data culled from the last millennium showed temperatures are climbing and spring thaws occur a week earlier and winter freezes commence a week later than they did 50 years ago. Numerous studies have shown that the last 2 decades of the 20th century were the hottest in 400 years and perhaps the warmest in several millennia.

Rapid ocean acidification, which increased by 30% in the past century, is another tipoff. The oceans are the world's carbon sink, absorbing about 50 times more CO_2 than the air does. But CO_2 forms carbonic acid when it dissolves in water. As a consequence, rising CO_2 emissions are fueling the growing acidity of the oceans, which is killing seafood species, coral reefs, and organisms at the foundation of the ocean food chain. By 2050, if carbon emissions continue at current rates, the alkalinity of the ocean will be lower than at any time in the last 20 million years, a change that is occurring 100 times faster than at any time since Earth was formed.

Industrialization, deforestation, and pollution have supercharged the concentration of greenhouse gases such as carbon dioxide, methane, and nitrous oxide in the upper atmosphere. These gases absorb extrasolar radiation and then release that excess heat into the lower atmosphere, inhibiting planetary cooling and creating a hothouse environment under the carbon canopy that amplifies temperatures on the Earth's surface. And all this has happened since the Industrial Revolution.

Effects of rising temperatures on the ecosystem. In the coming decades, as Marsa indicates, the higher temperatures will have numerous effects on our ecosystems: higher levels of ozone pollution in the air we breathe; more uncontrolled outbreaks of deadly infectious diseases as mosquitoes migrate to newly warm habitats; and more extreme weather events. Hot air holds more water so we will have more torrential rains, more ferocious hurricanes, and, conversely, more dry spells as a result of heat-induced changes in rainfall patterns. Rising temperatures could trigger pestilence, drought-induced food shortages, raging firestorms, massive migrations, political instability, and wars, even the return of bubonic plague, the Black Death that killed more than 25 million people in the Middle Ages. And then there are the debilitating injuries and deaths that come with increasingly violent and more frequent hurricanes, floods, and fires and the chronic illnesses exacerbated by being left untreated for lack of medical care after weather-related calamities. So, we must expect more of the likes of Hurricane Katrina, the tornado that hit Joplin, Missouri, and superstorm Sandy.

As Linda Marsa writes, "In the absence of meaningful mitigation and adaptive strategies, we are on the cusp of a terrifying and increasingly unhealthy future. . . . We are going to see incremental changes in the next 5 or 10 years but that might not compare to what we are going to see in the next 30 or 40 years."

According to a noted meteorologist, "It only took 1 degree to cause the 1930s Dust Bowl. Just 1 degree change in the surface temperature of the oceans cut off the pipeline of moisture that normally travels north from the Gulf of Mexico and triggered the long dry spell."

While there have been some noticeable fluctuations, according to Marsa, for the past 12,000 years, we have enjoyed a relatively stable climate that has allowed civilization to flourish. But we are now on the threshold of transformative changes in the weather. There is, however, a pervasive and falsely comforting belief that climate change will happen slowly, that the globe will heat up uniformly, and that the predicted devastation will not occur until long after the Baby Boomer generation has died of old age. The developing world—Africa, Asia, and South America—will bear the brunt of the toxic legacy of wealthier nations' addiction to fossil fuels. But even relatively affluent Americans will not be observing this seismic shift from a safe insulated distance. Studies from the Centers for Disease Control and Prevention (CDC) indicate that these climate changes will not be gradual but will appear as extreme events. The freak weather patterns occurring across the USA in recent times confirm that Earth is warming at a swifter pace than even the direst forecast predicted just a few years ago. Since the presidency of Kennedy, the USA has heated up more than 2°F, a change greater than the warming average for the whole planet. Winters are now shorter and warmer than they were 30 years ago, with the largest temperature rises of >7°F measured in the Midwest and northern Great Plains.

No matter how fast we move to reverse this trend by drastically cutting emissions, temperatures will continue to climb because of the heat-trapping carbon dioxide that has already been dumped into the environment. Carbon dioxide lingers in the atmosphere for centuries, while oceans absorb the heat by warming and releasing it back into the air for hundreds of years. Over the next century the thermostat will climb another 2°F to 11°F on average, a range that is contingent upon what we do to reduce greenhouse gases, according to projections from numerous governmental studies done both in the US and abroad. When the amount of carbon dioxide in the atmosphere climbs from the current 393 parts per million (PPM) (up from about 298 PPM in 1900) to 600 to 700 PPM and beyond by the end of this century, as climate modeling scenarios now anticipate, we will be living under a carbon blanket far worse than the suffocating cloud of smog that envelops today's most polluted megalopolises (Beijing and Shanghai). Conditions such as these will not only make breathing a chore, they will change the climate in ways so profound and cause such vast and far-reaching disruptions to our ecosystem's rainfall and water supplies that the world will be virtually unrecognizable.

Based on current projections by the National Center for Atmospheric Research, Earth's most populated areas—a huge expanse of land extending from northern Canada to the southern tip of South America, parts of Asia, and most of Australia and Africa—will be parched by drought by the century's end, drying up surface water and killing crops that hundreds of millions depend upon for survival. A 5% Fahrenheit rise is at the very outer edge of what we may be able to manage; anything higher than that raises serious questions about our survival as a species. Climatologist James Hansen, the chief climate scientist at NASA's Goddard Institute for Space Studies in Manhattan, stated, "Human-made climate change is almost certainly going to be the greatest moral issue of this century. . . . It's hard for people to recognize that we have a planetary emergency."

Many scientists now believe we are on the tipping point that could unleash unstoppable forces. Melting permafrost in Siberia could belch millions of tons of methane—a greenhouse gas 20 to 70 times more potent than carbon dioxide—into the atmosphere and change the climate abruptly and cataclysmically, and some areas, especially here in the USA, will be more impacted than others.

Newly industrialized developing nations such as Brazil, China, India, Indonesia, Mexico, and Turkey are rapidly creating a huge middle class that will demand more goods and create more pollution, putting additional pressures on a global ecosystem already buckling under the weight of human consumption. Vast stretches of the world could become virtually uninhabitable, forcing the exploding population—expected to reach 9 billion by 2050—to squeeze into ever smaller patches of livable land. The rule of thumb is that every 1°C rise in temperature (a little less than 2°F) decreases crop yields by 10%. Higher temperatures halt photosynthesis, prevent pollination, and lead to crop dehydration. How will we grow more food to feed all these extra people on a planet with more frequent droughts, floods, and heat waves? Food prices could double, pushing billions into starvation. Radically rising sea levels and the massive desertification of the grain baskets of the world, among other problems, will make it very hard for even the most developed economies to survive.

Rising temperatures and health. The World Health Organization (WHO) estimates that worldwide over the past 3 decades 150,000 people have died as a result of a warming planet—mainly from increased mortality due to high rates of malaria, diarrheal diseases, and floods—and 5 million cases of illness can be attributed to it annually. Up to 5 million deaths occur each year from air pollution, hunger, and disease as a result of climate change and emissions from carbon-intensive economies.

WHO has identified >30 new or resurgent diseases in the last 3 decades. The incidence of dengue fever, long thought eradicated in the USA and once close to being wiped out in South America, is now climbing in the Western hemisphere. The number of people hospitalized in the USA with it tripled between 2000 and 2007, according to the CDC, and the species of mosquito that spread dengue fever have established a firm foothold in the continental USA.

A hotter planet is also promoting the spread of numerous other vector-borne pathogens from ticks, mice, and other carriers of potentially deadly microbial hitchhikers surviving milder winters and fanning out across the country into newly suitable habitats, transmitting Rocky Mountain spotted fever, equine encephalitis, St. Louis encephalitis, and babesiosis, a once uncommon malaria-like infection. Lyme disease has migrated from Connecticut and New York to the Canadian border and westward to the Great Lakes region. The sweltering summer of 2012 saw the largest outbreak of West Nile virus ever in the USA, according to the CDC, with 38 states reporting 1118 cases, including 41 deaths.

Heat waves, like the one that killed >70,000 people in Europe in 2003 and 2005, are projected to become common. In 2010, Russia wilted under its most intense heat wave in 130 years of record-keeping with daily highs in Moscow hitting 100°F instead of the normal summer average of 75°F. Severe droughts ignited wildfires in the countryside, smothering Moscow in poisonous smog for 6 straight days. The combination of unprecedented heat and suffocating haze doubled the death rate to an average of 700 a day and >52,000 people overall.

Big cities will feel the heat more acutely because of their high concentration of asphalt, buildings, and pavement, which tend to absorb more heat in the day and radiate less heat into their immediate surroundings at night than rural areas do. Therefore, built-up areas get hotter and stay hotter, creating "urban heat islands" in which temperatures are 5° to 10°F warmer than surrounding areas. In the not-so-distant future, major metropolises like New York, Chicago, Philadelphia, and Phoenix could become uninhabitable hot zones for months at a stretch, triggering the deaths of thousands.

Allergies and asthma have reached epidemic proportions in industrialized nations. Asthma rates have increased by 50% in each decade for the last 40 years, and more than 300 million people worldwide now have asthma, while an additional 400 million have allergies. Already at least 50 million people in the US have allergies, and asthma affects 1 in 14 American adults and nearly 10% of our children, making it the leading cause of school absences. The incidences of both respiratory conditions are increasing partly because pollution and pollen worsen as the thermostat rises. Rising temperatures also have resulted in earlier and longer pollen seasons. More potent allergens, such as the pollen in ragweed, are being produced in higher quantities because of warmer temperatures and because the air contains higher concentrations of carbon dioxide.

Huge dust storms like the ones that recently blanketed Arizona, northern China, Australia, and other arid areas are also responsible for spreading lethal epidemics around the world. The airborne dust cloud can carry viruses like influenza or severe acute respiratory syndrome (SARS) and other potentially harmful bacteria, viruses, and fungal spores over thousands of miles. Storms across the Sahara Desert have been blamed for the spread of fungal meningitis spores, which infect more than 250,000 people a year. Domestically, higher temperatures and more intense storms are linked to coccidioidomycosis—Valley Fever—a sometimes fatal disease infecting >200,000 Americans annually that is contracted by breathing in a fungus found in soil in the southwest USA, Central America, and South America. In the past decade, the incidence of this illness has quadrupled in the drought-stricken Southwest.

Sociological trends also will exacerbate the spread of disease as the planet heats up. The drought-driven economic collapse occurring in many rural farming communities in developing countries has escalated migration to the world's megacities. The urban shanty towns that sprout up on the fringes of these giant metropolises tend to be filthy and overcrowded, making them breeding grounds for contagions. Increased global traffic has stepped up the transmission of tropical infectious diseases to industrialized nations. The speed with which SARS spread from pig farms in rural China to North America is just one example of how epidemics go global.

And then there is the psychological fallout of living through more frequent natural disasters—the breakdown in social cohesion, the lost income, debt, and property damage—that can spill over into mental health problems such as anxiety, depression, posttraumatic stress disorder, substance abuse, domestic violence, and suicide. These repeated natural disasters could lead to the collapse of our normally well functioning public health system. Katrina-like flooding, for example, stresses the health system to the breaking point where basic sanitation, uncontaminated food or water, and the ability to control communicable diseases disappear.

We must all drive less, fly less, eat less, consume less, and pollute less, and we must do it quickly or there will be less people to talk about it. There is much each of us can do now. An unhealthy planet means unhealthy people.

WILLIAM CLIFFORD ROBERTS, MD
6 November 2013

1. Yergin D. *The Prize: The Epic Quest for Oil, Money and Power.* New York: Simon & Schuster, 1991.
2. Yergin D. *The Quest: Energy, Security, and the Remaking of the Modern World.* New York: Penguin Books, 2012.
3. Marsa L. *Fevered: Why a Hotter Planet Will Hurt Our Health—and How We Can Save Ourselves.* New York: Rodale, 2013.

Chapter 14

April 2014

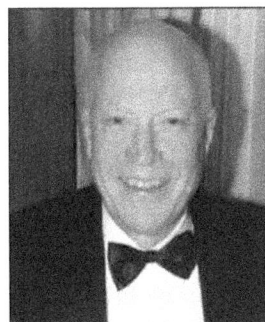

William C. Roberts, MD.

DEVELOPMENT OF INTERNAL MEDICINE

In 2003, Dr. H. Lawrence Wilsey gave me the book *Grand Rounds: One Hundred Years of Internal Medicine* edited by Russell C. Maulitz and Diana E. Long (1). The book was published in 1988 and includes chapters on general internal medicine and many of its subspecialties (infectious diseases, gastroenterology, rheumatology, nephrology, and cardiology). This book would appeal to any internist. The chapter that intrigued me the most was entitled "The Inner History of Internal Medicine" by Paul Beeson and Russell C. Maulitz. Paul Beeson is a favorite of mine, and maybe that is one reason I enjoyed so much his 40-page chapter. Beeson has many similarities to William Osler. Both were Canadians, both were chairmen of departments of medicine at prominent institutions (Osler: University of Pennsylvania and Johns Hopkins University; Beeson: Emory University and Yale University), both were Regius professors at Oxford University, United Kingdom, and both had biographies of them written by a neurosurgeon.

Beeson and Maulitz asked initially "What is internal medicine? And who is the internist?" The terms have been misunderstood by many in the public. American internists trace their ancestry back to the tiny Royal College elites granted monopoly rights by royal warrant beginning in the 16th century. The American College of Physicians professes a filial relationship with the Royal College of Physicians of London (now of England), empowered by Henry VIII in 1518. From there, Beeson and Maulitz developed the internist's world from the scientific, clinical, personal, and professional perspectives.

The process of demarcating new medical specialties first in Germany and soon after in the other industrial nations was fueled by two powerful engines: new technology (primarily diagnostic but also therapeutic) and an increased professional competition. Specialized fields like ophthalmology and otolaryngology found professional niches. Slightly later, old fields like surgery gained in professional power as they created their edifices on foundations of science.

The designation "internal medicine" seems to have originated around 1880 in Germany with the use of the modifying word *innere*. The term was employed to indicate a field of practice in which concepts were based on an emerging understanding of physiology, biochemistry, bacteriology, and pathology and in which surgical methods were not employed. The expression was intended to connote special knowledge and training rather than dogma, empty hypotheses, and mere observation of outward manifestations of disease. At that time, North America took most of its medical cues from Germany. Over a few decades, thousands of physicians and medical students flocked to the laboratories of polyclinics of Strasbourg, Berlin, and Vienna. Consequently, the expression "internal medicine" reflecting German institutional arrangements was adopted quickly in America. William Osler, incidentally, disputed its status as an incipient specialty but favored the good old name "physician" in contradiction to general practitioners, surgeons, and obstetricians and gynecologists. Osler tended to deemphasize the "specialized" aspect of the field and chose to stress its role as a gateway to other more limited specialties—domains of scientific knowledge or technical expertise now conventionally thought of as *sub*specialties. Most American internists preferred the phrase "internists" to Osler's "physician."

The chapter goes on to describe contributions made by American physicians and important events in the specialty: the development of the Association of American Physicians, the publication of the first edition of Osler's textbook, *Principles and Practice of Medicine* (1892), the founding of the Johns Hopkins Medical School (1893), the Flexner report on American medical education (1910), the development of the Rockefeller Institution, the making of clinical investigation scientific, the development of the full-time system, the explosion of medical research just before and after World War II, the changes in patient mix seen by internists over the decades, the changes in therapeutics in internal medicine, and the development of the various subspecialties in internal medicine.

KIDNEY TRANSPLANTS

According to Gary S. Becker and Julio J. Elias, writing in *The Wall Street Journal*, in 2012, 95,000 American men, women, and children were on the waiting list for a new kidney, the most commonly transplanted organ (2). Yet, only about 16,500 kidney transplant operations were performed that year. Taking into account the number of people who die while waiting for a transplant, this figure implies an average wait of 4.5 years for a kidney transplant in the USA. This situation surprisingly is far worse than it was just 10 years ago, when nearly 54,000 people were on the waiting list, with an average wait of 2.9 years. Finding a way to increase the supply of organs would of course reduce wait times and deaths, and it would greatly ease the suffering that many sick individuals now endure while they hope for a transplant. The most effective change, these authors believe, would be to provide compensation to people who give their organs.

The first kidney transplant and indeed the first successful organ transplant was in 1954 at the Brigham and Women's Hospital in Boston. Kidney transplantation did not really take off, however, until the 1970s with the development of immunosuppressive drugs that could prevent the rejection of transplanted organs. Since then, the number of kidney and other organ transplants, of course, has grown rapidly, but not nearly as rapidly as the growth in the number of people with defective organs who need transplants. Many of those waiting for kidneys are on dialysis, and life expectancy while on dialysis is not long. People, for example, aged 45 to 49 on average live an additional 8 years if they remain on dialysis, but they live an additional 23 years if they get a kidney transplant. Almost 4500 people died in 2012 while waiting for a kidney transplant, and most died because they were unable to replace their defective kidneys quickly enough. Most of those on dialysis cannot work, and the annual cost of dialysis averages about $80,000. The total cost over the average 4.5-year waiting period before receiving a kidney transplant is about $350,000, which is much larger than the $150,000 cost of the transplant itself.

Individuals can live a normal life with only one kidney, so about 35% of all kidneys used in transplants come from live donors. Most kidney transplants come from parents, children, siblings, and other relatives of those who need transplants. The rest come from individuals who want to help those in need of transplants.

Exhortations and other efforts to encourage more organ donations have failed to significantly close the large gap between supply and demand. Some countries use an implied consent approach, in which organs from cadavers are assumed to be available for transplant unless, before death, individuals indicate that they don't want their organs to be used. The US continues to use informed consent, requiring people to make an active declaration of their wish to donate. Switching to implied consent would unlikely lead to a large enough effect to eliminate the sizeable shortfall in the supply of organs in the US. That shortfall, however, is not just an American problem. It exists in most other countries as well, even when they use different methods to procure organs and have different cultures and traditions.

Paying donors for their organs would, in the authors' opinions, eliminate the supply-demand gap. In particular, sufficient payment to kidney donors would increase the supply of kidneys by a large percentage, without greatly increasing the total cost

of kidney transplantation. The authors opine that a very large number of both live and cadaveric kidney donations would be available by paying about $15,000 for each kidney. Few countries, however, have ever allowed the open purchase and sale of organs. Iran permits the sale of kidneys by living donors. The price there appears to be about $4000 per kidney, and the waiting time to get kidneys has been largely eliminated. (Iran's per capita income is one quarter that of the USA.) Since the number of kidneys available at a reasonable price would be far more than needed to close the gap between the demand and supply of kidneys, there would no longer be any significant waiting time to get a kidney transplant. The number of people on dialysis would decline dramatically, and deaths due to long waits for a transplant would essentially disappear. The system proposed by the authors would include payment to individuals who agree that their organs can be used after they die. This is important because transplantation for hearts and lungs and most livers only uses organs from the deceased. Under a new system, individuals would sell their organs "forward" (that is, for future use), with payment going to their heirs after their organs are harvested. Relatives sometimes refuse to have organs used even when a deceased family member has explicitly requested it, and they would be more inclined to honor such wishes if they received substantial compensation for their assent.

Whether paying donors is immoral because it involves the sale of organs is a much more subjective matter, but the two authors question this assertion given the very serious problems with the present system. Any claim about the supposed immorality of organ sales should be weighed against the morality of preventing thousands of deaths each year and improving the quality of life of those waiting for organs. How can paying for organs to increase their supply be more immoral than the justice of the present system?

Researchers in space have learned that stem cells grow super fast in that area (3). A CEO of a stem cell upstart (Zero Gravity Solutions) has indicated that a kidney can grow in space in 30 to 35 days. The organ shortage might be improved by space laboratories.

TRANSPLANTED WOMBS

Nine women in Sweden have successfully received transplanted wombs donated from relatives (4). The women with their new wombs will soon try to become pregnant. The nine women were born without a uterus or had it removed because of cervical cancer. Most are in their 30s. (In most European countries, including Sweden, using a surrogate to carry a pregnancy is not allowed.) There have been two previous attempts to transplant a womb—in Turkey and in Saudi Arabia—but both failed to produce babies. Some have raised concerns about whether it is ethical to use live donors for an experimental procedure that does not save lives. The womb transplants began in September 2012, and the nine womb recipients are all doing well. Many already had periods 6 weeks after the transplants, an early sign that the wombs are healthy and functioning. The transplant operations did not connect the women's uteruses to the Fallopian tubes, so they are unable to get pregnant naturally.

But all who received the womb have their own ovaries and can make eggs. Before the operation they had some eggs removed to create embryos through in vitro fertilization. The embryos were then frozen, and physicians plan to transfer them into the new wombs, allowing the women to carry their own biologic children.

WOMAN TO BIRTH GRANDCHILD

A 58-year-old Utah woman is set to give birth very soon to her first grandchild (5). She is serving as a gestational surrogate for her daughter and son-in-law after the couple struggled with fertility problems. The 32-year-old daughter has had about a dozen miscarriages, with the longest pregnancy lasting only 10 weeks. After she looked unsuccessfully for a surrogate, her mother volunteered. The baby girl was due in February 2014. This is not the first such incident. In 2012, a 53-year-old Iowa woman gave birth to her twin granddaughters, and in the same year a 49-year-old woman in Maine gave birth to her grandson.

INSOMNIA AIDS

According to a piece by Jennifer Alsever in *The Wall Street Journal*, Americans spent just over $32 billion in 2012 on sleep-related aids (6). According to an August 2013 study by The Centers for Disease Control and Prevention, 8.6 million people in the US reported taking medications before going to sleep. Falling asleep and staying asleep through the night is a constant struggle for many. Alsever described using an iPhone sleep app and a CD set based on audio brain research. There was also an MP3 download.

The Brainwave Music System was a 6-CD set created by Jeffrey Thompson, director of the Center for Neuroacoustic Research in Carlsbad, California. The CDs use music embedded with tones to make sleep come faster. The music apparently sounded somewhat dreamlike with low humming and piano melodies. Alsever tried two 30-minute sleep tracks and a 30-minute relaxation track. She played the relaxation track in the background while she performed regular activities before bedtime such as brushing her teeth, and she played the sleep CD at bedtime. She indicated that she fell asleep quickly and felt refreshed in the morning.

She also hired a relaxation coach who had taught corporate workshops and yoga and meditation classes. The bedtime packet cost $50 and included a custom recording of relaxing music with voice relaxation instructions and help with the development of a "sleep ritual." The American Institute of Stress in Fort Worth, Texas, offers referrals to stress-management professionals who can offer advice on how to wind down. The relaxation coach inquired about nightly habits, such as TV viewing and worry level at bedtime, and also preferences on relaxation sounds, such as wind chimes, Tibetan singing bowls, or seashore sounds. She advised to stop cleaning the house or working on the computer at night. The coach suggested creating a bedtime routine that brings down the level of activity, such as gentle stretching and a nighttime bath. The 27-minute relaxation track includes the relaxation coach's soft steady voice over the sound of Tibetan singing bowl music. The coach advised squeezing and relaxing

muscles, moving up from one's legs to one's eyes. Alsever indicated that she fell asleep 10 minutes into the track.

She also tried the SleepEasily MP3 package, a program by a Denver behavioral consultant. The five tracks didn't work well for Alsever. The download came with a 38-page PDF of instructions including how to use the ear plugs. On the sleep track the instructor advised thinking about calming your jaw muscles and opening your throat for an inner sleep breathe. In the 21-minute track, the instructors' words got slower and slower when talking about imagining sounds of seashells and lullabies.

Alsever also tested an iPhone and iPad app called "ABCs of Better Sleep" created by a British hypnotherapist. The app included tips on better sleep and a 23-minute hypnosis session for deep sleep. In a 12-minute practice session, the hypnotist explained what the ABCs of the program are: "A" stands for "Are my eyelids so relaxed that I couldn't open them if I tried?"; "B" stands for "breath" instructions—to take a deep breath, hold it, and then release it using every muscle; and "C" stands for "the sea," in which one imagines floating underwater. The app included a 23-minute audio clip with the main hypnosis session played in bed. Alsever fell asleep at the end of it and felt great the next day. The hypnotist indicated that once it was used for a week, the hypnosis session would no longer be needed.

OBESITY RATE

In the US the obesity rate appears to be leveling off, according to the National Center for Health Statistics (7). The percentage of adults in the USA who were obese (body mass index ≥ 30 kg/m^2) in 2008 through 2012 was about 35%. In 1960, it was 13% and in 1980, 15%. Thus presently in the US, about 80 million adults are overweight by at least 35 pounds (BMI ≥ 30). The prevalence of obesity increased dramatically in the 1980s and 1990s.

DECREASING CALORIES BY FOOD COMPANIES

Sixteen companies, including General Mills, Campbell's Soup, ConAgra Foods, Kraft Foods, Kellogg, Coca-Cola, PepsiCo, and Hershey, pledged to cut 1 trillion calories by 2012 and 1.5 trillion calories by 2015 in their products (8). A study sponsored by The Robert Wood Johnson Foundation evaluated the progress toward that goal and found that between 2007 and 2012, the companies had reduced their products' calories by the equivalent of 78 calories per person per day. The Robert Wood Johnson Foundation, which works to improve the nation's health, hired researchers at the University of North Carolina at Chapel Hill to count the calories in almost every packaged item in the grocery store. To do that, the researchers used the store-based scanner data of hundreds of thousands of foods, commercial databases, and nutritional-facts panels to calculate the calories the companies were selling. The investigators indicated that the companies have exceeded their own goals by a wide margin. As a consequence, many products now come in lower-calorie versions, are baked instead of fried, or are sold in miniature as well as larger versions. Smaller servings—100-calorie packs of popular snacks, for example—and smaller cans of sugary drinks may have contributed to the reduction in calories.

LATIN AMERICA'S FIGHT AGAINST JUNK FOOD

Since 2012, Peru, Uruguay, and Costa Rica have banned junk food from public schools (9). Ecuador recently mandated a nutritional label system that warns against high salt, sugar, and fat. Industrial food makers in Ecuador also will be banned from using images of animal characters, cartoon personalities, or celebrities to promote products high in salt, sugar, or fat. In 2013, Mexico passed a special tax of 8% on packaged foods like potato chips, and a per liter tax (about 8 US cents) on sugary beverages. (Mexico is Coca-Cola Company's second-biggest market in the world by volume sales.) Columbia is also considering a beverage tax. In contrast, in more developed countries, proposed soda taxes have failed.

Obesity has become a major problem in Latin America, and the trend coincides with Latin America's becoming an important growth region for multinational food and beverage corporations. (PepsiCo Inc.'s Latin American food volume sales soared 11% while contracting 1% in North America.) Mexicans presently allot 45% of their household food expenditures to packaged foods. Chileans are on par with Americans, spending 63% of their food budget on packaged products. In both Chile and Mexico, roughly 7 of 10 adults and nearly a third of children are overweight, and diabetes mellitus threatens to overwhelm the country's health system. Serious health problems correlate with high consumption of snacks, soda, and other industrialized foods. Good for Latin America!

SMOKING DECREASE

The war on smoking, now 5 decades old, is one of the nation's greatest public health success stories (10). In 1964, four in 10 adults in the US smoked; today, fewer than 2 in 10 smoke. In 1964, the number of cigarettes smoked in the US annually by adults was 4,195 and by 2011, the number had dropped by 70%. The first surgeon general's report on smoking and health appeared on January 11, 1964. Its statement that smoking is a cause of lung cancer and other disease was major news then. The report led to cigarette warning labels, a ban on TV ads, and eventually an antismoking movement that shifted the nation's attitude on smoking. Then, smokers were cool; today, many are outcasts (banished from restaurants, bars, public buildings, and their workplaces). The formula for success is no longer unclear: adopt tough warning labels, air public health ads, fund smoking cessation programs, impose smoke-free laws, and raise taxes on cigarettes. Few people start smoking after age 19!

High taxes kill smoking as surely as cigarettes kill smokers. The evidence that taxing decreases smoking is overwhelming. The 10 US states with the lowest adult smoking rates have an average tax of $2.42 on every pack, 3 times the average tax in the states with the highest smoking rates. New York has the highest cigarette tax in the country at $4.35 per pack, and just 12% of teens smoke in the state—far below the national average of 18%. In Kentucky, in contrast, the taxes are low (60¢ per pack), smoking restrictions are weak, and the teen smoking rate is double

New York's. Other low-tax states have similar dismal records. The effect of the cigarette taxes is amplified when the revenue is used to fund initiatives that help smokers quit or persuade teens not to smoke. The antismoking forces in the US in the last 50 years have helped to prevent 8 million premature deaths. But, as long as 3000 adolescents and teens take up smoking each day, the war against cigarettes is not over.

HOME HEALTH TESTING

Already tests are available at home to determine whether women are ovulating, to measure blood alcohol levels, to test for the presence of illegal drugs, to determine cholesterol and glucose values, and to find out whether one has HIV or hepatitis C (11).

MEDICAL SCHOOL APPLICATIONS

A record number of students applied to and enrolled in US medical schools in 2013 (12). The total number of applicants grew by 6.1% to 48,014, up from 45,266 in 2012, surpassing the previous record set in 1996 by 1049 students. The number of students enrolling in medical schools increased by 3% over last year at 20,055, exceeding 20,000 for the first time. The number of first-time applicants, an important indicator of interest in medicine, went up by 5.5% to 35,727. Overall, this surge in applicants continues a decade-long rise from a low of 33,624 in 2002. Since then, the number of applicants has risen each year to this new all-time high. Even though medical school enrollment is rising, unless Congress lifts the 16-year-old cap on federal support for residency training, there will be serious shortages of physicians across the board, geographically and across specialties. In 2013, four new medical schools welcomed their charter classes, accounting for about half of the enrollment increase. In addition, 14 medical schools increased their class sizes by more than 10%.

THE MAYO CLINIC AT 150 YEARS

On January 27, 1864, Dr. William Worrall Mayo ("Dr. W. W.") (1819–1911) announced in the area newspapers that he was opening a private medical practice in Rochester, Minnesota. He had been directed to Rochester 9 months earlier as the result of a short-lived appointment from President Abraham Lincoln to serve as an examining surgeon for the Union Army during the Civil War. From these beginnings, his independent private practice thrived and later experienced exponential growth when his sons, Dr. William James Mayo ("Dr. Will") (1861–1939) and Dr. Charles Horace Mayo ("Dr. Charlie") (1865–1939), joined after graduating from medical school in 1883 and 1888, respectively, to form a group practice that would later become Mayo Clinic (13). From these family origins, the small private practice on the remote prairie of southeastern Minnesota has evolved into an internationally recognized medical center.

The success of Mayo Clinic can be attributed to an organizational culture, begun by its founders, that provides cohesive values while inspiring innovation. This Mayo Clinic model of care has enabled Mayo Clinic to develop attributes and make discoveries that benefit people far beyond its patient base; it also positions the clinic to continue to lead well into the 21st century.

The mid-19th century educational background of Dr. W. W. was unique in that although not from a privileged background, he studied Latin and Greek, was a student of the physicist and chemist John Dalton (an early contributor to atomic theory and the medical description of color-blindness), attended college, and achieved two medical degrees. A strong advocate for lifetime learning, he was, as his eldest son, Dr. Will, eulogized him, "a man of hope and forward-looking mind." Among the oldest patient records is a ledger that Dr. W. W. used. His handwritten entry on January 8, 1866, "Left open for further thought and research," shows how he continually sought out new medical advances and was never satisfied with the status quo.

Dr. W. W.'s partnership with his two sons grew to become the first—and today, the largest—integrated, not-for-profit, private, multispecialty medical practice in the world. The values of Mayo Clinic are particularly informed by Rochester Franciscans, a Catholic order founded by Maria Alfred Moes ("Mother Alfred," 1828–1899) in Rochester, whose magnificent motherhouse, Assisi Heights, is slightly more than a mile from Mayo Clinic facilities. The Franciscans and the Mayos became partners in healing in response to a tornado that devastated Rochester in 1883. From this collaboration, Mother Alfred proposed that the sisters would fund construction of a hospital and serve as nurses if Dr. W. W. and his sons would provide surgical and medical care. As a result, St. Marys Hospital opened in 1889 and was an early adopter of Listerian aseptic and antiseptic principles. In addition to the Catholic values of the Franciscans and the scientific-humanistic values of the Protestant Mayo family, many cultures and traditions have contributed to the ethos of Mayo Clinic.

How has the Mayo Clinic become so successful? The core or primary value of Mayo Clinic is that "the needs of the patient come first." Generations of practitioners at Mayo Clinic have upheld this value. Strict adherence to this ethic affords daily purpose and meaning to the organization and its contributors. Such an environment, built over 150 years and focused on the welfare of the patient, has led to an ingrained commitment to excellence and ongoing continuous improvement for all activities that constitute the Mayo Clinic's approach to medical care. The unwavering commitment to the patient also is complemented by the discovery of new information and the translation and adaption of those discoveries to advance clinical care *(Table)*. Innovations in education also help inform all appropriate parties of new information, again with a focus on improving clinical care. The triple shield logo of Mayo Clinic—clinical care, education, and research—that is liberally displayed around Mayo Clinic campuses and other venues is an ongoing reminder of the philosophy and focus of the institution.

In 1919, the Mayo brothers and their wives signed a deed of gift donating most of their life savings and all of their assets in the Rochester medical practice (including land, buildings, and equipment) to an entity, the Mayo Properties Association, which would ensure the perpetuation of Mayo Clinic beyond the lifetimes of its founders. This gift from the Mayos, the

Table. Highlights of Mayo Clinic's many contributions to medicine*

- Intraoperative diagnosis using frozen sections of tissue specimens
- The world's first program in postgraduate medical education
- Reliable laboratory procedures for determining basal metabolic rate
- Broders index for tumor staging
- Goeckerman treatment for psoriasis
- The nation's first hospital-based blood bank
- Introduction of the postanesthesia recovery room to civilian hospitals
- Advocacy for the nutritional enrichment of flour
- The high-altitude oxygen mask and G-suit
- The pioneering use of streptomycin to treat tuberculosis
- The discovery and clinical application of cortisone (for which the investigators won the 1950 Nobel Prize in Physiology or Medicine)
- The first successful series of open heart surgical procedures using the heart-lung bypass machine
- Early development of the intensive care unit
- Early development of the radial nursing unit
- The Rochester/Olmsted County Epidemiology Project
- The first Food and Drug Administration–approved artificial hip joint replacement
- Introduction of computed tomography to North America
- Test for rapid diagnosis of anthrax poisoning following the September 11, 2001, terrorist attacks

*Reprinted with permission from Olsen KD, Dacy MD, 2014 (13).

equivalent of more than $100 million today, was accompanied by a statement that the ultimate success of Mayo Clinic, "past, present and future, must be measured largely by its contributions to the general good of humanity."

Teamwork has been a major emphasis since the beginning of the Mayo Clinic. Dr. W. W. stated, "No man is big enough to be independent of others." The Mayo brothers always spoke of their accomplishments in terms of "My brother and I." They encouraged medical subspecialization, and Mayo Clinic contributed to the establishment of many disciplines, including orthopedics, neurology, dermatology, thoracic surgery, anesthesiology, and pediatrics, yet the integrated team-oriented practice was always essential to Mayo Clinic's success.

Quality has been at the forefront of the Mayo Clinic. The first sentence in the Mayo Clinic model of care mentions high quality. A closed medical staff with fully integrated hospital care and outpatient clinics and a common medical record in an all-electronic environment are important factors that enhance safety and quality. Continuous professional training in quality and safety is mandatory for all staff. Five safety workplace behaviors are regularly discussed and incorporated: paying attention to detail, communicating clearly, having a questioning and receptive attitude, handing off effectively, and supporting each other. Mayo Clinic is proud to be at the top of all the main published quality indices and continues to set and define new standards of quality and safety.

Compensation of the physician staff focuses on quality, not quantity. All physicians at Mayo Clinic are salaried. Their salary range is approximately at the 70th percentile of market level with no productivity bonuses. It is the Mayo Clinic perspective that patients are not served well if physicians compete with each other. The highly productive work of the staff is maintained through careful staff selection for special expertise, proven excellence in patient care, and a strong work ethic. There are no employment contracts or tenured periods for physicians. The environment also promotes staff loyalty and stability, with low attrition. In recent years, only 2.4% of physicians and 4% of nurses left the institution after appointment to the staff.

And *cost* must be appropriate. Dr. Will described the never-ending number of patients who would seek out care at the Mayo Clinic if the clinic provided the best possible diagnostic and treatment outcomes at low cost, a concept now recognized as the value equation in health care. Mayo Clinic has taken a strong stance nationally that medical reimbursement should pay for value, not volume. Assessing and improving value is taken seriously and is defined by outcomes, quality, safety, and service divided by cost. Data from the *Dartmouth Atlas of Health Care* looking at total cost for patients in the last 2 years of life found that costs at Mayo Clinic were far less than at other major medical centers for similar patients. Factors contributing to these findings may include salaried physicians, efficiency of testing and procedures, ready access to a team of physicians, fast diagnoses, short hospitalizations and episodes of care, and fewer evaluations, tests, and consultations. Physicians at Mayo Clinic typically do not know the insurance status of their patients. Behind the practice structure at the clinic is a highly involved logistics system aimed at improving quality of care and reducing costs for all patients. This system is built on three goals: shortening the time for tests to be performed and results to be available, reducing the non–patient-related work for physicians, and optimizing the time that physicians spend with patients.

Comprehensive care has been a hallmark of the clinic. One provision of the Mayo Clinic model of care is the performance of a comprehensive evaluation. This is not necessary in all patients but remains a hallmark of the Mayo Clinic experience. Thorough evaluation includes attention to each patient's physical, emotional, psychological, and spiritual needs.

Scholarship and continuous improvement is a hallmark of the clinic. As an academic medical center, Mayo Clinic is committed to education and research, with a distinction being that these endeavors are ultimately focused on strengthening the standard of patient care. As such, at Mayo Clinic, all faculty participants, whether working primarily in clinical care, education, or research, are cognizant that they are part of a team effort focused on improving patient care, not just contributing to academic activity for its own sake.

The *rate of change in medical care, medical education, and medical research* is accelerating. In only the past 30 years, the institution has been transformed by Mayo Clinic's integration with St. Marys Hospital and Rochester Methodist Hospital in 1986; expansion of the Mayo model of care to group practices in Florida and Arizona in 1986 and 1987, respectively; creation of

the Mayo Clinic Health System in 1992; and the development of wide-ranging business endeavors to generate funds for the not-for-profit mission. Mayo Clinic now employees 4100 physicians/scientists and 53,600 allied health practitioners. Patients come to the Mayo Clinic from all 50 states and from many foreign countries. More than 1 million patients are seen each year, and more than 500 operations are performed daily. Revenue exceeds $8.8 billion per year. Mayo Clinic is not standing still. It continues to expand, discover, and create new knowledge, promote health, and deliver health care in new ways to patients and the public. Major initiatives include individualized medicine, regenerative medicine, and the science of health care delivery. A major area of research is individualized medicine with direct patient care impact from pharmacogenomics, gene therapy, proteinomics, metabolomics, and biomarker applications to predict and enhance therapeutics for cancer and other diseases. Mayo Clinic's leaders have announced the goal of touching 200 million lives annually by 2020. This will be undertaken by sharing and applying Mayo Clinic medical knowledge through print publications, websites, social media, and a variety of other products and services.

For patient care, Mayo Clinic tops the list.

ZONES ON PLANET EARTH WHERE PEOPLE COMMONLY LIVE 100 YEARS

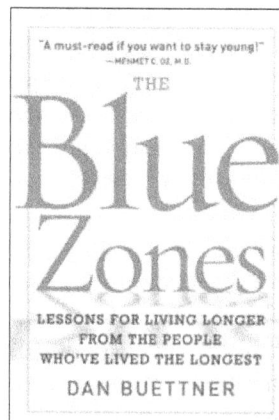

Dan Buettner has written a book entitled *The Blue Zones: Lessons for Living Longer from the People Who've Lived the Longest* (14). The Blue Zones are areas of the world with concentrations of some of the world's longest-lived people. When the author first set out to investigate human longevity, he recruited demographers and scientists at the National Institute on Aging to identify pockets around the world where people reached age 100 at rates significantly higher, and on average, lived longer, healthier lives than Americans do. The Blue Zones, the world's confirmed longevity hot spots, include Sardinia in Italy, Okinawa in Japan, Loma Linda in California, and the Nicoya Peninsula in Costa Rica. The author with his team traveled to these four Blue Zones where people have a 3 times better chance of living 100 years than does the average American and then described each of these places and the differing cultures that allowed longevity. Some studies have shown that about 25% of how long we live is dictated by genes and the other 75% by lifestyles and the everyday choices we make. This book provides a great deal of evidence that the way the people in the Blue Zones eat, interact with each other, shed stress, heal themselves, avoid disease, and view the world yields them many good years of life.

The Sardinian Blue Zone. The people of Sardinia have remained genetically distinct from the people in the rest of Europe. The Sardinians' lifestyle in the Blue Zone has not changed much since the time of Christ. The people there maintain not only their genetic features, but also their economic isolation and traditional social values, such as respect for elders, the importance of family, and the presence of unwritten laws. Genetic and cultural isolation appear to go hand in hand. Most male Sardinians are farmers or shepherds, and they can burn up to nearly 500 calories an hour. In the USA, only about 1 male in 20,000 reaches age 100. The chance of two centenarians in the same family is astronomically unlikely. In Sardinia, seeing more than one family member aged 100 or more is not an uncommon occurrence. The author found in the Sardinia Blue Zone 47 men and 44 women who lived past their 100th birthday in a population of just under 18,000, a rate of centenarians that exceeds that in the US by a factor of 30. More men than women lived to 100.

The diet of the shepherds and peasants in Sardinia is simple. Bread is by far the main food. Peasants leave early in the morning with a kilogram of bread in their saddlebag. At noon their meal consists only of bread with some cheese, occasionally an onion, a little fennel, or a bunch of radanelli. At dinner, the reunited family meal consists of vegetable soup (minestrone) with or without some pasta. Families eat meat about once a week, on Sunday. Fish does not figure prominently in their diet. The shepherds drink wine daily, usually only at the evening meal and no more than one quarter of the bottle. The wine is usually made from Cannonau grapes, resulting in a red wine with 2 to 3 times the level of flavonoids found in other wines. Goat's milk and mastic oil are other common foods.

In 1960, almost no one in Sardinia's Blue Zone was overweight; now 15% of adolescents are. Most unique longevity factors have disappeared or are disappearing quickly from residents' everyday life. The Sardinian wives are more sedentary than their husbands. Women tend to stay home caring for children, doing home repairs, and managing household finances. The Sardinian diet was largely lean and plant based with an emphasis on beans, whole wheat, and garden vegetables usually washed down by Cannonau wine. Goat's milk and mastic oil is far less common today in their diet than in the past.

The Blue Zone in Okinawa. This is in essence a Japanese Hawaii, an exotic laid-back group of islands with a warm temperate climate, palm trees, and white sandy beaches. For nearly a millennium, this Pacific archipelago, nearly 1000 miles from Tokyo, has maintained a reputation for extreme longevity. These islands for a long time were referred to as "the land of the immortals." Despite enduring years of Chinese and then Japanese domination, a devastating world war, famines, and typhoons, Okinawa can still claim to be the home of some of the world's longest-lived people. The Okinawan people enjoy what is probably the highest life expectancy on earth (in 2000 figures that was 78 years for men and 86 for women), the most years of healthy life (the Japanese have the greatest number of disability-free years at 72 for men and 78 for women), and one of the highest centenarian ratios (about 5 per 10,000). They suffer from diseases that kill Americans, but at much lower rates: a fifth the rate of cardiovascular disease, a fourth the rate of breast and prostate cancer, and a third the rate of dementia. In the USA or Europe, only about 15% of centenarians are independent in

their activities of daily living. Of 32 centenarians interviewed in Okinawa, all but four were functionally independent. According to governmental records, there are 700 centenarians among Okinawa's 1.3 million people.

The Okinawans grow vegetables in their gardens all year long. A family pig is butchered on certain holidays and cooked for a long time, the fat is skimmed off, and the rest of the animal is used in a stew-like dish. The Okinawan people historically have eaten meat only during ceremonial occasions. Before World War II, sweet potatoes were eaten for breakfast, lunch, and dinner. In 1900, Okinawans got 80% of their calories from sweet potatoes. Peasants tended to scrape out a living by cultivating millet, rice, and barley. The half dozen annual typhoons often wipe out or destroy their crops. The idea of retirement never occurred to the Okinawan peasants. To this day, there is not a word for retirement in their language. They eat vegetables, daikon, bitter melon, garlic, onion, peppers, and tomatoes, as well as some fish and tofu. They drink green tea. Before each meal, they say "*hara hachi bu*," meaning "Eat until you are 80% full." Okinawans may be the only human population that purposefully restricts how many calories they eat, and they do it by reminding themselves to eat only until they are 80% full. (It takes about 20 minutes for the stomach to tell the brain it is full.) Okinawans tend to have a positive outlook, are kind, and smile a lot. They avoid candy, cookies, and other sweets.

The notion of *moai,* which roughly means "meeting for a common purpose," originated as the village's financial support system. If a village member died or was depressed, neighbors visited. They create a safety net. The Okinawans tend to have close friends and watch after them. (In contrast, the average American adult has only two close friends he or she can count on, recently down from three.) Processed food is avoided. They eat a lot of mugwort, which tends to grow everywhere in Okinawa. Their food has a very low caloric density yet is very nutritious. The typical Okinawan meal—a tofu stir fry, miso soup, and some greens—has 3 or 4 times as much volume and more nutrients than the typical hamburger eaten in the USA, which has twice as many calories.

Okinawa's longevity lessons include embracing an *Ikigai* (having a purpose-imbued life that provides clear roles of responsibility and a feeling of being needed); relying on a plant-based diet (stir-fry vegetables, sweet potatoes, tofu, goya); gardening (almost all Okinawan centenarians grow or once grew a garden, a source of daily physical activity); eating more soy (tofu and miso); maintaining *moai* (secure social networks); enjoying the sunshine; staying active; planting a medicinal garden (mugwort, ginger, and turmeric); and having an attitude (an affable smugness).

Unfortunately, the Okinawan culture of longevity is beginning to disappear with the encroaching American food culture. Kentucky Fried Chicken and McDonalds were the last calamity to befall Okinawa; the fast-food invasion has threatened many of the positive behaviors that led to Okinawan longevity. Men under 55 in Okinawa are now among the most obese and do not live much longer than the Japanese average.

An American Blue Zone (Loma Linda, California). Loma Linda, which is Spanish for "lovely hill," is located about 60 miles east of Los Angeles and is the home of the Seventh-Day Adventists. Some of the most conservative Adventists do not believe in going to the theater or movies or indulging in any other form of popular culture. The Loma Linda University first embarked on a study of the dietary habits of 25,000 Adventists in California about 50 years ago. One key discovery of the Adventists health study was that approximately half of the Adventists were vegetarians or rarely ate meat. The Adventists who consumed nuts at least 5 times a week had about half the risk of heart disease of those who did not. This was true of men and women, vegetarians and nonvegetarians. Since that finding was published in 1992, at least four major studies have confirmed that eating nuts serves as a cardiovascular disease preventive. The study also found that consuming fruits, vegetables, and whole grains also was protective for a wide variety of cancers. They found, for example, that the Adventists who ate meat had a 65% increased risk of colon cancer compared with the vegetarian Adventists. Adventists who ate more legumes, like peas and beans, had a 30% to 40% reduction in colon cancer. Pancreatic, ovarian, and lung cancer frequencies were much lower in the vegetarian Adventists than in the flesh-eating Adventists. Being vegetarian, eating nuts, not smoking, being physically active, and having a normal body weight added as much as a decade to the lives of Adventists.

Being healthy has always been a fundamental part of the Adventists' message. One doesn't have to be an Adventist to admire how they have generated a Blue Zone out of whole cloth by sticking together and reinforcing the right behaviors for longevity. These include finding a sanctuary in time (the weekly 24-hour Sabbath, which provides a time to focus on family, God, camaraderie, and nature); staying lean; getting regular moderate exercise; spending time with like-minded friends; snacking on nuts; giving something back (helping others); eating meat in moderation; eating an early, light dinner ("eat breakfast like a king, lunch like a prince, and dinner like a pauper"); eating more fruits and vegetables; and drinking plenty of water.

Costa Rica's Blue Zone. In 2002, Louis Rosero-Bixby, a demographer working with Costa Rican population data, noticed that men living there seemed to be living longer than men in more developed countries around the world. This fact had gone unnoticed because in developing countries and in Central America—a part of the world notorious for malaria, dengue fever, and revolutions—most mortality studies did not even ask if anyone lived past age 80, which was considered well beyond the life expectancy of the area. Moreover, organizations like the United Nations had assumed that many Costa Ricans exaggerated their ages so that any finding would be considered invalid. Nevertheless, Louis Rosero-Bixby, the director of the Central American Population Center in San Jose, took a sampling of births recorded between 1890 and 1900 and then found the death records. From that he calculated the average age of death (life expectancy) and the chance of dying at any given age (mortality rate). Comparing these findings with data from developed countries, he figured that a Costa Rican man at age 60 had about twice the chance of reaching age 90 as did a man living in the US, France, or even Japan. He also found that if a man

reached 90, he could expect an average of another 4.4 years of life—again a life expectancy higher that than in most developed countries. Costa Rica spends only 15% of what America does on health care, yet its people live longer, seemingly healthier lives than people in other countries.

Rosero-Bixby identified a group of villages around the Nicoya Peninsula in Costa Rica where the proportion of the oldest people was significantly higher than in the rest of the country. The Nicoya Peninsula, until very recently, was one of the most isolated parts of Costa Rica. Buettner and his colleagues learned that Nicoya, like all of Costa Rica, has the best public health system in Central America—with good sewage systems, immunization programs, and clinics in almost every village. The investigators learned that Nicoyans had lived in relative isolation for the last 4 centuries, so their culture developed differently from that of the rest of Costa Rica, although they are not genetically different. They have the country's lowest rates of cancer. The authors' colleagues interviewed about 20 of the oldest Nicoyans, asking them about diet and hours of sleep, taking their blood pressure and heart rate, and putting them through short physical tests. After considerable investigation and facts learned from the 1958 book entitled *Nicoya: A Cultural Geography* by Phillip Wagner, the investigators concluded that Nicoyans ate the emblematic low-caloric, low-fat, plant-based diet rich in legumes. But, unlike in other Blue Zones, the Nicoyan diet featured portions of corn tortillas at almost every meal and huge quantities of tropical fruit. The water that Nicoyans drank had calcium and magnesium contents higher than anywhere else in Costa Rica. The investigators calculated that if the average Nicoyan consumed (through drinking, cooking, or making coffee) 6 liters of water daily, he or she would ingest a gram a day of calcium. (The World Health Organization had previously found that populations drinking hard water had 25% fewer deaths from heart disease than populations drinking soft water.) Thus, Costa Rica's longevity secrets include having a *plan de vita* (a strong sense of purpose); drinking hard water (with a high calcium content); keeping a focus on family; eating a light dinner; maintaining social networks; keeping hard at work; getting some sensible sunlight; and embracing a common history (modern Nicoyans' roots to the indigenous Chorotega and their traditions have enabled them to remain relatively free of stress). Their traditional diet of fortified maize and beans may be the best nutritional combination for longevity the world has ever known.

Previous areas of the world believed to be similar to the Blue Zones described by Buettner, including the longevity claims made decades ago about populations in Georgia in the Soviet Union, in Pakistan's Hunza Valley, and in Ecuador's Vilcabamba Valley, all turned out to be overstated and based on faulty data, according to Buettner.

For those of us living in non–Blue Zone areas, Buettner recommends the following: natural movement (be active without having to think about it); *hara hachi bu* (painlessly cut calories by 20%); plant slant (avoid meat and processed food); purpose now (take time to see the big picture); downshift (take time to relieve stress); belong (participate in a spiritual community); loved ones first (make family a priority); and right tribe (be surrounded by those who share Blue Zone values).

MUSINGS ON MORTALITY

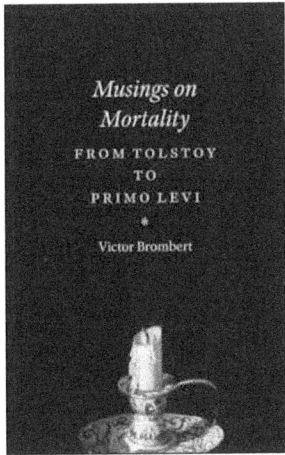

Victor Brombert, a 90-year-old emeritus professor of literature at Yale and Princeton, who escaped Hitler and fought as a young American soldier on Omaha Beach, has written *Musings on Mortality: From Tolstoy to Primo Levi*, which examines how eight major 20th-century authors wrote about death (15). Since physicians face the end of life rather frequently with their patients and themselves, the book may be of interest. It includes the thoughts regarding this topic of Leo Tolstoy *(The Death of Ivan Ilych)*; Thomas Mann *(Death in Venice, The Magic Mountain, Mario and the Magician)*; Franz Kafka *(The Death Journey in the Everlasting Present)*; Virginia Woolf *(To the Lighthouse, Between the Acts, Jacob's Room, Mrs. Dalloway, The Waves, The Years, The Common Reader, A Room of One's Own, Orlando, Elegy)*; Albert Camus *(The Stranger, The Plague, The First Man, A Happy Death, Nuptials, The Myth of Sisyphus, The Wind of Djémila, The Fall, The Exile and the Kingdom)*; Giorgio Basani *(The Garden of the Finzi-Continis, The Gold-Rimmed Spectacles, Five Stories of Ferrara, The Heron, "The Cardplayers")*; J. M. Coetzee *(Waiting for the Barbarians, Boyhood, Elizabeth Costello, Dusklands, In the Heart of the Country, Slow Man, The Good Soldier, Foe, Youth, Age of Iron, Disgrace, The Master of Petersburg)*; and Primo Levi *(The Search for Roots, The Wrench, The Periodic Table, The Sixth Day, The Drowned and the Saved, Lager, Survival in Auschwitz, If Not Now, When?, The Truce, If This Is a Man)*.

In the epilogue, Brombert emphasizes that *Musings on Mortality* is not to be mistaken for meditations on death or obsessions with it. Confronting mortality implies being alive, questioning how to live, or raising moral issues. He affirms that the need to live fully is "prompted by the recurrent sense of the transitory and the perishable." Thus, he stresses that we should savor whatever hours we are granted, for soon enough the eternal barman will announce with finality the last call.

THE PASSENGER PIGEON

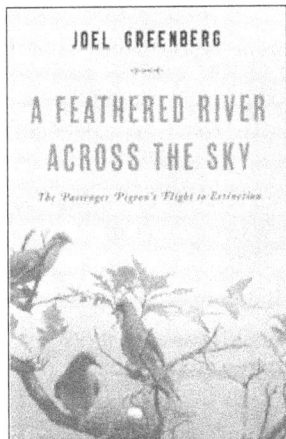

Joel Greenberg has written *A Feathered River Across the Sky* about the disappearance of the passenger pigeon (16). Two hundred years ago, the passenger pigeon was one of North America's greatest natural wonders. One hundred years later it was gone, as lost as the dinosaurs. Greenberg's book tells the sad story of how this singular species, once the most numerous bird on the planet, became extinct. The passenger pigeon, a relative of the common city pigeon, but larger and more brightly colored with a long tail, once flew in America's skies in flocks of astonishing size. Around 1860, an English naturalist visiting the US wrote:

> Early in the morning . . . I was perfectly amazed to behold the air filled, the sun obscured by millions of pigeons . . . in a vast mass a mile or more in breadth, and stretching before and behind as far as the eye could reach. . . . It was late afternoon before any decrease in the mass was perceptible. . . . The column (allowing a probable velocity of sixty miles an hour) could not have been less than 300 miles in length. That suggests there were more than 3.7 billion birds in that flock—only a portion of the entire continental population.

This report was not an outlier. Such distinguished ornithologists as Alexander Wilson and John James Audubon reported similar sightings, as did many others.

But, on September 1, 1914, Martha, a denizen of the Cincinnati Zoo, was found dead in her cage. She was the last of her kind. Stuffed and mounted, she is in the Smithsonian, although not currently on display. What could have driven a bird so abundant as to blot out the sun into extinction in only half a century? Joel Greenberg makes clear it was the combination of three factors: the species' peculiar nesting habits, the Industrial Revolution, and human ignorance.

The passenger pigeon was a child of the once vast eastern North American forest, a forest that stretched unbroken from the Atlantic to well past the Mississippi River. The nut trees of this forest, such as oak and beech, produced mast in prodigious quantities, which animals like the passenger pigeon would feed on, but mast is produced irregularly. One year in one area there is a bumper crop; the next year that area will likely produce next to none. So passenger pigeons not only migrated in mass numbers, they also nestled that way, flocking to an area where lots of mast had been produced the previous fall. These nesting areas could themselves be almost unimaginably huge. One in Wisconsin in 1872 covered 850 square miles of forest. A single tree might contain a hundred nesting pairs or more. Some observers reported trees with as many as 600 nests.

In the morning, the males would leave the nesting area to forage, returning at midday, when the females would leave. About 2 weeks after the eggs hatched, the adults abandoned the well-fed, indeed roly-poly squabs, who would flutter down to the ground and begin feeding for themselves. After a few days they would be strong enough to fly away.

Mass nesting in unpredictable locations was an effective reproductive strategy for the passenger pigeon as a species. Predators who happened to be nearby would have a field day, but with so many pigeons and squabs, they could hardly make a dent in the total numbers. Even in the early days of European settlement, when settlers armed with shotguns discovered they could bring down a dozen or more pigeons with a single blast, human hunters weren't numerous enough to be a threat to the birds.

But in the 19th century, the burgeoning population of the US surged westward, and the forest was increasingly turned to farmland. The big eastern cities, growing in size, needed inexpensive food, and nothing was more plentiful and inexpensive than the pigeon, which could be cooked like chicken, then a semi-luxury dish. But it was the railroad and telegraph, which began to spread across the landscape in the 1830s and 1840s, that proved lethal to the species.

Previously, hunters' inability to predict where passenger pigeons would nest in a given year protected the creatures. With the telegraph, however, the news of a major nesting could move at the speed of light. With the railroad, market hunters could converge in a few days and then send the slaughtered pigeons to market. And slaughtered they were. Greenberg quotes one pigeoner at the great Wisconsin nesting of 1872 attacking the departing males in the morning.

> Hundreds, yes thousands, dropped in the open fields below. . . . The slaughter was terrible beyond any description. Our guns became so hot by rapid discharges we were afraid to load them. . . . Below the scene was truly pitiable. Not less than 2,500 birds covered the ground.

Having killed as many of the males as they could, the hunters moved in on the females and the squabs, who, unable to fly yet, were easy pickings. Greenberg reported one estimate that at least a hundred barrels, each holding 300 birds, were shipped daily during the 40 days that the hunt lasted. That doesn't count the birds shipped alive, consumed locally, or just left to rot. Nor does it count the myriad squabs that starved to death in the nests because their parents had been killed.

Besides guns, nets were used. Designed like vast mouse traps, they would be baited with corn and other grains and with tame birds to lure the wild ones. (This was the origin of the term "stool pigeon" because the birds were tethered to a small platform called a stool.) When enough birds had gathered, the trap would be sprung and snapped over the victims. The catch would be enormous. One spring of a trap in Wisconsin yielded 35,000 birds. A three-man team in 1878 netted more than 50,000 birds during the hunting season.

With this sort of predation, the number of passenger pigeons declined rapidly. As it did so, the market hunters converged on the remaining flocks, and the population crashed. By the 1890s, the flocks were too scattered and too few to be worth pursuing anymore. By that time it was too late. The last definite specimen to be shot in the wild died in 1898. The last birds seen in the wild were observed about a decade later. By 1912, only a few birds, all captive, remained. Will humans survive our increasing population proliferation, nuclear weapons, and our rapidly changing environment?

WAR ON POVERTY

January 2014 was the 50th anniversary of President Lyndon B. Johnson's declaration of the war on poverty. As Thomas G. Donlan writes in *Barron's,* "From it came Medicare, Medicaid, Head Start, Community Action, and many other antipoverty programs," numbering at least 126 (17). "The poverty rate," as Donlan continues, "in 1964 was 19% and in 2013, 16%." At that rate, Donlan calculated that the poor will still be poor in 2264. The federal and state governments' spending amounted to more than $16 trillion (adjusted for inflation) over 50 years.

Did all that money improve the economic potential of the people who live in poverty? Donlan answers "yes." Antipoverty spending, now about $600 billion a year in our $3.4 trillion federal budget and another $230 billion in antipoverty spending by the states, makes life in poverty less painful than in 1964, especially for the sick, aged, and children. That money, however, has not brought meaningful education, positive attitudes, or better employment. The amount of money that the US has spent on fighting poverty is close to the size of the national debt.

The amount of money spent in 2013 on fighting poverty in the US would have been enough to send every poor person a check for $11,000, which is the annual US measure of poverty for an individual. Many of the 46 million people in poverty were pushed there by sickness, so more than half of the money spent on fighting poverty goes through the Medicaid program. Thus, poor people in ill health would still be needy if they received an annual check for $11,000.

Donlan indicates that the 16% poverty rate is an annual summation, but most people become poor temporarily and then recover. The Census Bureau indicates that nearly 32% of the nation's households were in poverty for at least 2 months from 2009 through 2011. It also indicates that only 3.5% of households were in poverty for the whole 3 years.

Surprisingly, the standard government data on the income of people in poverty does not include the value of poverty-fighting benefits, the largest of which include the food people buy with food stamps and other food subsidies, home-heating subsidies, the earned income tax credit, the premium for private health insurance that would substitute for Medicaid, free and reduced-priced school lunches, and public housing and housing subsidies.

The Census Bureau's statisticians of poverty developed an alternative poverty rate a few years ago that accounts for government programs as income. It also estimates expenses for out-of-pocket health care, work-related expenses, and child care expenses. For 2012, the overall poverty rate was slightly higher, 16% for the supplemental poverty measure vs. 15.1% with the official poverty measure in 2012. The supplemental poverty measure shows that if there were no government programs, the US would have a poverty rate of nearly 30%.

DEFINING "PUBLIC SERVANTS"

Peggy Noonan, who usually has a piece in Saturday editions of *The Wall Street Journal,* recently had a piece on selfishness in our political life (18). I was struck by the following paragraph:

> There's an increasing sense in our political life that in both parties politicians call themselves public servants but act like bosses who think the voters work for them. Physicians who routinely help the needy and the uninsured do not call themselves servants. They get to be the 1%. Politicians who jerk around doctors, nurses and health systems call themselves servants, when of course they look more like little kings and queens instructing the grudging peasants in how to arrange their affairs.

OPPORTUNITY ON MARS

On January 24, 2004, the rover Opportunity landed on the Martian surface, and 10 years later it is still going strong (19). Opportunity has finally spotted a place where the conditions were once hospitable to living organisms. The first such site, a complex of lake beds and streams, was revealed by NASA's Curiosity rover that landed on Mars in mid 2012. It is just unbelievable to me that this rover is still roving 10 years after it started on Mars. These kinds of accomplishments humble medicine.

WILLIAM CLIFFORD ROBERTS, MD
10 February 2014

1. Beeson PB, Maulitz RC. The inner history of internal medicine. In Maulitz RC, Long DE, eds. *Grand Rounds: One Hundred Years of Internal Medicine.* Philadelphia: University of Pennsylvania Press, 1988:15–54.
2. Becker GS, Elias JJ. Cash for kidneys. *Wall Street Journal,* January 18–19, 2014.
3. Vance A. It's faster to grow a kidney up here than down there. *Bloomberg,* December 2–8, 2013.
4. Associated Press. Nine receive transplanted wombs. *Dallas Morning News,* January 14, 2014.
5. Associated Press. Woman, 58, to give birth to grandchild. *Dallas Morning News,* January 9, 2014.
6. Alsever J. Trouble falling asleep? Ways to wind down faster. *Wall Street Journal,* January 14, 2014.
7. Hellmich N. Obesity rate in USA levels off. *USA Today,* October 18, 2013.
8. Jalonick MC. Favorite foods are getting less fattening. *Dallas Morning News,* January 2, 2014.
9. Guthrie A. Latin America's public enemy #1: junk food. *Wall Street Journal,* December 28–29, 2013.
10. 50 years later, war against smoking aims at teens. *USA Today,* January 9, 2014.
11. Chretien K. Lessons from 23andMe home tests: self-testing is the future. *USA Today,* January 9, 2014.
12. Mann S. Record number of students apply, enroll in medical school in 2013. *AAMC Reporter,* November 2013.
13. Olsen KD, Dacy MD. Mayo Clinic—150 years of serving humanity through hope and healing. *Mayo Clin Proc* 2014;89(1):8–15.
14. Buettner D. *The Blue Zones: Lessons for Living Longer from the People Who've Lived the Longest.* Washington, DC: National Geographic Society, 2008 (277 pp.).
15. Brombert V. *Musings on Mortality: From Tolstoy to Primo Levi.* Chicago: University of Chicago Press, 2013 (188 pp.).
16. Greenberg J. *A Feathered River Across the Sky: The Passenger Pigeon's Flight to Extinction.* New York: Bloomsbury, 2014 (304 pp.).
17. Donlan TG. Poverty and measurement. *Barron's,* January 13, 2014.
18. Noonan P. Our selfish 'public servants.' *Wall Street Journal,* January 18–19, 2014.
19. Watson T. Opportunity still rocking and roving on Red Planet. *USA Today,* January 24, 2014.

Chapter 15

July 2014

MICROBES

Sam Kean recently reviewed two books, *The Amoeba in the Room* by Nicholas P. Money and *Missing Microbes* by Martin J. Blaser (1). Kean begins by telling how geneticist Craig Venter took a sailing trip to Bermuda and while there decided to do a little research. He hauled up 50 gallons of the Sargasso Sea and began trawling it for DNA. The water was cold and appeared sterile, but Venter found 1.2 million distinct genes in his sample, all new to science. Based on previous research, he knew that none of the DNA came from fish or plants or any other visible life form. It was all microbial. For perspective, human beings have 23,000 genes; Venter had uncovered perhaps thousands of new microbes without even trying.

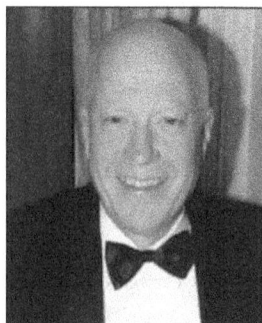

William C. Roberts, MD.

This Bermuda experiment underlined something biologists have argued for years: that we know virtually nothing about the world of microbes. By every fair reckoning, viruses, bacteria, and other one-celled organisms dominate life on Earth. Bacteria outnumber all plants and animals by several orders of magnitude, and viruses outnumber bacteria. Microbes also outweigh people. Just the bacteria found in the ocean weigh more than all the elephants on Earth—millions of times more. Yet, we have not even been able to grow most microbes in the lab to study them.

In *The Amoeba in the Room*, Money, a mycologist at Miami University in Ohio, deploys several strategies to enlarge our appreciation of the microscopic. He indicates that "a pinch of soil may seem inert but it contains 1 billion bacteria and tens of millions of fungi and protists. Ten thousand bacteria could be squeezed inside the period at the end of this sentence, and one gram of pure bacteria contains 2 trillion cells." And microbes are tough. Some species live in the pH equivalent of battery acid, while others prefer bleach. Some live at depths of 36,000 feet in the Pacific Ocean; others waft miles above the atmosphere. Some have colonized Chernobyl.

Missing Microbes, by Martin Blaser, an infectious disease specialist at New York University, focuses on a profound concern: the damage that modern life inflicts on the vast number of microbes that all of us, even healthy people, carry inside us at all times. A human being consists of 30 trillion cells but 100 trillion microbes, and they colonize every niche inside us. We are conditioned to think of microbes as dirty parasites. Most microbes, however, are harmless, and many perform vital metabolic functions. Some digest carbohydrates; others help absorb nutrients like salt and water. Some regulate our blood sugar and still others manufacture vitamin K. We would die without these microbial partners, and at some point the distinction between "us" and "them" becomes meaningless. Blaser compares this "microbiome" to a full-fledged internal organ—one that weighs 3 pounds, as much as a human brain. And just like a kidney or liver, a microbiome can fail.

Blaser describes a vivid anecdote involving his daughter. While an infant, she suffered from ear infections and was given strong antibiotics. Over the next few years she developed mild asthma and a mango allergy. In her teens and 20s, she began traveling widely in Latin America where she inevitably battled diarrhea. Another course of antibiotics cleared it up, but she soon began suffering from chronic stomach pains. Several years of misery later, a specialist finally diagnosed celiac disease—even though she had never had trouble eating gluten before.

Although it may have been a coincidence that his daughter's asthma and her food allergies both first appeared after she took antibiotics, Blaser suspects otherwise. He argues that while effective in clearing up her acute infections, the drugs also caused collateral damage, wiping out essential microbes and somehow inducing these chronic conditions. He doesn't limit himself to these elements either. He blames the rise of autism, juvenile diabetes, obesity, and Crohn's disease—each of which have skyrocketed in recent decades—on missing microbes.

Although to a person with a microscope, every disease looks microbial, research does lend some support. Mouse studies have linked disruptions in the microbiome to a number of medical scourges, including obesity. And modern medicine, as well as factory farming, exposes us to more and more powerful antibiotics. Because antibiotics are blunt, killing friend and foe alike, prescribing strong doses to children might well disturb the establishment of a proper microbiome early in life. A rise in Caesarean sections also cheats a newborn of exposure to a mother's vagina, which houses several essential microbes.

When it comes to microbes, our ignorance runs deep: we barely know what we don't know. Both *Missing Microbes* and *The Amoeba in the Room,* for all their differences, lay out the disturbing consequences of that fact. As one microbe researcher has put it: "I make no apologies for putting microorganisms on a pedestal above all other living things. . . . Killing all certain species of microbes would spell doom for us and perhaps the whole planet."

PATH TO HAPPINESS

Hugh Hewitt has just published *The Happiest Life*, his 15th book (2). Hewitt is a renaissance man, the host of a nationally syndicated coast-to-coast show called the *Hugh Hewitt Show*, Monday through Friday from 6:00 to 9:00 PM Eastern. He also is a professor of law and a lawyer in private practice. He writes weekly for the *Washington Examiner* and www.TownHall.com and lectures frequently at colleges and universities. In his radio and television activities, he has interviewed far more than 10,000 people, perhaps double that number, and, therefore, has acquainted himself with numerous points of view.

His latest book describes the seven gifts for happiness and the characteristics of the seven givers. The seven gifts he describes are *encouragement, energy, enthusiasm, empathy, good humor, graciousness,* and *gratitude*. Each is preceded, he cautions, by generosity. He also uses the phrase "for the most part," indicating that nobody gets out of here without pain or sorrow along the way. Hardship and grief, he emphasizes, are inevitable in all of our lives and are crucial to the happiness that the seven gifts he discusses make possible.

Hewitt obviously has talked to a number of friends and interviewees about happiness and the path to happiness. Interestingly, money is not discussed at all. One of his interviewees, citing numerous studies by the best academics in the world, argued that having at least two or three of the big four—namely, faith, family, community, and fulfilling work—was usually enough, but having all four increases the odds of happiness. And bad things still happen to good people; illness and accident, of course, can upset even the happiest of lives. Hewitt argues to sacrifice everything for family, and not just immediate family but the extended family. Keep them close, he advises; spend time with them. Always put them first.

Friends matter a lot, and we should value and serve them. Seek new ones and cling to old ones. Work alongside them for the good of the community. Do not betray them or neglect them. And find something to do that you enjoy doing, adjusting your consumption to your income so that you can do work that gives you pleasure and fulfillment. All these things, he concludes, add up to "earned success," and earned success is the essential ingredient of happiness.

He recommends watching out for the period in life that men and women are most likely to be unhappy. For men, the unhappiest period is at the age of 45, and not because of dropping testosterone levels. At that age, men realize they may have missed the "off ramp" to happiness. They may have driven past the chance for family, for deep friendship, for the sort of work that saw them spring up in the morning eager to begin a new

day, and for a real relationship with God. Of course, this age thing may be a false premise, because many people find faith or friends, renewed family bonds, or a new career after age 45, but it is harder to do because of previous choices.

Hewitt also stresses that human happiness is inextricably bound with doing good. Because we are born with a conscience, actions opposite that produce profound unhappiness. The best way to achieve happiness is to do good for others—starting with the seven gifts. The best guarantee of deep unhappiness is to do injury. In truth, all one has to do to ensure misery is to be stingy with the seven gifts. The other most common destroyer of happiness is addiction.

Doing good, he emphasizes, means sometimes doing very hard things, as soldiers do in combat or police do in their work. But even the hardest things, he argues, can bring satisfaction and deep happiness if done rightly for the right reasons. Hewitt explains that he has known many soldiers, sailors, airmen, and Marines. Among them are some of the happiest, most fulfilled people he has ever met. Theirs are lives of high honor and incredible sacrifice, and they have often given more than any civilian can even imagine and seen suffering on a scale that would stun the most cynical man or woman. Hewitt also argues that living in the midst of great sacrifice and incredible suffering for the longest period of time is what made George Washington and Abraham Lincoln our greatest Americans, and is how Winston Churchill defined greatness in the 20th century. Their "earned success" was in the midst of the greatest drama possible—the fate of their entire country—but their choices came down to the same decisions every person makes about selflessness every day, earning their own success every day. Few people outside of combat have the opportunity to lay down their life for a friend, but everyone has the opportunity to give these incredible gifts.

Hugh Hewitt went to his Harvard alumni gathering 35 years after he had graduated. He asked many of his fellow reunion-goers what made them, the alumni of such an incredible institution, happy. The most common answer he received was family and friends, with faith figuring into many accounts of genuine happiness. None of those he asked mentioned money or assets. None would count material accomplishment as that which brought them happiness! These Harvard alumni represent a pretty large cross-section of people from a very diverse set of backgrounds who have pursued a great variety of careers in places all over the country and indeed the world. None of them, he emphasizes, would say that their greatest happiness came from the things they had gotten. All of them point to the people and institutions to which they had given. Hewitt concludes that "it is all about giving."

SOME EDWARD O. WILSON THOUGHTS

In an interview of biologist Edward O. Wilson, the 85-year-old author of 30 books, Harvard professor of comparative zoology, and the world's authority on ants, happiness was a topic of conversation (3). Wilson emphasized that humans are just one of 8 million species on planet Earth. He calls for an end of the "age of man," meaning that humans should take a cautionary step back and think how we can cede more of the Earth to nature, to help stabilize the ecosystem. He worries that if we don't, the planet will come to look like a spaceship run by technical geniuses. He opines that humans do not know what we are doing, that we have no goal. "You can say we want less war, or we want everybody to be happy, or we want everybody to have long lives and have good health…, but what kind of goal is that? That is the goal of the family dog." He opines that what human beings really want is grace. "We want understanding, we want to be surrounded by beauty, and we want to be surprised constantly by discoveries of something unlike ourselves." It is another reason we should leave more of the world to nature, he argues, along with "the shield that biodiversity provides us against catastrophe." A fully functional ecosystem could help protect humans from pathogens and parasites that are kept in check by biodiversity.

Wilson's most famous book was his 1975 *Sociobiology*, now considered a pioneering work in the field. In his 2012 book, *The Social Conquest of Earth,* Wilson challenged the idea of kin selection—the long-held theory that individuals display altruistic, self-sacrificing behavior toward their relatives, with the aim of perpetuating their own genes. He put forth a theory of group selection, a kind of natural selection that acts on all members of a group rather than just related members and ultimately evolves the fitness of the entire group. I hope Dr. Wilson stays around many more years.

RATING MARRIAGE

Elizabeth Bernstein (4) developed a mini-test to help couples get a sense of the strength and weakness of their marriage. She developed statements for couples to answer on a scale from 1 to 5. (For the full 40-question quiz, go to www.WSJ.com/Wellness.) Sample items include the following. *Trust:* There is a sense of trust in my relationship. *Companionship:* My partner and I feel connected when we are together even when we are not saying much. *Intimacy:* My partner and I have a good sex life. *Validation:* I listen and hear my partner; my partner listens and hears me. *Conflict:* When there is conflict, my partner and I can usually compromise; my partner and I are able to focus on the conflict at hand rather than bringing in other issues and escalating our disagreement. *Assistance:* My partner celebrates with me when something good happens to me; I celebrate with my partner when something good happens to my partner. *Teamwork:* My partner and I agree on financial budgeting. *Boredom:* My partner and I like to try new hobbies and activities together.

For couples seeking help for a troubled relationship, a rating serves as a baseline, a point from which to move upward. What does it mean when the partners' scores don't match? At least 25% of couples disagree on the score. In those cases the spouse who rates the marriage very low often has already mentally detached himself/herself from the relationship, while the spouse who rates it high is "totally clueless."

Why is it so hard to clearly see and analyze the health of one's own marriage? One reason is we don't have many role models. We don't know very much about other people's marriages; the only one we ever see from the "inside" is our parents'. Each person brings different expectations to the partnership, and most people, even our closest friends, don't usually publicly air their marital problems, so we have no idea how our relationship

stacks up next to other relationships. She advises refraining from comparing your marriage to other couples' marriages. "Evaluate your own expectations…. We often compare what we are getting in a relationship to what we think we should be getting. To the extent that what we are getting exceeds our expectations, we are going to be happier."

PLATO TODAY

Rebecca Newberger Goldstein recently published *Plato at the Googleplex* (5). In the book Goldstein imagines Plato traveling on a speaking tour to places such as Google's headquarters, a cable news show, and a neuroscience laboratory. Although Plato lived >2000 years ago, his beliefs, she says, are more relevant than ever. "We are rethinking what virtue is and what it is to live a good life," she says. For a long time, she argues, "The notion of virtue was monopolized by monotheism, by Judeo-Christian theology, but the Greeks were pre-monotheistic and they were really consumed with the question of what it is to live a life that matters. The ancient Greeks had religion but you didn't want the attention of the Gods. They were terrible. So the Greeks approached virtue from a secular standpoint as many people do now." Many of the questions people have today are similar to ones that came up during Plato's time, such as whether life's purpose is to gain fame, power, or happiness. Goldstein thinks that while our culture of self-help may sometimes stand in for religion, philosophy is much better suited to answer life's questions.

According to Goldstein, Plato would have had strong opinions on today's ethical questions. She believes that Plato would urge people to seek moral excellence over fame and fortune. He would also promote "flourishing," which she describes as stepping outside oneself and learning about the world over pursuing happiness.

In the book, Plato starts his tour at Google because Goldstein thinks that tech entrepreneurs "may be the new philosopher kings." They are the new "elite." At first, her Plato approves of the way technology has democratized information. Then Plato realizes that everybody is going to the sources that agree with them, which she argues is dangerous for democracy. Goldstein says she now forces herself to read news from sources she disagrees with, which has helped her to change her stance on a few issues. With technology, everyone has more of a voice, but it is broadening our minds or narrowing our minds. Reading Plato convinced her of the need to be able to change her own mind, even about Plato himself. The most important lesson from Plato's teaching, she says, is the need to look outside oneself. Your life is ever expanding the more you take in of the world. "It's a kind of paradoxical idea that to be truly committed to yourself you have to be really committed to other things."

Dr. Goldstein first became interested in philosophy after reading books by Bertrand Russell, Will Durant, and eventually Plato. "Reading them gave me the sense that I know nothing and I want to know something." She soon moved on to Baruch Spinoza. "We all want to be saved one way or another whether it's through God or philosophy or politics." Still she thinks that philosophy can be uncomfortable. "It is supposed to shake you up," she says. "It's very hard for us to know the truth and when you think you know it you have to think again."

THE DIVINE COMEDY—A SELF-HELP BOOK

Rod Dreher has characterized *The Divine Comedy* as a self-help book, and surprisingly that's how Dante Alighieri himself saw it (6). In a letter to his patron, Cangrande della Scala, the poet said that the goal of his trilogy—*Inferno, Purgatory,* and *Paradise*—is "to remove those living in this life from the state of misery and lead them to the state of bliss." *The Divine Comedy* does this by inviting readers to reflect on their own failings, showing them how to fix things and regain a sense of direction, and ultimately how to live and love in harmony with God and others.

The Divine Comedy arose from the rubble of Dante's life. He had been an accomplished poet, an important civic leader in Florence at the height of that city's powers. But he wound up on the losing side of a fierce political struggle with the pope and, in 1302, fled rather than accept a death sentence. He lost everything and spent the rest of his life as a refugee.

The comedy, which Dante wrote in exile, tells the story of his symbolic death, rebirth, and ascension to a higher state of being. It is set on Easter weekend to emphasize his allegorical connection with Christ's story, but Dante also draws on classical sources. Dante's masterpiece is an archetypal story of journey and heroic quest. Its message speaks to readers, whether faithful or faithless, who are searching for moral knowledge and a sense of hope and direction. In its day, the poem was a pop-culture blockbuster. Dante wrote it not in the customary Latin but in Florentine dialect to make it widely accessible. He was not writing for scholars and connoisseurs; he was writing for commoners, and it was a hit. According to historian Barbara Tuckman, "In Dante's lifetime, his verse was chanted by blacksmiths and mule-drivers."

Few realize the surprisingly accessible beauty of Dante's verse in modern translation. Nor will they grasp how useful his poem can be to modern people who find themselves caught in a personal crisis from which there seems no escape. Dante's search for deliverance propels him on a purpose-driven pilgrimage from chaos to order, from despair to hope, from darkness to light, and from the prison of self to the liberty of self-mastery.

DIFFICULT TWO-LETTER WORD

Saying "no" is sometimes quite difficult (7). In the past, pharmaceutical companies sponsored many educational activities for physicians with visiting speakers of prominence often providing the presentations. Many physicians responding to a pharmaceutical representative's request to attend the meeting might answer "yes" or "I'll do my best to be there." The latter, I have learned, is simply a rather "gracious" way of saying no. Many of those meetings I have attended through the years have half-empty rooms, and who is paying for those empty chairs? The patients! If physicians and others had simply declined the invitation, there would not have been empty chairs at the meeting. Just like the three-letter word "net" may be the most important word in business, the two-letter word "no" may be the most important word to keep one's life in good balance. Some people have to practice saying the word. When a request takes one by surprise, a version of "I'll think about it" might be a ready answer. Delaying an answer, however, usually means an unstated no.

HISTORY OF EXERCISE

According to Amanda Foreman (8), the ancients knew well that people would use any excuse to avoid exercise, bad weather being among the most popular. To counteract the natural human tendency toward inertia (only 1 in 6 American adults does anything like the recommended amount of physical activity), the Greeks had their Olympics, the Chinese their tai chi, and the Indians their yoga. The Romans made exercise a legal requirement for all male citizens aged 17 to 60 years. With some exceptions, like Thomas Aquinas, who was colossally fat, lack of exercise was rarely a problem in the Middle Ages. Few people had time for aerobics when survival was the common thought. The early American settlers were too busy chopping wood and dodging arrows to worry about their overall fitness. By the federal era, things had changed. Thomas Jefferson was appalled by the sedentary habits of his countrymen. "If the body be feeble, the mind will not be strong," he warned, adding: "Not less than two hours a day should be devoted to exercise and the weather should be little regarded." His words, however, did little to stop the trend toward indolence. A century later, when the US entered World War I in 1917, military authorities were shocked to discover that one of three draftees was unfit for combat. Washington, DC, responded with a raft of new laws, mandating that physical education be part of every school curriculum. Nevertheless, in the early 1950s, almost 60% of US children failed at least one component, compared with only 9% of children in European countries.

Many poets and prose writers advocated walking. Wordsworth, Coleridge, and Shelley were all noted walkers. The 19th century essayist Thomas De Quincey believed that Wordsworth's daily walk was responsible for "much of what is excellent in his writings." Similarly, a 2-mile stroll is said to have inspired John Keats to write his greatest poem, "Ode to Autumn." Charles Dickens was another great walker, routinely covering 20 miles in a day. During his last trip to the US, he devised a 13-mile walking race for his friends George Dolby and James Osgood. On that February 29, 1868, race day, heavy snow fell. Icicles formed on the men's beards. Both Osgood and Dolby braved the storm, urged on by Dickens from the comfort of his carriage. He rewarded them afterwards with a "very splendid dinner" with guests including Oliver Wendell Holmes and Henry Wadsworth Longfellow. Dickens repeated often: "Walk and be happy, walk and be healthy. The best way to lengthen out our days is to walk steadily and with a purpose."

YEARS REMAINING

The Centers for Disease Control and Prevention website provides tables that estimate what happens to Americans from birth to death (9). Starting with 100,000 births, the tables estimate the total number of person-years of life for the group (a person-year is 1 year of life by one person), the number of deaths each year, and the number of person-years remaining at the end of each year. The table stops at age 100. Therefore, the maximum possible number would be 10 million person-years (100 years times 100,000 lives). Even the starting number tells something: instead of 10 million, it is 7,851,473 person-years, a gigantic improvement from the 5,358,122 person-years of 1910. We have gained a stunning 2,493,335 person-years in the last century! Beginning from the 7,851,473 person-years of life, the remaining person-years decline year by year. By age 40, we have used 51% of our person-years, and only 49% remain. By 65, we have used 78.5% of our person-years, with only 21.5% remaining. By 75, we have 11.5% of our person-years remaining. By age 85, we have used 96% of our person-years. By 95, only 0.1% of our person-years remain. By age 100, only 4785 person-years remain.

CREMATION ON THE RISE

The percentage of US deaths in which remains were cremated in 1960 was 3.6% and in 2012 it was 43.2% (10). That rate is projected to reach 49% by 2017 and 57% by 2025. The tradition of families staying in one town or one state and then being buried in the same place is becoming increasingly less common. Mississippi has the lowest cremation rate at 17%, followed by Alabama, 20%; Kentucky, 22%; Louisiana, 23%; and West Virginia, 26%. The five states with the highest cremation rates are Nevada, 74%; Washington, 73%; Oregon, 71%; Hawaii, 70%; and Maine, 69%. Texas has a cremation rate of 37%. Funeral directors say that many social and religious drawbacks that once kept cremation in check no longer hold sway. The Catholic Church, which once frowned upon cremation, now seems all but resigned to the massive shift in the public's attitude toward cremation. Although the Catholic Church doesn't favor cremation, because it believes in the resurrection of the body after death and therefore prefers burial, it does not prohibit the growing practice. The Cremation Association of North America cites five primary reasons why people say they prefer cremation: it saves money (30%), it saves land (13%), it is simpler (8%), the body is not in the earth (6%), and it is a personal preference (6%). Money is clearly the biggest motivation. An average adult funeral cost about $710 in 1960; in 2012, not taking inflation into account, the average funeral was just over $7000. Adding the typically required vault raises the price to nearly $8500. Cremations are less than half the cost of a funeral.

SHAM SURGERY

In a landmark study of a new cardiovascular device unveiled in January 2014, patients received anesthetics, had a large-bore catheter inserted into one of their major arteries, and had contrast material injected into their bloodstream (11). The physicians worked on them for about an hour, with unnecessary pokes and prods, while a monitor displayed the false progress. The patients were not being treated. They had agreed to undergo the angiographic procedure without knowing if they got the real treatment. They were part of the Food and Drug Administration (FDA)–approved study of a new medical device from Medtronic to treat refractory high blood pressure that is resistant to conventional medicines. Some patients were randomly assigned to this sham procedure (placebo group). Was their sacrifice worth it? That question many may want to consider as the FDA insists on a new study methodology with uncertain benefits. The methodology's high cost means that some new products may be delayed for many years. The goal is to isolate the observed effect of a new treatment from other factors that could affect the results. The

blood pressure device works by destroying small nerves in arteries that supply the kidneys. The activity of these nerves contributes to hypertension. The FDA wants to learn if the psychological influence of the procedure, rather than the new device, may lower the blood pressure.

Preliminary results from the sham study suggest that the device might not deliver the hoped-for benefits. While some people think the problem was not with the device but more with the way the procedure was designed in that trial, the negative results are already emboldening proponents of sham studies.

Yet, research that introduces harm or risk with no opportunity for benefit would seem to conflict with the principle governing research on humans. Some of these principles are reflected in the Declaration of Helsinki, an international treaty concerned with the conduct of medical research. Other experiments using sham surgery are obligating patients to undergo unnecessary anesthetics, radiation, abdominal incisions, endoscopy, and injections into the rectum, to mention a few examples. The FDA tries to address ethical issues by letting patients who get sham treatments eventually join the real treatment group, but this often requires a second operation. The sham trials also can be costly because they involve unnecessary procedures. They are hard to recruit for when patients know they may get a false unnecessary operation. All of this raises development costs and encourages firms to skip the US market and commercialize new products overseas. This obviously can suppress innovation. Instead of clinging to inflexible testing requirements, Scott Gottlieb suggests that the FDA should allow trials that are feasible, reflect clinical practice, and are morally defensible. There are methods for evaluating science that do not require such contrived experiments on people.

ATTENTION DEFICIT HYPERACTIVITY DISORDER

The Centers for Disease Control and Prevention released data in March 2013 showing that 11% of school-aged children in the US—6.4 million kids—had received the medical diagnosis of attention deficit hyperactivity disorder (ADHD), a 41% increase in the past decade (12). Over two-thirds of kids with an ADHD diagnosis received prescriptions for stimulants like amphetamine (Adderall) or methylphenidate (Ritalin). The data sparked a debate about whether American children were being overdiagnosed and overmedicated for ADHD.

The diagnosis and treatment of ADHD are spreading globally. In 2010, in Israel, methylphenidate use increased by 76%. The following year a study by Israel's Health Care Services found that as many as 1 in 5 Israeli children were prescribed stimulants without a proper ADHD diagnosis. Growing awareness of ADHD combined with increasing pressure on children to achieve academically in countries like China, India, South Korea, and Saudi Arabia has led to surging numbers of diagnoses and prescriptions worldwide. Between 2000 and 2010, global ADHD medication sales soared 26% a year to more than $8 billion. The total is projected to reach as high as $14 billion in the next 2 years.

Substantial evidence now shows that ADHD medication, when truly warranted, not only boosts attention but also improves academic performance and a child's quality of life. But even as global sales surge, evidence accumulates that stimulants are no silver bullets. Hundreds of controlled clinical trials have found that while ADHD medications have clear benefits in the short term (measured in months or a few years), the long-term effects are not clear. Prolonged use may in some cases promote brain growth but in other cases alter brain chemistry, eliminating some of the medications' initial effectiveness.

The pressure to treat ADHD is growing particularly fast in China and South Korea, which are making a strong push to improve academic performance. Many elementary and secondary schools in China force children to sit for hours, attending lectures and cramming for tests. It is only natural that children in these circumstances need help to remain focused. There are signs of some resistance to this trend in Europe. Their health officials advise physicians to resort to medication only after trying behavioral therapy.

MULTIPLE SCLEROSIS AND STATINS

Chataway and colleagues (13) in London studied 70 patients with multiple sclerosis (MS) who took a statin (simvastatin) and found that brain shrinkage, which usually averages 0.6% annually in MS patients, fell to about 0.3% annually, and neurologic function improved after 2 years on 80 mg of simvastatin. The trial suggests another possible benefit of the statin class of drugs.

A RAISE FOR CUBAN PHYSICIANS

Beginning June 1, 2014, hundreds of thousands of medical workers in Cuba will get raises, in some cases exceeding 100% (14). Physicians with two specialties will see their salary go from the equivalent of $26 a month to $67, while a new nurse will make $25 a month. The Communist Party keeps the salaries very low.

DISCOVERIES, INVENTIONS, AND ENVIRONMENTAL CHANGE

In 1858, Edwin Drake began his effort to extract oil from the ground, at a time when all of America relied on whale oil to light its lamps and to lubricate the new machines of the industrial world (15). The USA dominated the whaling industry, which sent its ships on multiyear 10,000-mile journeys from its Massachusetts base of operations around the tip of South America and into the Pacific in pursuit of humpbacks and sperm whales. The blubber from the butchered beasts, melted down into oil, earned New Bedford, Massachusetts, the title of "The City that Lit the World." The whaling villages of Honolulu and Lahaina in the Hawaiian Islands welcomed 100 to 800 ships a year, until a century of unceasing slaughter depleted the whale populations.

At the same time, tinkerers and entrepreneurs in Pennsylvania began developing petroleum-based lamp oil as a cheaper alternative to the increasingly limited supplies from whaling. In 1851, Samuel Kier began collecting crude oil from puddles and springs near his salt mines. He refined it into the newly patented "kerosene," inventing a lamp to accommodate his product, promising better and cheaper illumination than whale oil.

But it remained for Drake, a former railroad conductor, to devise a way to get more of the petroleum from below the earth's surface. His well near Titusville, mocked as "Drake's Folly," took almost a month to reach a depth of 70 feet. It employed Drake's revolutionary concept of using piping in the bore hole so rocks

surrounding the drill shaft wouldn't collapse and close the bore hole. He never patented the process and died in poverty 22 years later. But his engineering genius saved the whales!

Oil drilling facilitated the mass production of kerosene, which quickly replaced whale oil as the fuel of choice for lighting. The mighty whaling industry, which employed an estimated 70,000 persons at its peak, dwindled to near extinction, saving the shrinking whale populations from near-certain extinction. The emerging oil industry eventually added 100 times the jobs of the whaling business it replaced. Meanwhile, automobiles fed by the extracted oil made their own huge contribution to environmental enhancement. Though reviled today as sources of air pollution and global warming, cars initially replaced the millions of horses whose prodigious droppings and rotting carcasses fouled every major 19th century city with a potent and indelible stench.

In the same way, according to Michael Medved, a raft of yet unforeseen breakthroughs, providing the promise of profit for their intrepid developers, will do more to address our environmental challenges than even the most sweeping legislation or the most anguished pleas for conservation.

EMPLOYED VS. UNEMPLOYED

We all know about the unemployment rate, but there is relatively little discussion about the employment rate or the employment-to-population ratio, which measures the share of all potential workers who have a job (16, 17). This measure in 2007 was 62% on average, 60% in 2009, and 59% in 2013. The jobless rate has fallen to nearly 6% from 10% in October 2009, and the private economy for the first time has regained all the jobs lost to the financial panic. But the unemployment rate underestimates the jobs problem, because people who stop looking for a job no longer count as "unemployed" in the official tables. In a normal economy, the employment and unemployment rates have an inverse relation: when one rises the other falls and vice versa. But in the current economy, the unemployment rate is falling but the employment rate has fallen too. Former workers are simply leaving the economy or sitting on the sidelines. The labor force participation rate, which measures the active portion of available workers not including dropouts, now stands at just over 63%, a level last seen in 1978.

Many attribute the decline of work in America to the wave of baby boomers heading into retirement and the fact that the population at large is getting older. This view is probably amplified by workers who retire earlier because they lost their job and cannot find a comparable one. Yet, the decline in work is also affecting those between the prime working ages of 25 and 54 years! The employment rate for those workers rose steadily in the postwar period, dipping during recessions but always returning to an upward climb. The rate reached an all-time high in 1999 at 82%, dipped in the early 21st century, and was recovering until the recessionary collapse. At just under 77% today, this measure of work has only recently returned to the 2009 levels. That's roughly where it last hovered in 1984 and 1985 before climbing amid the Reagan growth surge. So, after a 2% annual economic growth since 2009, the share of mid-career workers in their best earning years who are on the job is still historically low. In recent years incentives to not work have also accentuated the problem—it is easier to get

Social Security Disability and food stamps, for example. All of this, of course, harms the country through loss of the gross domestic product that the missing workers would contribute and by spending far more on social programs. People who want a job are losing a paycheck, and the dignity of work and the larger US culture of work could be eroding.

Figure 1. Three institutional journals.

HEROIN RESURGENCE

A conference of >200 officials, organized by the Police Executive Research Forum, met in Washington, DC, in April 2014 to discuss the resurgence of heroin after its former popularity in the 1950s and 1960s (18). A survey by the Police Executive Research Forum of 170 US police agencies cited heroin as their communities' top drug problem: heroin, 36%; marijuana, 23%; methamphetamine, 20%; prescription pills, 7%; and crack cocaine, 6%. Heroin and other opiates are now claiming more lives in many communities than violent crime and car crashes. Several reasons appear to account for its new popularity: it's more available and more pure than previously, and it is less expensive than prescription opiates, costing from $4 a bag in some places to $20 in others, making it an attractive drug of choice. In New York City in 2012, there were 730 drug overdose fatalities, with half of those estimated to be related to heroin and prescription opiates, nearly double the number of homicides. The National Drug Threat Assessment rates heroin as the second greatest drug risk, after the abuse of methamphetamine. Attorney General Eric Holder speaking at the conference stressed that the heroin problem was national and urged police and other first responders to carry the drug naloxone, more commonly known as Narcan, that helps resuscitate victims from potentially deadly overdoses.

SYNTHETIC MARIJUANA

Thirty-eight patients came to Dallas' hospitals in a 2-day period in April 2013 with signs of severe intoxication and psychosis and were suspected of marijuana overdose (19). Some of the patients had to be sedated, and others were restrained and carried into the emergency room by hospital personnel. Some of the patients had increased aggression and tachycardia. Fifteen other patients were treated in a single day in Austin during the same week for suspected synthetic marijuana overdose. A new danger!

INSTITUTIONAL GENERAL MEDICAL AND SURGICAL JOURNALS

Through the years, many institutions at one time or another had their own medical journals, but most with time vanished, most commonly for lack of financial support. One of the oldest and most successful was the *Bulletin of the Johns Hopkins Hospital,* which began in 1889 (3 years before the hospital opened) and continued under that name until 1949, when the name

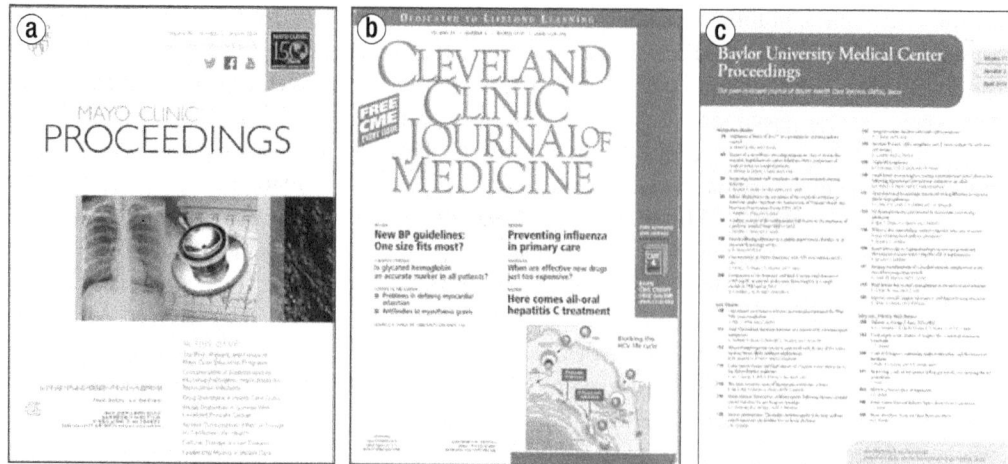

was changed to *The Johns Hopkins Medical Journal* which, to my great disappointment, was discontinued in 1966. A number of classic medical articles were published in its pages.

The *Proceedings of the Staff Meetings of the Mayo Clinic (Figure 1a)* began in 1926 (about 4 decades after the clinic started). Its name was changed to *Mayo Clinic Proceedings* in 1964, and it continues going strong. It too has published its share of classic articles through the years. The monthly issues are now published by Elsevier.

The *Cleveland Clinic Journal of Medicine (Figure 1b)* was started in 1931, 10 years after the clinic's founding, and it has been going strong ever since. Like the Mayo Clinic journal, the *Cleveland Clinic Journal of Medicine* goes to >100,000 physicians and is widely read.

The *Baylor University Medical Center Proceedings (Figure 1c)* is a recent addition, having started in 1988 by Dr. George J. Race, 85 years after the hospital was founded. Nevertheless, it now goes to >7000 physicians and is indexed in PubMed and as a consequence it receives 2 million internet "hits" yearly. The number of articles published in the *BUMC Proceedings* now exceeds the number of articles published in a 3-month period in the *Cleveland Clinic Journal of Medicine* and is not far behind that of the *Mayo Clinic Proceedings*.

CERTIFICATION BOARD SCAMS

In May 2014, I received a letter from the American Board of Cardiology Committee on Honors and Awards, dated May 9, 2014, and signed by A. J. Alaa Windsor, MD *(Figure 2)*. I was a bit surprised and transiently honored when I read the letter until I got to the second page, which indicated that there were actually three engraved award plaques: one read *The American Board of Cardiology Award of Honor for 2014*; another *The Distinguished Master Laureate of the American Board of Cardiology*; and the third *Senior Consultant to the American Board of Cardiology*. Under each of these was the option to order a number of plaques. Near the bottom of the second page was the following: "Please assist in the funding of this program of recommendation of excellence. Please enclose registration fee of $300 made to: American Board of Cardiology. Please enclose engraving and preparation fee of $70 for each 10″ × 8″ engraved plaque and $15 for shipping

AMERICAN BOARD OF CARDIOLOGY
COMMITTEE ON HONORS AND AWARDS
304 NEWBURY STREET
SUITE 309
BOSTON, MA 02115

May 9, 2014

Dear Doctor Roberts,

On the basis of your outstanding record as a Cardiologist and Educator, Distinguished Member of the Association of University Professors of Cardiology, Master Educator at one of America's finest medical schools, and as a physician respected for excellence of knowledge and experience and willingness to share knowledge with future cardiologists and medical students, we wish to honor you for the excellence and humanitarian work that has been your life's accomplishment to the benefit of mankind.

After decisions at meetings in Las Vegas, Nevada, this week, we wish to bestow the 2014 Award of Honor. It is a very great pleasure and honor for me to notify you of the award and to express our deep respect for the excellence that you bring to the medical specialty of Cardiology. We are pleased to designate you as a Distinguished Master Laureate of the American Board of Cardiology.

The American Board of Cardiology considers the designation as Laureate to be a higher level than Diplomate. The Laureate has the distinction of being exemplary as a humanitarian, as well as being excellent in knowledge and professional excellence in the specialty of Cardiology. Designation as Master Laureate is our very highest designation. Master Laureates are named Senior Consultant to the American Board of Cardiology.

Awarding is based on outstanding dedication as a medical educator, profound excellence in the specialty of Cardiology, and humanitarian aspects of medical practice including highest ethics, compassion, and the most noble qualities of a true healer.

At your earliest convenience, please send written acknowledgement of your acceptance of the award of the American Board of Cardiology, and indicate preferred exact spelling of your name and degree for proper engraving of certificates and for plaque engraving.

Very Truly,

A. J. Alaa Windsor, M.D
Acting Director, Committee on Honors and Awards

Founded as Not For Profit NV Corporation

Figure 2. Scam award notification letter.

and handling of each plaque." Also at the top of this second page is a declaration related to acceptance of the award:

> I hereby accept the American Board of Cardiology Award of Honor and the designation as Master Laureate and Senior Consultant of the American Board of Cardiology. I promise to continue to uphold the centuries old traditions of excellence and humanitarianism in medicine and shall continue to practice medicine in accordance with the Oath of Hippocrates, the Ten Commandments, and the Golden Rule to treat others as I would have others treat me. And I will continue to always faithfully work to support and promote excellence, education, compassion, kindness and truest humanitarianism in medicine.

I thought about this particular document overnight and became leery, and the next day searched for A. J. Alaa Windsor, MD, on Google and could not find one thing on him. My assistant, Becky Banks, found that the American Board of Internal Medicine (ABIM) provided the following scam warning on its website:

> ABIM has received reports from several of our diplomates regarding letters and solicitations they have received from groups offering "certification" in Geriatric Medicine, Cardiology and Hospital Medicine, among other things. ABIM is concerned about the welfare of patients who may choose doctors representing themselves as "board certified" based on their possession of a certificate from unaccredited "boards" that award certificates but require no accredited training, testing or medical background review. . . . If you hear from them, or receive any certification information that seems suspicious, ABIM would like to know about it (abim.org/news/scam-certification-boards.aspx).

William Clifford Roberts, MD
12 May 2014

1. Kean S. The zoo in you. *Wall Street Journal*, April 19–20, 2014.
2. Hewitt H. *The Happiest Life: Seven Gifts, Seven Givers and the Secret to Genuine Success*. Nashville, TN: Nelson Books, 2013 (178 pp.).
3. Wolfe A. E. O. Wilson: The noted biologist on courting controversy and the end of the age of man. *Wall Street Journal*, April 19–20, 2014.
4. Bernstein E. How happy is your marriage? *Wall Street Journal*, December 3, 2013.
5. Goldstein R. *Plato at the Googleplex: Why Philosophy Won't Go Away*. New York: Pantheon Books, 2014 (464 pp.).
6. Dreher R. Dante's path to paradise. *Wall Street Journal*, April 19–20, 2014.
7. Bernstein E. The right answer is 'no.' *Wall Street Journal*, March 11, 2014.
8. Foreman A. A brief history of avoiding exercise. *Wall Street Journal*, February 22–23, 2014.
9. Burns S. How much of your life remains? *Dallas Morning News*, April 6, 2014.
10. Ragland J. The American way of death is changing. *Dallas Morning News*, April 12, 2014.
11. Gottlieb S. The FDA wants you for a sham surgery. *Wall Street Journal*, February 19, 2014.
12. Hinshaw SP, Scheffler RM. How attention-deficit disorder went global. *Wall Street Journal*, March 12, 2014.
13. Chataway J, Schuerer N, Alsanousi A, Chan D, Macmanus D, Hunter K, Anderson V, Bangham CR, Clegg S, Nielsen C, Fox NC, Wilkie D, Nicholas JM, Calder VL, Greenwood J, Frost C, Nicholas R. Effect of high-dose simvastatin on brain atrophy and disability in secondary progressive multiple sclerosis (MS-STAT): a randomised, placebo-controlled, phase 2 trial. *Lancet* 2014 Mar 18 [Epub ahead of print].
14. Associated Press. Cuban doctors will get raises to $67 a month. *Dallas Morning News*, March 22, 2014.
15. Medved M. Innovation will heal the planet. *USA Today*, February 19, 2014.
16. Hubbard G. Where have all the workers gone? *Wall Street Journal*, April 5–6, 2014.
17. The decline of work. *Wall Street Journal*, April 5–6, 2014.
18. Johnson K. Heroin a growing threat across USA, police say. *USA Today*, April 17, 2014.
19. Fancher J. Synthetic marijuana suspected in overdoses. *Dallas Morning News*, May 3, 2014.

Chapter 16

October 2014

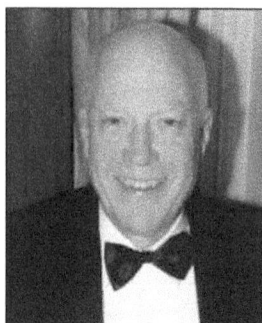

William C. Roberts, MD.

DOCTORS OF ANOTHER CALLING

Dr. David K. C. Cooper has edited a splendid book describing in detail 35 physicians who became famous not in medicine but in a nonmedical arena (1). Each chapter describes one of these distinguished men (no women were among the 35), and an appendix entitled "Who Could Have Been Chosen" provides a lengthy list of physician writers, entertainers, explorers, athletes, politicians, military men, humanitarians, and educators, as well as a philanthropist, a few criminals, and prominent scientists in areas other than medicine.

The book begins with *St. Luke*, the most widely read physician, called by St. Paul "the beloved physician." It then describes other famous physicians. *Dante Alighieri* (1265–1321), a physician in Florence, Italy, was exiled by political rivals in 1302 and never allowed to return. He devoted the remaining 19 years of his life to writing his famous trilogy, *The Divine Comedy*. *Nicholas Copernicus* (1473–1543), the Polish celestial physician, demonstrated that the Earth, rather than being the center of the universe, orbited around the sun. Thus, this physician is tied to the origins of astronomy and astrophysics. *John Locke* (1632–1704) was one of the greatest minds of the 17th century, a philosopher and political theorist but also a pragmatic and progressive physician. *Hans Sloane* (1660–1753) collected plants, animals, minerals, antique coins, and many other objects that became the foundation for the British Museum and later the Natural History Museum of London. *Thomas Dover* (1660–1742) made a fortune as a buccaneer and returned to practice in England thereafter and popularized Dover powder, which made him another fortune. Five physicians signed the Declaration of Independence and were prominent practitioners in their day. *Mongo Park* (1771–1806), a Scottish physician, led two expeditions into the heart of West Africa. *Thomas Young* (1773–1829) was stated to be the smartest person ever and contributed vastly to many areas of science, engineering, and numerous other fields. *Peter Mark Roget* (1779–1869) produced the thesaurus after he retired from his medical practice.

Several physicians became poets, including *John Keats* (1795–1821) and *Oliver Wendell Holmes* (1809–1894). Other writers included *Conan Doyle* (1859–1930), who created Sherlock Holmes; *Anton Chekhov* (1860–1904), the famous Russian writer; *W. Somerset Maugham* (1874–1965), whose plays were seen by tens of thousands and whose books sold in the millions; *Archibald Joseph Cronin* (1896–1981), a bestselling novelist; *Khaled Hosseini* (1965–), an acclaimed novelist and humanitarian; and *Abraham Verghese* (1955–), professor of medicine at Stanford University and the author of *My Own Country*, *The Tennis Partner*, and *Cutting for Stone*. And then there were the famous explorers: *David Livingston* (1813–1873) and *Edward Wilson* (1872–1912), Antarctic explorer, painter, and naturalist. The military leaders included *Leonard Wood* (1860–1927) and *Ernesto "Che" Guevara* (1928–1967). Other physicians were prominent in business, including *Abraham Gesner* (1797–1864), the Canadian father of the petroleum industry, and *Armand Hammer* (1898–1990), an entrepreneur, diplomat, and philanthropist. *Jules Stein* (1896–1981) was a visionary extraordinaire—and his chapter was written by our own Marvin J. Stone and his son, Rob. Athletes included *Roger Bannister* (1929), who completed the first 4-minute mile while a medical student in London. He went on to have a distinguished career as a neurologist and subsequently was the head of an Oxford College. *Henry Stallard* (1901–1973) was a 1924 Olympics middle-distance runner (1500 meters) immortalized in the 1981 epic British film *Chariots of Fire*. He went on to have a distinguished career in ophthalmology.

This is a splendid book making one proud to be a physician. Many of the authors of the individual chapters are members of the American Osler Society.

BANNING THE HANDSHAKE IN MEDICAL CENTERS

The handshake represents a deeply established social custom. In recent years, however, there has been increasing recognition of the importance of hands as vectors for infection, leading to formal recommendations and policies regarding hand hygiene in hospitals and other health care facilities (2). Such programs have been limited by variable compliance and efficacy. Regulations to restrict the handshake from the health care setting, in conjunction with more robust hand hygiene programs, may help limit the spread of disease and thus could potentially decrease the clinical and economic burden associated with hospital-acquired infections and antimicrobial resistance. Given the profound social role of the handshake, a suitable replacement gesture may need to be adopted and then promoted with widespread media and educational programs. With the tremendous social and economic burden of hospital-acquired infections and antimicrobial resistance and the variable success of current approaches to hand hygiene in the health care environment, it would be a mistake to dismiss, out of hand, such a promising, intuitive, and affordable ban.

ANNUAL PHYSICAL EXAMINATION

The Society of General Internal Medicine argues against routine health checks (3). Despite its recommendation, an annual physical examination is the most common reason for visiting a primary care physician. During these visits, patients, physicians, and private insurers all expect a physical examination. In actuality, the value of an annual physical examination has not been tested. These annual examinations may introduce the danger of overdiagnosis. There is always a small possibility that this examination might detect some silent, potentially deadly cancer or aneurysm. Unfortunately, for the patients, these serendipitous, lifesaving events are much less common than the false-positive findings that lead to invasive and potentially life-threatening tests.

Almost nothing in the complete annual examination is based on evidence. For a generally healthy older person, the physical examination could reasonably be limited to blood pressure measurement and assessment of body mass index. As Michael B. Rothberg, MD, indicates, so many examination elements, such as testicular or thyroid exams to detect cancer, actually have evidence to recommend against them. But most simply have insufficient evidence to recommend for or against. Medicare, which has traditionally refused to pay for routine physicals, now covers an annual wellness visit. The physician exam component, however, is limited to measurement of blood pressure and body mass index. The rest of the visit includes updating medical history, testing for cognitive impairment, assessing risk factors, performing evidence-based screening (e.g., for colorectal cancer or diabetes mellitus), and providing personalized health advice.

VACCINE COSTS

Vaccination costs have gone from single digits to sometimes triple digits in the last 2 decades (4). Some physicians have stopped offering immunizations because they say they cannot afford to buy these potentially life-saving preventive treatments that insurance often reimburses poorly, sometimes even at a loss. Childhood immunizations are so vital to public health that the Affordable Care Act mandates their coverage without an out-of-pocket cost, and they are generally required for school entry. Once a loss leader for manufacturers, because they are usually more expensive to produce than conventional drugs, vaccines now can be very profitable. Old vaccines now cost more; new ones have entered the market at once unthinkable prices. Since 1986, the average cost to fully vaccinate a child with private insurance to the age of 18 has increased from

$100 to $2200, according to the Centers for Disease Control and Prevention (CDC). Even with deep discounts, the costs for the federal government, which buys half of all vaccines for the nation's children, have increased 15-fold since 1986. The most expensive shot for young children is Prevnar 13, which prevents diseases caused by pneumococcal bacteria from ear infections to pneumonia. Like many vaccines, Prevnar requires multiple jabs. Each shot is priced at $135, and every child in the US is required to get four doses before entering school. Pfizer, the sole manufacturer, had revenue of nearly $4 billion from the Prevnar vaccine line last year. Prevnar 13, which protects against 13 strains, has gone up 6% each year since it was approved by the Food and Drug Administration in 2010. There are some good reasons vaccines like Prevnar are more expensive than previous offerings. Vaccine trials, which once included thousands of volunteers, must now include tens or hundreds of thousands, as fears about side effects such as autism have grown. Additionally, some of the new vaccines are complicated to manufacture.

CIGARETTE SMOKING

According to the CDC, 18% of US adults, or 42 million, were cigarette smokers in 2012, down from 28% in 1992 (5). Smoking rates vary regionally: Kentucky, a major tobacco producer, had the highest smoking rate in the country in 2013, 30%, followed by West Virginia and Mississippi. Utah had the lowest rate (12%), followed by California and Minnesota. Smoking rates among lesbians, gays, and bisexuals are 28% compared to 17% among heterosexuals. According to Legacy, the higher smoking rates are tied to greater social stress, more frequent visits to bars, and higher rates of alcohol use. The adult smoking rate among Americans below the poverty line was 28% in 2012, compared to 17% for those above the poverty line. The smoking rate in households with annual incomes above $100,000 is 9%.

Cigarettes cost less in heavy smoking states. The 10 states with the highest smoking rates had an average cigarette tax of 82¢ a pack in 2012, compared with $2.42 in the 10 states with the lowest smoking rates. About 70% of American smokers say they want to quit, and about 50% try to quit every year. Many smokers indicate that they are ashamed of the habit, but kicking the habit remains tough. Only about 1 in 20 who try to quit actually succeed.

Forty-two million is still a lot of people. In some states a pack of cigarettes is now over $10. If one put $10 in the bank every day of the year from age 18 to 65, one would be quite well off when retiring, if still alive.

HIGH SCHOOL SMOKING

In 2013, just 16% of high school students in the US smoked cigarettes, down from 36% in the peak year of 1997, according to the CDC (6, 7). Other news from the survey of >13,000 teens: 25% of students were in physical fights in 2013, down from 42% in 1991; and 32% watched 3 hours of TV daily, down from 43% in 1999. Some of that time shifted to computers, with 41% using a computer for nonschool reasons at least 3 hours a day, up from 22% in 2003. In addition, 27%

had at least one soda a day, down from 34% in 2007; 41% of those who drove admitted to texting or emailing while driving; 2.3% had used heroin, but in some large urban school districts that usage was up to 7.4%. The share of students threatened or injured with a gun, knife, or other weapon on school property dropped to 7% from a peak of 9% in 2003. Condom use among the sexually active (about one-third of teens) was down to 59% from a peak of 63% in 2003. A once-rapid decline in cigar use has slowed, leaving cigars as popular as cigarettes with high school boys. Unfortunately, there are still 2.7 million high school students who smoke.

HIV DIAGNOSIS RATE FALLING

The US HIV diagnosis rate fell to 16.1 per 100,000 persons in 2011, down from 24.1 a decade earlier (8). The World Health Organization estimates that 35 million people globally have the virus that causes AIDS. In the US, 1.1 million people are believed to be infected. The diagnosis rate is a direct measure of when people actually tested positive for the virus. The diagnosis rates dropped even as the amount of testing rose. In 2006, the CDC recommended routine HIV testing for all Americans aged 13 to 64, saying an HIV test should be as common as a cholesterol test. The percent of adults ever tested for AIDS increased from 37% in 2000 to 45% in 2010, according to CDC data.

TOO MANY POUNDS GLOBALLY

The obesity epidemic is global: 2.1 billion people, or about 29% of the world's population, were either overweight (body mass index 26–30 kg/m²) or obese (body mass index >30) (9). The prevalence of overweight and obese people rose nearly 28% for adults and 42% for children between 1980 and 2013. In 1980, 857 million of the world's population was overweight or obese. (Obese people are also overweight, of course, but this is the terminology now used everywhere.) These data involved 183 countries. No country reported a decrease in obesity during that period! In 2013, 24% of boys and 23% of girls were overweight or obese in developed countries; in developing countries, 13% of boys and 13% of girls were overweight or obese. The number of obese people in 1913, in millions, were as follows: USA, 87; China, 62; India, 40; Russia, 29; Brazil, 26; Mexico, 25; Egypt, 24; Germany, 17; Pakistan, 17; and Indonesia, 15. Body weight is not a good thing for the USA to lead the world in.

POULTRY, PORK, AND BEEF CONSUMPTION

According to the Organization for Economic Cooperation and Development, pork (porcine muscle) is the world's most consumed meat, but in the next 5 years it is almost certain that poultry will become number one (10). By 2020, global meat consumption in millions of metric tons annually is expected to be the following: chickens, 134; pigs, 129; and cows, 75. The trend is expected to hold true for just about every region and country, developed or developing. Chicken is the cheapest and most accessible meat in the world. Both bovine and porcine meat prices are expected to well outpace prices for chicken. Poultry is also free of the sort of cultural barriers that affect

pork. Some of the world's largest chicken-eating countries per capita are those that consume almost no pork, namely Malaysia, Israel, and Saudi Arabia.

The good news is that the poultry industry is much kinder to the environment than the porcine or bovine industries. Per kilogram consumed, chicken's carbon footprint is roughly half that of pork, a quarter that of beef, and nearly a seventh of lamb. According to a spokesman of the Environmental Working Group, "If every American stopped eating beef tomorrow and started eating chicken instead, that would be the equivalent of taking 26 million cars off the road!"

A 125-POUND WOMAN DOWNS 144 OUNCES OF BOVINE MUSCLE IN 15 MINUTES

At the Interstate 40 landmark in Amarillo, Texas, the Big Texan Steak Ranch, Molly Schuyler—a professional competitive eater who this year also broke the world record for consuming huge quantities of chicken wings in a certain amount of time—ate the first 72-ounce steak dinner with all the trimmings in 5 minutes, and a second 72-ounce steak dinner with all the trimmings in <10 minutes. Amazing! I wonder how she felt the next day.

LIFE EXPECTANCY

People around the world are living longer, according to the World Health Organization (11). The average girl born in 2012 can expect to reach 73 years and the average boy, 68. That gives them an average of 6 more years of life than children born in 1990. The US does better than average, with a female life expectancy now of 81 and a male life expectancy of 76. Nevertheless, the US ranks 37th overall and does not make the top 10 for either gender. The life expectancy of the top 10 countries for females in years are the following: Japan, 87.0; Spain, 85.1; Switzerland, 85.1; Singapore, 85.1; Italy, 85.0; France, 84.9; Australia, 84.6; Republic of Korea, 84.6; Luxembourg, 84.1; and Portugal, 84.0. The top 10 countries for male life expectancy in years: Iceland, 81.2; Switzerland, 80.7; Australia, 80.5; Israel, 80.2; Singapore, 80.2; New Zealand, 80.2; Italy, 80.2; Japan, 80.0; Sweden, 80.0; and Luxembourg, 79.7.

OPTIMAL NIGHT'S SLEEP

Several sleep studies, according to Somathi Reddy (12), have found that 7 hours—not 8 hours—is the optimal amount of sleep when it comes to certain cognitive and health markers. Other recent studies have shown that skipping on a full-night's sleep, even by 20 minutes, impairs performance and memory the next day. And, getting too much sleep, not just too little, is associated with health problems including diabetes mellitus, obesity, and certain cardiovascular diseases, as well as higher rates of death. The lowest mortality and morbidity is with 7 hours! The CDC is helping to fund a panel of medical specialists to review the scientific data on sleep and develop new recommendations, probably by 2015.

A study by Kripke and colleagues (13) in 2002 tracked over a 6-year period data on 1.1 million people who participated in a large cancer study. People who reported that they slept 6.5 to

7.4 hours had a lower mortality rate than those with shorter or longer periods of sleep. In that study, 32 health factors were controlled for, including medications. Another study, also by Kripke and associates (14) in 2011, recorded the sleep activity of about 450 older women using devices on their wrist for a week. Some 10 years later, the investigators found that those who slept <5 hours or >6.5 hours had a higher mortality.

Studies based on people reporting their own sleep patterns may have some inaccuracies. Timothy Morgenthaler, president of the American Academy of Sleep Medicine and professor of medicine at the Mayo Clinic Center for Sleep Medicine, advises patients to aim for 7 to 8 hours of sleep a night and to evaluate how they feel. Sleep needs vary between individuals, largely due to cultural and genetic differences. People should be able to figure out their optimal amount of sleep in a trial of 3 to 7 days, ideally while on a vacation. An alarm clock should not be used. Go to sleep when you get tired. Avoid too much caffeine or alcohol. Stay off electronic devices a couple of hours before going to bed. These investigators advise that during the trial, you should track your sleep with a diary or a device that records your actual sleep time. If you feel refreshed and awake during the day, you've probably discovered your optimal sleep time.

The new sleep guidelines will be drawn by a panel of experts being assembled by the American Academy of Sleep Medicine, the Sleep Research Society, and the CDC. Another group, the National Sleep Foundation, has also assembled an expert panel that expects to release updated recommendations for sleep times in January 2015. These groups currently recommend 7 to 9 hours of nightly sleep for healthy adults. The National Heart, Lung, and Blood Institute recommends 7 to 8 hours. Most current guidelines say school-aged children should get at least 10 hours of sleep a night and teenagers, 9 to 10.

The average American adult sleeps 6 hours 31 minutes on an average weekday and 7 hours 22 minutes on weekends. About 70% of Americans get less sleep on workdays than they say they need. Sleeping with a partner is preferred by 60% of adults. About 20% of American adults sleep with a pet. Pajamas are worn by 73% of American adults and 12% sleep nude. A third of adults sleep with one pillow, 40% with two, and 15% with four or more pillows.

FROM BABY DIAPERS TO ADULT DIAPERS

In the past 4 years, sales of baby diapers in the US have fallen 8% and sales of adult incontinent products have increased 20% (15). Births peaked in the US at 4.32 million in 2007 and declined for 5 years before leveling off recently. Some 3.96 million babies were born in the US in 2013, up slightly from 2012. The country's fertility rate has dropped to a record low of 63 births per 1000 women of childbearing age. At the same time, >3 million Americans are now turning 65 years every year. Over the past 15 years, US sales of incontinence products have roughly tripled to around $1.5 billion annually. Globally, sales of these incontinence products are growing at a rate of 84% annually, faster than paper-based household products. As many as 25 million Americans, or about 1 in 10 adults, have some form of urinary incontinence that can range from occasional small leaks

when they cough or sneeze to a complete loss of bladder control. While most infants and toddlers use diapers for 2 to 3 years, incontinence users typically have to buy products for much longer periods, as the problem seldom goes away. The average user spends about $80 a month. Retiring baby boomers—Americans born between 1946 and 1964—are driving a surge in the US population aged ≥65, which is expected to nearly double to 84 million by 2050 and make up 20% of the country.

KARL FRIEDRICH MEYER (1884–1974)

My introduction to Dr. Meyer was via a recent article published in *Lancet* by Mark Honigsbaum (16). Meyer was born in Basel, Switzerland and began his research studies at the University of Basel in 1902, where he concentrated on biology, zoology, histology, and laboratory techniques. In 1909, he received a doctorate of veterinary medicine from the University of Zurich, and in 1924 during a sabbatical from the University of California, he obtained a PhD in bacteriology from the University of Zurich. His first employment was in South Africa, but in 1910 he moved to the Veterinary School of Pennsylvania, where he soon rose to full professor. There he worked on *glanders*, a bacterial disease in horses, mules, etc., which first affects the mucous membranes. It may be lethal and is dangerous to humans. He also helped elucidate the transmission of the bacteria causing a contagious abortion disease of cattle and also affecting humans via unsterilized milk, causing possibly lethal fever. This disease was called *Brucellosis*. In 1914, he moved to San Francisco and the University of California at Berkeley, where he stayed the rest of his life.

In 1950, *Reader's Digest* invited Paul De Kruif to pen a tribute to his friend, veterinarian and bacteriologist Karl Friedrich Meyer. In 1926, when Sinclair Lewis was casting around for a real-life disease detective with which to populate his novel *Arrowsmith,* it is said De Kruif suggested Meyer as the model for Gustaf Sondelius, Lewis's Swedish plague-hunter. In 1928, De Kruif, a Dutchman who had worked at the Rockefeller Institute, published *Microbe Hunters, a History of the "Great Men" of Medical Microbiology.* De Kruif called Meyer "the most versatile microbe hunter since Pasteur." He described how Meyer from his laboratory in San Francisco had gone in search of the hidden factors of a series of deadly food-borne, animal-borne, and arthropod-borne diseases. In a career spanning over 3 decades, Meyer showed that *botulism* was a highly resistant spore found in soils across the USA; that *psittacosis* or "parrot fever" was an ornithosis spread by some 50 species of birds; and that the mysterious outbreaks of "staggers" seen in horses in the American Midwest during the 1930s and 1940s were due to *equine encephalitis*, a virus transmitted by mosquitoes that bred along irrigation ditches.

Just as in the 21st century concerns about food and security, climate change, and the incursion of humans into the natural habitats have led to the recognition of new emerging infectious diseases, so in the 1930s California's rapid population growth and the incursion of settlers into valleys and deserts teeming with arthropod-bearing parasites and exotic fungi presented public health workers with new and unexpected disease challenges. To solve these problems, Meyer ventured far from his laboratory, enlisting the aid of experts in entomology, animal ecology, and soil and climate science. At the same time, drawing on his expertise as a comparative pathologist, he had to convince often skeptical public health officials of the threat that animals, whether in the form of dairy herds (*Brucellosis*), parakeets (*psittacosis*), or ground squirrels (*sylvatic plague*), posed to human populations at a time when the importance of latent "infections" and "animal reservoirs" popularized by Meyer were not widely appreciated. This was no easy task. Thus, Meyer was an important bridge figure in mid-20th century medical research that sought to link microbial behavior to broader bacteriological, environmental, and social factors that affect host-pathogen interactions and the mechanisms of disease control.

As Honigsbaum describes, Meyer made many contributions to the burgeoning field, and one can get a sense of his methodology in changing thinking on disease from his investigation, particularly of psittacosis. Today, few people recall the hysteria about the parrot fever epidemics of the 1930s, but in the preantibiotic era, psittacosis was a disease that, like avian influenza or severe acute respiratory syndrome today, could provoke widespread panic. This was particularly the case in the US, where lurid stories about diseased Argentinean parrots were taken up by the prominent magazine *American Weekly* and the illness of the wife of a prominent US senator prompted Herbert Hoover to ban the interstate transport of lovebirds.

Although by 1930, it was known that psittacosis was transmitted by parrots, before Meyer, no one appreciated the extent to which the disease was also spread by parakeets, or that the large proportion of budgerigars bred in American aviaries harbored the "virus" (actually a small intracellular bacterium, *Chlamydia psittaci*) without displaying signs of illness. These silent infections were a particular problem in California where, during the Depression, many people supplemented their incomes by breeding budgerigars in backyard aviaries.

The urgent need for a study of psittacosis had been brought home to Meyer in December 1931, when three elderly California women had taken ill at a coffee club, dying soon thereafter. Meyer quickly established that the women had been infected by a pet budgerigar and that the bird had come from an aviary in Los Angeles. Meyer found that psittacosis was endemic to aviaries in the city, prompting the question of how the disease had been first introduced to southern California. To find out, Meyer paid a barber on a Pacific liner to bring him 200 wild shell parakeets from Australia. On arrival in San Francisco, these birds were placed in quarantine while Meyer waited to see what would happen. When one of the birds died 4 weeks later, Meyer did an autopsy. To his astonishment, he found typical lesions of psittacosis in the bird's spleen, the same as had been observed in California budgerigars. Meyer immediately shared the information with Charles Kellaway, who was in San Francisco at the time, and on his return to Australia Kellaway alerted Frank Macfarlane Burnet, who launched his own study in which he found that psittacosis was an endemic infection of wild parakeets and had probably been enzootic among Australian parrots for centuries. Burnet, who later was

awarded the Nobel Prize, postulated that while the wild young birds were infected in the nest, these natural, mild infections could flare up under the stress of close confinement, resulting in the birds' losing their acquired resistance and shedding the virus. By questioning importers, Meyer established that it was common practice for shippers to throw wild unbanded birds into the same pens as clean birds, greatly facilitating the spread of the virus. He concluded that in the wild these virus strains were highly adapted to their avian hosts, but conditions in shipping containers in California aviaries had greatly increased their virulence—hence, the frequent spillovers of enzootic psittacosis infections into humans.

By 1934, Meyer had tested nearly 30,000 parakeets and certified 185 California aviaries as psittacosis-free. Although he insisted that test animals at his laboratory be kept in a special isolation room and that his laboratory workers wear rubber gloves and masks at all times, the rules were not always observed. In 1935, Meyer himself breached protocol when he removed his rubber gloves to take a phone call and developed psittacosis. Meyer fortunately made a full recovery. A fascinating investigator.

ARNOLD S. RELMAN, MD (1923–2014)

Dr. Marvin Stone recently called my attention to an article in *The New York Review of Books* entitled "On Breaking One's Neck" by Arnold Relman (17). Dr. Relman served as editor in chief of the *New England Journal of Medicine* from 1977 through 1991 and before that was a renowned clinician and investigator (in nephrology). He was professor of medicine and director of the Boston University Medical Services at Boston City Hospital and, later, chair of the department of medicine at the University of Pennsylvania School of Medicine. He also was editor of the *Journal of Clinical Investigation* from 1962 through 1967 and was a member of the Institute of Medicine of the National Academy of Sciences.

The essay "On Breaking One's Neck" by Dr. Relman describes his hospital experiences after an accident on June 27, 2013, 10 days after his 90th birthday, when he suddenly and disastrously fell down the stairs of his home, broke his neck, and nearly died. Subsequently, he made an astonishing recovery, in the course of which he learned how it feels to be a helpless patient close to death. He also learned some things about the US medical care system that he had not fully appreciated, even though it was a subject that he had studied and written about for many years. His essay regarding his own treatment and his impressions thereof is a fascinating read. Just a few months after his injury, he began to resume his previous activities and enjoy life again.

He called his recovery astonishing, and it would never have happened without the superb emergency treatment he received at the Massachusetts General Hospital and the rehabilitative care that followed in another institution. But as he indicated, he was convinced that other factors contributed to his survival: his family support, a strong body, an intact brain, and very good luck. He also believed that his previous medical training helped because it made him aware of the dangers of pneumonia and other infections from contamination of catheters and tubes, so he pushed to have the latter removed as soon as possible and took as few sedatives and painkillers as possible. But there was something else that helped to sustain him: he wanted to stay around as long as possible to see what was going to happen to his family, to the country, and to the health care system that he had studied so closely. Unfortunately, on June 17, 2014, about a year after his fall, he died from complications of advanced malignant melanoma (18, 19).

ALIEN SPECIES INVADING THE USA

As Bryan Walsh (20) indicates, Burmese pythons began appearing regularly in South Florida >15 years ago. It is likely pythons, brought in as pets, either escaped or were released into the wild and then like so many retirees before them, fell in love with the Sunshine State's climate. Today, as many as 100,000 Burmese pythons may be living amid the wetlands of South Florida, though no one knows for sure. Scientists have linked a drastic decline in small mammals in South Florida's Everglades National Park to the pythons, which can lay up to 100 eggs at a time, grow more than 7 feet in their first 2 years, and now face no natural predators.

The pythons are not alone. On nearly every border, the US is under biological invasion. A quarter of the wildlife in South Florida is exotic, more than anywhere else in the US, and the region has one of the highest number of alien plants in the world. There are more than 50,000 alien species in the US, where they often compete or simply eat native flora and fauna. Invasive species are probably the second biggest threat to endangered animals after habitat loss. One study suggested that invasives could cost the US as much as $120 billion a year in damages. In Texas, *feral hogs* rampage through farmers' fields; in the Northeast, *Emerald Ash borers* turn trees into kindling; in the Great Lakes, *zebra mussels* encrust pipes and valves, rendering power plants worthless. On July 1, 2014, authorities at Los Angeles International Airport seized 67 live invasive *giant African snails* that were apparently intended for human consumption (20).

The problem seems to be getting worse (20). Most invasive species have been brought into the country by human beings either on purpose, in the case of exotic pets or plants, or accidentally with alien species hitching a ride to new habitats. During any 24-hour period, some 10,000 species are moving around in the ballast water of cargo ships. Climate changes are forcing species to move as they adapt to rising temperatures. The planet is becoming a giant mixing bowl, one that could end up numbingly homogenized as invasives spread across the globe. A biologist in Canada calls what's happening "global swarming." The balance of nature—an ideal state in which every species is in its right place—is seemingly being upended.

Life has always been on the move, but until recently that mobility was limited by oceans, mountains, and other geographic barriers. That separation allowed life to evolve into as many as 8.7 million separate species, if not far more. But then *Homo sapiens* arrived. As humans spread around the globe, they brought their favorite plants and animals with them, along with stowaways like black rats, which originated in tropical Asia before infesting the planet from the holds of sailing ships.

For a long time there was little concern about the effects of introducing alien species to new ecosystems; they were sometimes even sought after. It is not surprising that the growth of invasive species has closely followed the growth of global trade. As canoes and clippers gave way to container ships and jumbo jets, it became easier to move species around the globe. The sheer speed in which things move around the planet gives species coming from one part of the planet a much better chance to arrive alive, happy, and ready to reproduce in another part. Since the St. Lawrence Seaway was opened in 1959, oceangoing vessels have been able to sail into the lakes, bringing alien species with them. That is how the zebra mussel, one of the most tenacious aquatic invasives, found a home in the Great Lakes. There are now millions of the mussels in the Great Lakes; clusters encrust anchors and docks and disrupt the marine food chain. Zebra mussels can grow so plentiful that they block the intake valves of power plants and industrial facilities, causing hundreds of millions of dollars in damage. The mussels take all the plankton out of the water, pulling the rug out from under the entire ecosystem.

The reality is that we already live in a deeply invaded world. Alien species are everywhere. Almost all of the grasses in American lawns come from somewhere else, including Kentucky Blue Grass. More than one-quarter of the plants in Vermont and more than one-third in Massachusetts come from outside those states (20).

Invasive plants and animals have flocked to Florida for some of the same reasons that more than 600 people a day move there: the sunny climate, the plentiful land, and a generally welcoming attitude toward newcomers. And like the new human arrivals, invasive wildlife enters the state through the sprawling Miami International Airport, which ranks first in the US in international freight shipments and live-animal traffic, with about 3000 live wildlife shipments every month. While border control officials check cargo for invasive species, the sheer number of alien species entering Florida on any given day and a climate that seems designed to turbocharge the growth of anything living tilts the odds in the species' favor.

Invasion biology has become a sprawling discipline with its own journals, academic centers, and graduate programs (20). Just because a plant or animal is alien does not automatically mean it will become a dangerous invasive. But all else being equal, it is better for nature if species stay at home, and it is worth spending billions of dollars worldwide to prosecute a war against aliens. Even though the spread of invasives can actually lead to an increase in local diversity, North America has an estimated 20% more species now than it did before European colonization. On a global scale, unchecked invasions can lead to planetary homogenization. Just as global trade has allowed megabrands like Wal-Mart and McDonald's to spread around the world, crushing local mom and pop shops, human activity has allowed jellyfish and Argentine ants to invade new territory, displacing natives along the way.

Human beings, of course, have become the dominant force on the planet, so much so that many scientists believe we have entered an entirely new geologic epoch: *the Anthropocene*. We have already been shaping the planet unintentionally, through greenhouse gas emissions and global trade and every other facet of modern existence. The challenge now is to take responsibility for that power over the planet and use it for the right ends. There is one species that can claim to be the most dominant invasive of all time. From its origins in Africa, this species has spread to every corner of the world and every kind of climate. Everywhere it goes, it displaces natives, leaving extinction in its wake, altering habitats to suit its needs, with little regard for the ecological impact. Its numbers have grown nearly a million-fold and its spread shows no sign of stopping. That invasive species of course is us!

BUNDLED HOSPITAL PAYMENTS

Traditionally, hospitals have charged patients separately for every service and supply they use (21). Fees for surgeons, anesthesiologists, and other providers come in complex bills of their own. Now, more hospitals see so-called "bundled" payments as the wave of the future. In bundled care, patients or insurers are charged one overall price for everything involved in, say, a hip replacement or coronary bypass—from the preoperative tests to postoperative care, for as long as 120 days after the surgery. If the hospital delivers that care for less than the stated price, it keeps the savings. If complications occur and the patient needs more care, the hospital absorbs the extra cost. Proponents say bundled payments, unlike fee-for-service billing, provide strong incentives for physicians and hospitals to work together to keep costs and complications low. Patients and insurers also know upfront what care will cost, which is usually much less than the sum of all those separate bills. The concept began with heart surgery and joint replacement and is expanding to cancer care and chronic conditions, such as diabetes mellitus. According to Melinda Beck, some 350 health care organizations are participating in pilot bundled-payment programs with Medicare, covering 48 health conditions. Several states are experimenting with bundles in their Medicaid programs.

Promising to deliver quality care at a specific price does put physicians and hospitals at risk, so agreeing on what the bundle includes and how to price it is critical. Geisinger Health System, a bundling pioneer, redesigned its procedures and eliminated unjustified variation in care, and outcomes improved and costs decreased. In its first 2 years, Geisinger's coronary bypass bundle decreased costs by 5% and reduced the mortality rate by 67%. Its perinatal program reduced the rate of Cesarean sections by 36% and the average stay in the neonatal intensive care unit by 1.5 days. To date, however, the only health plan using Geisinger's care bundle is its own, a nonprofit health maintenance organization with nearly 450,000 members. Commercial insurers have been slow to embrace bundled care because it requires them to process claims differently. More than 100 hospitals initially involved in Medicare's pilot program decided not to continue, mainly due to administrative issues. Bundled payments pose significant challenges—including how hospitals should set prices, manage costs, distribute savings, and get physicians to think about delivering integrated care, rather than isolated care.

INTERNAL MEDICINE FELLOWSHIPS

The percentage of internal medicine specialty fellowships filled for positions starting in July 2014 were the following: cardiovascular disease, 99.6%; pulmonary disease/critical care, 99.4%; gastroenterology, 98.0%; hematology/oncology, 97.1%; rheumatology, 91.7%; endocrinology/diabetes and metabolism, 91.2%; infectious disease, 77.4%; nephrology, 75.9%; and geriatric medicine, 42.1%.

GRADUATE MEDICAL EDUCATION

As Chandra and colleagues (22) pose it, "A central health care–related policy question for the United States is whether the federal government's role in financing graduate medical education (GME) increases the number of physicians trained and influences their specialty choices by subsidizing the cost of training." As these authors indicate, total federal GME funding amounts to nearly $16 billion annually. Medicare's contribution to GME is $9.5 billion, nearly $3 billion for direct medical education to pay the salaries of residents and supervising physicians, and about $6.5 billion for indirect medical education to subsidize the high cost that hospitals incur when they run training programs. Federal Medicaid spending adds another $2 billion for GME, and an additional $4 billion comes from the Veterans Health Administration and the Health Resources and Services Administration. States support GME through nearly $4 billion in Medicaid spending. These authors argue that direct medical education funding does little to offset the training of physicians; residents essentially pay the full cost of their training, while the direct medical education program simply transfers money to recipient hospitals. Indirect medical education is more controversial in terms of both the accuracy of the costs that are reimbursed and the underlying concept: paying institutions more because they spend more, rather than because they provide higher value. Such cost-based reimbursement runs counter to the direction that health care reimbursement is heading.

If the policy goal of federal funding for GME training is to alleviate physician indebtedness or to encourage more medical school graduates to go into primary care practice, other strategies may be more effective, such as offering selective loan forgiveness or vouchers to offset tuition for trainees who opt for careers in primary care. Such strategies, these authors argue, directly benefit the recipient physician instead of the training institution. Alternatively, if the current training system is not preparing residents adequately to practice using team-based strategies or to focus efficiently on improving health care outcomes, GME monies could be targeted for activities directed toward these goals, with appropriate metrics verifying the outcomes of the training.

WASHINGTON LOBBYING

From 1999 through 2013, 20 different interest groups or individual firms spent at least $150 million to influence Congress and executive branch agencies (23). The biggest spender was the US Chamber of Commerce, spending $1,066,810,680; number 2 was the American Medical Association, which spent $306,077,500; the American Heart Association was number 5, with $259,177,661; number 6 was the Pharmaceutical Research and Manufacturers of America, with $255,146,420; and Blue Cross Blue Shield was number 8, at $231,835,532. The totals for the US Chamber were not limited to what was spent to lobby federal officials, but also included spending to influence state and local governments. The biggest spenders in 2013 included pharmaceuticals/health products, $226,114,456; followed by insurance, oil, and gas, computers/Internet, electric utilities, and TV/movies/music. These lobbying expenses do not include political donations to various candidates.

THE ATHENA DOCTRINE

The subtitle to this book by John Gerzema and Michael D'Antonio is "How Women (and the Men Who Think Like Them) Will Rule the Future" (24). These authors surveyed 64,000 people in 13 nations; two-thirds said the world would be a better place if men thought more like women. The sentiment was the same across the planet: "We've had enough of the winner-takes-all masculine approach to getting things done; it's time for something better."

In 2010, these authors wrote the book *Spend Shift*, and during the year afterwards they traveled the country and heard from many people who agreed with the thesis that a quiet revolution had taken place in "the way we buy, sell, and live" and applauded how individuals, families, businesses, and organizations were adapting to tougher economic conditions. These authors stressed the theme of adaptation and not merely survival because they saw that the effects of the "Great Recession" that began in 2008 would not be reversed quickly. Despite low interest rates, government spending, government cutbacks, and bank bailouts, full recovery seemed elusive. A growth did return, of course, to the US economy, but its pace was anemic and the previously high employment rates have not returned. Although the immediate insights offered in *Spend Thrift* were clear, these authors learned more as they presented them to audiences around the world and began to notice something they had not fully appreciated. Most of the traits exhibited by the successful entrepreneurs, leaders, organizers, and creators whom they profiled seemed to come from aspects of human nature that are widely regarded as feminine. That was not to say that these innovators were mainly women—indeed, they were not—or that they believed that human equality belonged primarily to one gender or the other. It was simply that time and again these authors heard people say the skills required to thrive in today's world—such as honesty, empathy, communication, and collaboration—come more naturally to women. The authors decided that they needed to conduct research to discover how people in various parts of the world define traditionally masculine and feminine traits. Then the authors had to discover if the feminine qualities were more highly valued. If the answer turned out to be yes, then they could search for case studies to show that the trend worked in the real world.

To better define masculine and feminine, the authors sampled 32,000 people to classify 125 different behavioral traits as masculine, feminine, or neither. They chose words like *selfless*, *trustworthy*, *curious*, and *kind* from previous empirical studies in behavioral psychology and gender-related research. They found a strong consistency across countries in what was perceived as feminine, masculine, or neither. Some words defining masculine included *rugged*, *dominant*, *strong*, *arrogant*, *rigid*, *leader*, *analytical*, *proud*, *decisive*, *ambitious*, *overbearing*, *hardworking*, *logical*, *aggressive*, *brave*, *daring*, *competitive*, *gutsy*, *stubborn*, *assertive*, *driven*, and *direct*. Words defining feminine included *free-spirited*, *charming*, *trustworthy*, *articulate*, *reliable*, *dedicated*, *dependable*, *reasonable*, *nimble*, *adaptable*, *obliging*, *healthy*, *popular*, *passive*, *committed*, *helpful*, *creative*, *flexible*, *intuitive*, *social*, *sincere*, *passionate*, *kind*, *supportive*, *giving*, *good listener*, *gentle*, *vulnerable*, *emotional*, *involved*, *friendly*, *selfless*, *empathetic*, *understanding*, *patient*, *poised*, and *trendy*. After defining their terms, the authors developed a statistical model for how masculine and feminine traits related to solving today's challenges. After getting the data, they saw that across age, gender, culture, and country, feminine traits correlated more strongly with making the world a better place than did masculine traits.

The authors found that many of the qualities of an ideal modern leader are considered feminine. We seek a more expressive style of leader, one who shares feelings and emotions more openly and honestly. Across the globe, societies want those in power to connect more personally—an understandable response to the hidden agendas and tightly wound power circles often associated with men. They found that an ideal leader must be a long-term thinker who plans for the future to bring about sustainable solutions, rather than posturing for expediency. The qualities of being decisive and resilient (identified as more masculine) are both important, but the definition of "winning" is changing. It is becoming a more inclusive construct rather than a zero-sum game. In a highly interconnected and interdependent economy, masculine traits like aggression and control, which are largely seen as "independent," are considered less effective than the feminine values of collaboration and sharing credit. They found that being cause-focused rather than self-focused was a more valued leadership trait. This perhaps indicated that being loyal (feminine) was more important than being proud (masculine). We want our leaders to be more intuitive, more understanding of others' feelings, and more able to access various angles of a problem or consequences of an action before taking action. They also found that being flexible is an essential modern skill. It permits people to listen, learn, and build consensus to get things done. They found that over 80% of their respondents said that relationships and respect of others count more toward success than money. When they explored the concept of morality, they found that it was strongly associated with loyalty, reason, empathy, and selflessness—all feminine traits. The value placed on this trait reflects society's outrage over the greed, corruption, and self-interest of our times.

They found that in every country respondents were most in agreement when it came to linking feminine traits and values to happiness. Again, many of the same virtues such as patience, loyalty, reason, and flexibility underscored the emphasis on adapting to a new world. They found that knowledge and influence were replacing traditional materialistic status symbols driven by masculine concepts of power and esteem. They found that none of the most highly masculine traits (rugged, aggressive, dominant, brave, arrogant) were among the most valued when it came to being either a great leader or a more moral or happy person. Those masculine attributes that did register as important to leadership, morality, or happiness—decisive and confident—fell toward the bottom of the rankings for what it means to be masculine.

It is the age of Athena!

MEGACITIES

There are now 30 cities on planet Earth with populations of ≥10 million: Tokyo has 38 million; Delhi, 25; Shanghai, 23; Mexico City, 21; San Paulo, 21; Mumbai, 21; Osaka, 20; Beijing, 20; New York, 19; Cairo, 18, Dhaka, 17; Karachi, 16; Buenos Aires, 15; Kokata, 15; Istanbul, 14; Chongqing, 13; Rio de Janeiro, 13; Manila, 13; Lagos, 13; Los Angeles, 12; Moscow, 12; Guangzhou, 12; Kinshasa, 11; Tianjin, 11; Paris, 11; Shenzhen, 11; London, 10; Jakarta, 10; Seoul, 10; and Lima, 10. Of these megacities, only two are located in the US, six are in China, and three in India (25).

Eight of the 30 largest cities are in countries that the World Bank defines as high-income. By 2030, the United Nations projects that only 4 of the 30 largest cities will be in nations viewed as high income: Tokyo, Osaka, New York, and Los Angeles. In 1950, New York was the largest urban area in the world, with just over 12 million residents. Now, it has nearly 19 million but ranks only ninth. In 1950, only New York and Tokyo had more than 10 million people.

KEVIN DURANT

What a guy! He saluted his mother while accepting the National Basketball Association's *Most Valuable Player* award in May 2014 (26). Durant responded to the trophy presentation by talking about how much his mom sacrificed, moving the family from apartment to apartment and working long hours to make ends meet. Yet, she always found time to tell her sons that she loved them. She was, said Durant, at his games and his practices and involved in his life in ways that money couldn't cover—in ways that only a mother's heart could provide. He fought back tears as he detailed many of those tough moments. He declared that his mother, Wanda Pratt, was "the real MVP." Her son's teammates and fans gave her an emotional standing ovation. In Durant's case, he is all too aware of what his mom selflessly endured to make him a responsible man as she fought the odds of raising a family alone in Washington. "We weren't supposed to be here," a sobbing Durant said. "You made us believe, and kept us off the streets, put clothes on our backs, and food on the table. When you didn't eat, you made sure we ate. You went to sleep hungry. You sacrificed for us." What a guy and what a mother!

GARRISON KEILLOR

A *Prairie Home Companion* is the live radio variety show founded and hosted by Mr. Keillor 40 years ago (27). He is a storyteller extraordinaire and his latest work, *The Keillor Reader*, is a treat. Some brief quotes: "Half of all people are below average." "Whoever increases knowledge, increases sorrow." "The rivers run into the sea and yet the sea is not full." "The race is not to the swift nor the battle to the strong nor riches to men of understanding, but time and chance happeneth to them all."

SAFEST FORM OF TRANSPORTATION: THE AIRPLANE

In 2013, out of 36.4 million flights, there were 81 accidents and 210 fatalities, down from 90 accidents and 685 fatalities in 2009, according to the International Air Transport Association.

ADVICE FROM A CURMUDGEON

In 2014, Charles Murray, PhD, published *The Curmudgeon's Guide to Getting Ahead: Dos and Don'ts of Right Behavior, Tough Thinking, Clear Writing, and Living a Good Life* (28). I believe this is Dr. Murray's 15th book. Charles Alan Murray (born 1943) is an American paleo conservative and a paleo libertarian-leaning political scientist, author, columnist, and pundit currently working as a fellow at the American Enterprise Institute, a conservative think tank in Washington, DC. He is best known for his controversial book *The Bell Curve*, coauthored with Richard Herrnstein in 1994, which argues that class and race are linked with intelligence. He first became well known for his book *Losing Ground: American Social Policy 1950–1980*, which appeared in 1984 and discussed the American welfare system. His articles have appeared in *Commentary Magazine*, *The New Criterion*, *The Weekly Standard*, *The Washington Post*, *The Wall Street Journal*, and *The New York Times*. Dr. Murray was born in Newton, Iowa, and because of his high SAT score was accepted into Harvard University, where he graduated in history in 1965. His PhD was received in 1974 from Massachusetts Institute of Technology in political science.

The latest book, *The Curmudgeon's Guide to Getting Ahead*, is written mainly for young people who have recently graduated from college or have just received some type of postgraduate degree, and he advises on how to get ahead in life and how to have a happy one. The book is divided into four basic sections with anywhere from 6 to 13 chapters under each section. The first major section, entitled **"On the Presentation of Self in the Workplace,"** has the following titles: Don't suck up; Don't use first names with people considerably older than you until asked, and sometimes not even then; Excise the word *like* from your spoken English; Stop "reaching out" and "sharing" and other prohibitions; On the proper use of strong language; On piercings, tattoos, and hair of a color not known to nature; Negotiating the minefield of contemporary office dress; Office emails are not texts to friends; What to do if you have a bad boss; The unentitled shall inherit the earth; Manners at the office and in general; Standing out isn't as hard as you think. Under the heading **"On Thinking and Writing Well"** are the following chapters: Putting together your basic writing tool kit; A bare bones usage primer; Writing when you already know what you want to say; Writing when you don't know what you want to say; Don't wait for the muse; and Learn to love rigor. **"On the Formation of Who You Are"** has the following chapters: Leave home; Recalibrate your perspective on time; Get real jobs; Confront your inner hothouse flower; Think about what kind of itches need scratching; Being judgmental is good and you don't have a choice anyway; Come to grips with the distinction between *can do* and *may do*; Come to grips with the difference between being nice and being good; Don't ruin your love affair with yourself. In the section **"On the Pursuit of Happiness"** are the following chapters: Show up; Take the clichés about fame and fortune seriously; Take religion seriously especially if you have been socialized not to; Take the clichés about marriage seriously; Be open to a start-up marriage instead of a merger marriage; Watch *Groundhog Day* repeatedly; and That's it! Try hard. Be true. Enjoy. Godspeed.

I love this book and I think we all can get a good deal from it.

WILLIAM CLIFFORD ROBERTS, MD
August 11, 2014

1. Cooper DKC, ed. *Doctors of Another Calling: Physicians Who Are Best Known in Fields Other Than Medicine*. Newark, NJ: University of Delaware Press, 2014.
2. Sklansky M, Nadkarni N, Ramirez-Avila L. Banning the handshake from the health care setting. *JAMA* 2014;311(24):2477–2478.
3. Rothberg MB. The $50,000 physical. *JAMA* 2014;311(21):2175–2176.
4. Rosenthal E. Doctors, patients feel pinch of shot costs. *Dallas Morning News*, July 5, 2014.
5. Esterl M, Mehrotra K, Bauerlein V. America's smokers: still 40 million strong. *Wall Street Journal*, July 16, 2014.
6. Painter K. Teen smoking hits record low. *USA Today Weekend*, June 13–15, 2014.
7. Esterl M. Less smoking, more texting. *Wall Street Journal*, June 13, 2014.
8. Stobbe M. HIV rate falls over decade. *Dallas Morning News*, July 20, 2014.
9. McKay B. About 29% of the world is overweight. *Wall Street Journal*, May 30, 2014.
10. Washington Post. Chicken about ready to rule the roost. *Dallas Morning News*, July 20, 2014.
11. Painter K. Life expectancy up; Japanese females living longest of all. *USA Today*, May 15, 2014.
12. Reddy S. Sleep experts close in on the optimal night's sleep. *Wall Street Journal*, July 22, 2014.
13. Kripke DF, Garfinkel L, Wingard DL, Klauber MR, Marler MR. Mortality associated with sleep duration and insomnia. *Arch Gen Psychiatry* 2002;59(2):131–136.
14. Kripke DF, Langer RD, Elliott JA, Klauber MR, Rex KM. Mortality related to actigraphic long and short sleep. *Sleep Med* 2011;12(1):28–33.
15. Ng S. As births slow, P&G turns to adult diapers. *Wall Street Journal*, July 17, 2014.
16. Honigsbaum M. In search of sick parrots: Karl Friedrich Meyer, disease detective. *Lancet* 2014;383:1880–1881.
17. Relman A. "On Breaking One's Neck." *New York Review of Books* 2014;61(2):26–29.
18. Angeli M. On Arnold Relman (1923–2014). *New York Review of Books*, August 14, 2014.
19. Arnold S. Relman, 1923–2014. *N Engl J Med* 2014;371(4):368–369.
20. Walsh B. Invasive species: from giant snails to Asian carp, alien wildlife is on the move. *Time*, July 28, 2014, pp. 20–26.
21. Beck M. Hospitals promote bundled payments as wave of the future. *Wall Street Journal*, June 9, 2014.
22. Chandra A, Khullar D, Wilensky GR. The economics of graduate medical education. *N Engl J Med* 2014;370(25):2357–2360.
23. Lindenberger MA. The cost of being heard in Washington, D.C. *Dallas Morning News*, June 23, 2014.
24. Gerzema J, D'Antonio M. *The Athena Doctrine: How Women (and the Men Who Think Like Them) Will Rule the Future*. San Francisco: Jossey Bass, 2013.
25. Norris F. Urbanization shifts population centers. *Dallas Morning News*, July 20, 2014.
26. "You're the real MVP." Durant's speech is a Mother's Day card for the ages. *Dallas Morning News*, May 11, 2014.
27. Keillor G. Finding Lake Wobegon. *AARP Bulletin*, May 2014.
28. Murray C. *The Curmudgeon's Guide to Getting Ahead: Dos and Don'ts of Right Behavior, Tough Thinking, Clear Writing, and Living a Good Life*. New York: Crown Business, 2014.

Chapter 17

January 2015

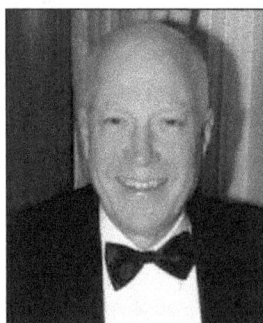

William C. Roberts, MD.

LIPID LEVELS IN PATIENTS WITH CORONARY HEART DISEASE

Sachdeva and colleagues (1) from 6 US medical centers described admission lipid levels in 136,905 patients hospitalized with coronary artery disease from 2000 to 2006. The mean lipid levels were as follows: low-density lipoprotein (LDL) cholesterol, 105 ± 40; high-density lipoprotein (HDL) cholesterol, 40 ± 13; and triglycerides, 161 ± 128 mg/dL. LDL cholesterol <70 mg/dL was observed in 18% of the patients, and ideal levels (LDL <70 with HDL ≥60 mg/dL) in only 1% of patients. HDL cholesterol was <40 mg/dL in 55% of the patients. Before admission, 28,944 (21%) of the patients were receiving lipid-lowering medications. Thus, almost half of patients hospitalized with coronary artery disease had admission LDL cholesterol levels <100 mg/dL; more than half had admission HDL levels <40 mg/dL; and <10% had HDL levels >60 mg/dL. To prevent coronary disease, it is likely that the serum LDL cholesterol will need to be <50 mg/dL.

HYDROCODONE

The most prescribed drugs in the USA are painkillers containing addictive opioids, and they are also driving the deadliest drug problem in the USA (2). On average, 46 people a day die from painkiller overdoses, and 1150 enter emergency rooms each day. Deaths from illegal drugs do not even come close to this number. In 2013 alone, physicians wrote about 180 million prescriptions for hydrocodone and oxycodone, nearly one for every adult in the USA. After underplaying the problem for years, the US Food and Drug Administration (FDA) recommended restrictions on access to drugs containing hydrocodone, which is highly addictive. The changes, which limit refills and mandate more frequent visits to physicians to obtain prescriptions, went into effect in October 2014.

Just one day later, the FDA approved Zohydro ER (hydrocodone bitartrate), a new drug that is pure hydrocodone (3). Unlike other hydrocodone drugs, Zohydro contains no acetaminophen, which in high does can cause liver damage. Zohydro comes without the abuse-resistant measures now common in most narcotic painkillers, such as hardened shells which make them difficult to crush. In capsule form, Zohydro can be easily crushed to be snorted or injected. In the Zohydro case, the FDA flouted the recommendation of its own expert panel, which had voted 11-2 against approval. Overriding a panel is not unheard of but is infrequently done. The FDA's safety mission ought to be broad enough to preclude placing an easily abused painkiller on the market amid an abuse epidemic. An unsigned editorial in *USA Today* (September 30, 2014) opined that the FDA should reconsider Zohydro and should encourage other approaches to curbing painkiller abuse as well. It advised state monitoring systems that can prevent doctor shopping by patients seeking multiple prescriptions.

The FDA commissioner, Dr. Margaret A. Hamburg, emphasized that the FDA reviews drugs using a scientific approach within our legal framework and considers not only those who abuse opioids, but also those who use them responsibly. She continued, "While we appreciate the concerns surrounding our recent approval of Zohydro, it should be recognized that Zohydro is a time-released analgesic that, without the added risk of acetaminophen, fills a need for pain patients who respond best to hydrocodone." She indicated that the problem of opioid overdose is largely driven by inappropriate prescribing, use, and diversion of these drugs. FDA is part of a broader administration-wide strategy to combat overdose. She concluded: "Opioid abuse in this country can only be brought under control by concerted effort from many prescribers, pharmacists, scientists, public health officials, law enforcement, patients and their families. FDA will continue to do its part to overcome this public health crisis."

OBESITY AND CANCER

The American Society of Clinical Oncology recently indicated that obesity is now implicated in as many as 1 in 5 cancer deaths—about the same rate as cancers linked to smoking (4). Yet, most people aren't aware of this link. A poll released in 2013 found that only 7% of Americans realized there was a link between obesity and cancer. Obesity-related cancers have contributed to increased health care spending. The price per patient of cancer treatments has gone up about 35% since 1996, and the number of people with cancer has risen from 9.2 to 16.1 million. Together, price and incidence have pushed cancer spending from $38 to $89 billion. In Texas, about 18% of adults smoke, a significant drop from smoking rates 40 years ago. Since 1990, however, the incidence of obesity (body mass index >30 kg/m^2) has climbed to more than 30%. The nationwide obesity rate now is 35%. Obesity also appears to cause more aggressive breast cancer in postmenopausal women and prostate cancer in older men than in the nonobese victims of these cancers. Obesity also has been implicated in several other cancers. Texas Oncology, a major cancer treatment group, opined that obesity and lack of exercise are factors in cancer of the colon, uterus, gallbladder, pancreas, thyroid gland, and esophagus. The prevention: lose some pounds.

TEXAS'S OBESITY

In 1990, just 24 years ago, only 1 in 10 Texas adults were obese; by 2013, nearly 1 in 3 were obese (5). American adults today on average weigh 24 more pounds than they did in 1960. In 2010, 1.26 million Texans had heart disease; it is projected that 5.7 million will have heart disease by 2030. The national obesity rate for Latinos is 42.5%. The report estimated that Texas cases of adult-onset diabetes mellitus could rise from about 2 million in 2010 to nearly 3 million by 2030. Cases of obesity-related cancer in the state could climb from approximately 330,000 to just over 800,000 by 2030. Six states had increases in obesity in 2013, and none of the 52 states or territories had a decrease in the frequency of obesity! In Texas, in 2011, 16% of high school students were obese. If all American adults lost 10 pounds, our health would skyrocket.

GERMS IN THE WORKPLACE

Sumathi Reddy (6) described a study performed by some University of Arizona researchers at an office building with 80 employees. The researchers contaminated a push-plate door at the building's entrance with a virus called bacteriophage MS-2. (The virus does not infect people yet it is similar in shape, size, and survivability to common cold and stomach flu viruses.) Within 2 hours the virus had contaminated the break room—coffee pot, microwave button, fridge door handle—and then spread to restrooms, individual offices, and cubicles. There the virus had heavily contaminated phones, desks, and computers. By 4 hours they found the virus on more than 50% of the commonly touched surfaces and on the hands of about half of the employees in the offices. Most of the people did not know each other. The studies were funded by Kimberly-Clark, the Irving, Texas, maker of consumer brands including Kleenex and Huggies.

In an intervention, the Arizona researchers then gave about half of the employees hand sanitizer and disinfectant wipes to use. After the intervention, detection of the virus on people's hands went from about 30% to 10%. The results were similar to an experiment in which the researchers infected a single employee with a droplet containing an artificial virus that did not cause illness. Within 4 hours, half of the commonly touched surfaces and the hands of half of the employees were infected with at least one virus.

Studies indicate that average adults bring their hands to their nose, mouth, or eyes about 16 times an hour! For children aged 2 to 5, the number can be up to 50 times an hour. The researchers calculated that employees would have had a 30% chance of infection if the organism experimented with affected humans. Just because we are exposed to a virus or bacterium does not mean we will get sick. Much depends on the dose or number of virus particles that we are exposed to, whether we have been exposed to the germ before, and our overall susceptibility and health. Many people have devised low-tech methods of avoiding germs. One can use his or her elbow or knuckle in the elevator rather than the fingertips. The use of a paper towel in one's hand to open the door in any public restroom is helpful.

Different viruses, of course, have different lifespans, and they also are dependent on factors such as temperature and the material where they are harboring. Some viruses are more infectious than others. Our bodies harbor viruses all the time. The average person harbors trillions of bacteria and dozens of virus species. The norovirus, the most common cause of infectious diarrhea, is super infectious, while others may be less infectious or more difficult to catch. Studies conducted at day care centers have found that 30% to 40% of children without symptoms have respiratory viruses on them. Pathogens have survival rates ranging from seconds to months. Most respiratory viruses can survive a minimum of 2 to 4 days. Some viruses die at high temperatures. Microbes survive differently on different materials. Microbes on porous surfaces, such as carpeting and upholstery, have better survival rates on synthetic fibers like polyester than on cotton. Pathogens are readily transferred on stainless steel surfaces although certain metals such as copper tend to have an antimicrobial effect, and germs will not be able to survive on them more than a few hours. Microbes have comparatively good survival on plastic or Formica. Anything with textured grooves or connection points, like a keyboard or a child's toy, will have a tendency to collect dirt, which can help survival.

While the University of Arizona researchers believe the use of hand sanitizers and disinfecting wipes can sharply reduce the spread of viruses, not all experts agree. Dr. Martin J. Blaser, director of the Human Microbiome Program at New York University's Langone Medical Center, says he generally does not recommend hand sanitizers and disinfectant wipes because they kill good bacteria, which can help protect against bad bacteria. Exceptions, he says, are in hospitals and during the flu season. Of course, a handshake can transfer from 10 to 20 times the bacteria as a fist bump.

The University of Arizona researchers have also conducted experiments in hotels, schools, and health care facilities. They found that infecting one hotel room with the virus led to the infection of nearby rooms. They speculated that cleaning tools, like mops and towels, spread the germs. The virus also spread to the conference room. Their next study will involve restrooms.

MYTHS ABOUT GERMS ON AIRCRAFTS

Everett Potter described 5 myths about germs on aircrafts (7):

1) *The most dangerous health hazard in the air is the cabin air itself.* No. The real problems lie on the chair upholstery, the tray table, the arm rest, and the toilet handle, where bacteria such as methicillin-resistant *Staphylococcus aureus* and *Escherichia*

coli can live for up to a week on airplanes that aren't properly cleaned. Tray tables have the highest levels of bacteria, and seatbelts and arm rests also are places where bacteria like to survive.

2) *Bagged pillows and blankets are okay to use.* Blankets sealed in plastic are okay, but only for the lower legs. Pillows should be avoided because the pillowcases are not changed.

3) *The aircraft is cleaned between flights.* How often and well an aircraft is "cleaned" is something of a secret. Removing trash and magazines is routine, but most industry watchers say a proper cleaning occurs infrequently. The Federal Aviation Administration does not regulate cleaning, so the frequency and thoroughness of cleaning are left to the airlines. An aircraft is supposed to be completely wiped down every 30 days of service or at 100 flying-hour intervals, but that means an aircraft can be used for dozens of flights between deep cleanings.

4) *Airlines have taken steps to ensure that passengers can't contract diseases like the Ebola virus in the aircraft.* There have not been any reported cases of the Ebola virus spreading within the confines of an aircraft cabin so far. Ebola, of course, is not an airborne virus but is spread through bodily fluids. Still, passengers should adhere to rigorous hygiene practices.

5) *There is not much we can do to protect ourselves when trapped in an aircraft cabin.* Not true. There are multiple steps that every passenger can take to prevent the spread of bacteria when flying. First, travel with and use an alcohol-based hand sanitizer. Also travel with a pack of disinfectant wipes. Wipe the armrest and the table tray. Stay hydrated. Use a tissue or paper towel to open bathroom doorknobs and touch toilet handles. The most vulnerable area may be the eyes. Keep your hands away from your eyes, as tear ducts are a fast route for germs to the nose and throat.

SIMPLE STEPS TO LIVE LONGER

Leslie Barker (8), writing in *The Dallas Morning News,* provided 10 simple steps to add time and quality to our lives:

1) *Floss.* Flossing removes plaque, the bacterial film that forms along our gum line. It might even lessen our chances of heart disease, Alzheimer's disease, and some forms of cancer.

2) *Get a colonoscopy.* Nine out of 10 people whose colon cancer is discovered early will still be alive in 10 years.

3) *Stop eating before you are full.* Being 100 pounds overweight can subtract at least a decade from your life.

4) *Use sunscreen.* In 2014, 3.5 million people in the US will get skin cancer, and 76,000 more will develop melanoma. Only about one-third of adults in the US use sunscreen.

5) *Stop smoking.* If you quit at age 30, you can increase your life by 10 years; at age 40, 9 years; at age 50, 6 years; and at age 60, 3 years.

6) *Get enough sleep.* Not getting enough sleep has been linked to memory problems, hearing problems, anger, high blood pressure, stroke, depression, vehicle accidents, and obesity.

7) *Exercise.* People who exercise 15 minutes a day add 3 years to their life. Every minute we exercise adds 7 minutes to our lives!

8) *Eat produce.* Eating 5 or more servings per day reduces our risk of stroke by about 25%. Seventh-day Adventists who typically follow a vegetarian diet outlive those who do not by 3 to 7 years.

9) *Cultivate healthy relationships.* People with friends and people in healthy relationships tend to live longer.

10) *Be grateful.* Be positive and complimentary. Those actions may not lengthen life, but they make it more enjoyable.

HOW LONG IS ENOUGH?

Ezekiel J. Emanuel, who helped write the Affordable Care Act and who is a brother to Chicago's mayor, says that 75 years is enough (9). That is how long he wants to live. He indicated that by the time he reaches 75, he will have lived a complete life:

I will have loved and been loved. My children will be grown and in the midst of their own rich lives. I will have seen my grandchildren born and beginning their lives. I will have pursued my life's projects and made whatever contributions, important or not, I am going to make. And, hopefully I will not have too many mental and physical limitations.

He is now 18 years short of 75. He will have plenty of time to change his mind. He explained:

I am talking about how long I *want* to live and the kind and amount of health care I will consent to after 75. Americans seem to be obsessed with exercising, doing mental puzzles, consuming various juice and protein concoctions, sticking to strict diets and popping vitamins and supplements, all in a valiant effort to cheat death and prolong life as long as possible. This has become so persuasive that it now defines a cultural type: what I call the American Immortal. I reject this aspiration. I think this maniac desperation to endlessly extend life is misguided and potentially destructive. For many reasons, 75 is a pretty good age to stop. Americans may live longer than their parents, but they are likely to be more incapacitated. Does that sound very desirable? Not to me. What are those reasons? Let's begin with demography. We are growing old, and our older years are not of high quality. Since the mid-19th century Americans have been living longer. In 1900 the life expectancy of an average American at birth was approximately 47 years. Today, a newborn can expect to live about 79 years.

Ezekiel Emanuel indicated that his view has practical implications. He stated that once he has lived to 75, he will not actively end his life but he will not try to prolong it. He indicated that at age 75 and beyond, he will need a good reason to even visit a physician and take any medical tests or treatment, no matter how routine and painless. And that good reason is not "it will prolong your life." He will stipulate a do-not-resuscitate order and a complete advance directive indicating no ventilators, dialysis, surgery, antibiotics, or any other medication—nothing except palliative care. He went on:

Again, let me be clear: I am not saying that those who want to live as long as possible are unethical or wrong. I am certainly not scorning or dismissing people who want to live on despite their physical and mental limitations. I'm not even trying to convince anyone I'm right. Indeed, I often advise people in this age group on how to get the best medical care available in the United States for their ailments. That is their choice and I want to support them. And I am not abdicating 75 as the official statistic of a complete, good life in order to save resources, ration health care or address public-policy issues arising from the increases in life expectancy. What I am trying to do is delineate my views for a good life and make my friends and others think about how they want to live as they grow older. I want them to think of an alternative to succumbing to that slow constriction of activities and aspirations perceptively imposed by aging.

I hope that I am around in 2032, the year Ezekiel Emanuel reaches age 75, to see whether he still believes his ideas generated 18 years earlier.

TRAFFIC FATALITIES

In 2002, highway deaths totaled 38,491; in 2012, they totaled 30,800 (10). During those 12 years, a number of cars were added to the road, so in proportion to the increased number, the decrease is rather remarkable. Wearing a seatbelt is another way to lengthen survival and increase life's quality.

FOOTBALL INJURIES, CHRONIC TRAUMATIC ENCEPHALOPATHY, AND THE NATIONAL FOOTBALL LEAGUE

Each week, *The Dallas Morning News* publishes the Dallas Cowboys' injury toll. In 2013, 15 of the 40 team players missed one or more games, and one missed all 16 season games. So far in 2014, 8 players have missed one or more games, including 1 who has missed all 8 so far. And Tony Romo with 2 back operations was recently injured again (as of October 2014).

Steve Almond has published *Against Football: One Fan's Reluctant Manifesto* (11). Professional football has displaced baseball as America's number 1 fan sport. Almond, who used to be a major National Football League (NFL) fan, has now turned his back on the game. He asks fans to consider their own complicity in ignoring and even encouraging the darker side of the sport. He indicated that "the reason ferocious hits get broadcast over and over, often in slow motion, is because fans love to see them." The TV people, of course, know the fans' appetite.

Almond reported on the effects of head injuries and on a form of dementia called chronic traumatic encephalopathy (CTE), common in former football players. The NFL has not just been slow to react to these findings; it has employed junk science to muddy the debate. Even more chilling is how little we know about the effects of football on brains that are still developing. Almond cited a Purdue University study that showed that high school football players experience diminished brain function even in the absence of concussions.

A chapter on NFL's business practices could make the most ardent pigskin fan bristle. The NFL has created what amounts to a risk-free business environment where taxpayers get bilked. Almond provided plenty of blood-boiling examples, like the NFL's tax-exempt status—unique among major sports leagues—and the now commonplace arrangement that sees taxpayers fund NFL stadiums while team owners reap the economic rewards.

The New Orleans Saints even receive an "inducement payment" of up to $6 million a year just to keep the franchise in the city. That's on top of the $200 million that taxpayers forked over for renovating the Mercedes-Benz Superdome. They will see none of the $50 to $60 million the team received in naming rights from the carmaker. NFL Commissioner Roger Goodall's salary in 2013 was $35 million. Between the recent domestic violence scandals and the stream of medical research revealing that football is more dangerous than previously thought, the sport that Goodall oversees has garnered plenty of negative headlines. But will the bad press ever cause fans to stop enriching America's most popular pastime?

The thought of any large-scale exodus of fans is unlikely. TV ratings are up again this season from already astronomical levels. The continued popularity, as Almond pointed out, is due in part to the way the sports media promote rather than cover the games. "Sports represent one of the few growth sectors for the corporate media," he observed. "It's far more profitable to cover football as a glorious diversion than as a sobering news story."

The decline of boxing from one of America's popular sports might have seemed equally impossible. The steady supply of future gridiron warriors is already starting to thin. High school football participation has fallen 2% since 2008, and the drop is more pronounced for younger players. While falling participation might bring about football's decline, Almond dared fans to consider how long they could continue to ignore football's obvious flaws to preserve their weekend ritual. The average age of death of former NFL players is 55 years!

A proposed $765 million settlement of concussion lawsuits against the NFL is presently on the table (12). There are approximately 19,500 retired NFL players, and 6000 (28%) are expected to develop Alzheimer's disease or at least moderate dementia. Dozens more will be diagnosed with amyotrophic lateral sclerosis (Lou Gehrig's disease) or Parkinson's disease during their lives. That is nearly 3 in 10 former players who will develop these debilitating brain conditions earlier than and at least twice as often as the general population. The NFL's calculations show that players <50 years had a 0.8% chance of developing Alzheimer's and dementia, compared with <0.1% for the general population. For players 50 to 54, the rate was 14% compared with <0.1% for the general population. The gap between the players and the general population grows wider with increasing age. The proposed settlement includes $765 million for player awards, $75 million for baseline assessments, $10 million for research, and $5 million for public notice. The settlement would not cover current players.

Some have argued that the NFL's offering is a pittance given its $10 billion in annual revenue. Critics also lament that the settlement plan offers no awards to anyone diagnosed with CTE in the future and that the Alzheimer's and dementia awards are cut by 75% for players who also suffered strokes. The plan would pay up to $5 million for players with amyotrophic lateral sclerosis, $4 million for deaths involving CTE, $3.5 million for Alzheimer's disease, and $3 million for moderate dementia and other neurologic problems. Only men under 45 who spent at least 5 years in the league would get these maximum payouts.

The awards are reduced on a sliding scale if the men played fewer years or were diagnosed later in life. The players' data, therefore, predicts the average payout in today's dollars to be $2.1 million for ALS, $1.4 million for death involving CTE, and $190,000 for Alzheimer's disease or moderate dementia. Only 60% of those eligible for awards are expected to enter the program. My daughter does not allow her 2 boys to play football. It's understandable.

A NONMEDICAL EBOLA CZAR

Thomas G. Donlan (13), writing in *Barron's,* said that "the mere use of the word czar ought to be considered a sign of approaching futility." He indicated that "the services of at least 149 czars have been appointed in the USA since 1918, including for example AIDS czar, Asian carp czar, bank czar, bioethics czar, bird flu czar, car czar, climate czar, copyright czar, cyber securities czar, democracy czar, drug czar, economic czar, energy czar, food czar, green jobs czar, health czar, homeland security czar, homelessness czar, inflation czar, information czar, intelligence czar, and on through the alphabet to the weatherization czar." The Ebola czar Ron Klain is the latest in the long dynastic succession, but Donlan indicated that these czars are essentially unable to perform miraculous feats of organizational efficiency. The American czars have responsibility without power.

Donlan indicated that scientists and drug companies have neglected the development, testing, and marketing of vaccines, including the Ebola vaccines, because there is no money for them in doing so. Sixty years ago, Dr. Jonas Salk devised his own trial for his vaccine to protect against polio. Salk simply asked parents to sign consent forms for the kids to participate in a double-blind study in which neither the children nor the parents nor the people administering the injections would know if a hypodermic needle contained a vaccine or a placebo. About 2 million children participated. Today, a drug company would not be allowed to do that in Africa or in the USA. An Ebola vaccine that is 100% effective at preventing the disease in monkeys was developed 10 years ago but never tested in humans according to Donlan. But we commonly hear the drug companies blamed for the supposed lack of a vaccine. Drug companies have resisted spending the enormous sums needed to develop products useful mostly in countries with little ability to pay. As Donlan said, "This produces two choices: either drug companies must be allowed to raise prices on their other drugs to create a surplus for charity work or the government must raise taxes and borrowing to pay for vaccines and orphan drugs."

Donlan indicated that the real problem could be the enormous expense created by a safety and regulatory system imposed on the world by the FDA and its counterparts in Western Europe and also by a small corps of professional ethicists who have excessive concern for informed consent in drug trials and insufficient concern for scientific progress to aid victims of dreaded diseases.

Donlan concluded as follows: "Given a choice between the regulatory protection of 2014 and the mass vaccine testing of 1954, we'll take the system that worked to fight disease. And we would like to take the one that doesn't crown a czar." Donlan also indicated that "too often we forget that the real czar— of all the Russians—was deposed, imprisoned, and executed. Nicholas II is an inappropriate symbol of power or wisdom, and remains so."

DRUGSTORE CEASES SELLING CIGARETTES

CVS Caremark stopped selling cigarettes in September 2014 (14). It has 7700 retail locations and is the second largest drugstore chain in the US behind Walgreens. It manages the pharmacy benefits for 65 million Americans and has 900 walk-in medical clinics. Its tobacco sales total about $2 billion a year. Good for CVS!

UNDERAGE ALCOHOLISM

In 2012 the National Institute on Alcohol Abuse and Alcoholism reported that 855,000 people between ages 12 and 17 years struggled with alcohol dependence or abused alcohol (15). And 5.9 million people aged 12 to 20 consider themselves binge drinkers. According to a piece by Stephanie Embree in *The Dallas Morning News,* 6 times as many young adults die from alcohol abuse than from any other substance. No one knows whether that first drink is the beginning of alcoholism or not.

MARKETING DRUGS

The system is changing (16). When physicians were mainly in private practice, pharmaceutical representatives visited them frequently urging use of drugs manufactured by their company. Today, 42% of physicians practice as salaried employees of hospital systems, up from 24% in 2004. As a result, the pharmaceutical industry is shifting its sales efforts from physicians to the institutions they work for. In 2005, drug companies employed about 102,000 US sales representatives, who mostly pitched to physicians. By mid-2014, their numbers were down to about 63,000. Stepping in are so-called "key-account managers" who build relationships with hospital administrators. The 20 biggest drug companies employ roughly 600 key-account managers, 3 times the number 5 years ago. The trend is in early stages. Sales representatives still account for the bulk of drug sales, but companies are increasingly deploying key-account managers in regions where hospitals have moved more quickly to buy practices.

Eli Lilly & Company, for example, last year scrapped its old sales-rep approach in 6 metropolitan areas including Boston and Salt Lake City in favor of key-account teams. The pharmaceutical companies are asking how they can get health system adoption. Getting a drug on the hospital system's formulary can mean potentially millions of dollars in sales from thousands of physicians' prescriptions. Drug companies used to send armies of sales reps to woo individual physicians after introducing new drugs. The reps would sometimes take physicians to sports events or cater lunches for their offices, and they usually left samples. Physicians were often more interested in a drug's clinical trial results than costs. Reps could generate hundreds of millions of dollars over the few months after a drug's introduction.

But physicians are losing influence. Hospital systems are growing more powerful as they bulk up by buying physician practices, nursing homes, urgent care centers, and other hospitals. Insurers and the federal health care overhaul are squeezing hospitals and physician payments and shifting reimbursements from how much care is given to how effective it is. To manage costs, hospital systems are taking control of what drugs their physicians can prescribe. Many limit physician contact with sales people. The gatekeepers are committees and administrators. Today's key-account managers can spend many months trying to persuade administrators to put a drug on the formulary. And big systems have more negotiating power over price than small systems. At health systems, the sales emphasis has shifted to not just how the medicine works but also how it lowers the total cost of managing disease. Formulary committees in the hospital systems decide what drugs to recommend based on evidence of effectiveness, toxicity, and cost. A committee in one hospital recently standardized treatment of certain colorectal cancer patients around the use of the drug Vectibix, which costs about $38,000 for a 16-week course, removing a drug from its list that was found to be similar but cost about 15% more. It says that physicians working in its 21 hospitals follow the cancer drug-prescribing protocols about 80% of the time.

For drug companies, health systems' expanding control not only can slow new drug acceptance but may also hurt profits by limiting a drug's peak sales and by driving down prices as systems use their increasing control over what physicians prescribe to press for discounts. For patients, the trend can be a mixed blessing. They are more likely to get drugs that evidence shows will keep them healthy and out of the hospital, but patients may face more restrictions on their choice of drugs. Physicians are finding the trend mixed. Physicians are losing their ability to negotiate with insurers. Some systems bar physicians from meeting drug sales reps during office hours and the systems are crafting formularies that will direct what their physicians can prescribe. The good side from the physician standpoint is that more time is available to spend on patient care. But, it is harder to learn about new drugs.

BOVINES AND METHANE

Cows have long been castigated for their methane-belching, manure-producing ways, one of agriculture's top contributors to climate change (17). The Environmental Protection Agency has fingered the methane emissions of "enteric fermentation"—the digestive process of animals with multichambered stomachs—as second only to emissions from natural gas and petroleum systems in greenhouse gas emissions. Our president has proposed cutting methane emissions from the US dairy industry by 25% by 2020. The US dairy industry has pledged the same goal. They call it the "Cow of the Future" project. The aim is a super-cow that produces far less methane and far more milk. A farmer enters data, including the cow's age and size, what kind of barn she is in, whether she's ever in the pasture or mud, and even how hot the weather is. Out pops the optimal feed formulation for the 100 or so pounds of food each cow eats in a day, washed down by 30 gallons of water. Cows in their prime get milked

3 times a day instead of twice. This more closely resembles a natural cycle and results in 10% to 15% higher milk production. Many farmers use bovine hormones to extend the peak of a cow's lactation. One farmer indicated that "we take the feed out of the fields and get two products—milk and manure. Milk goes to the consumer. The manure we store and reapply as fertilizer. We are analyzing all of it" so it stays in balance.

The cows are treated pretty nicely these days. In many farms the cows lounge on beds of soft sand. They are cooled by spritzers of water and breezes generated by fans. They eat a custom-blended diet of gourmet grains that a computer determines will suit them best. Each cow wears a collar with a computer chip that keeps track of her milk production, which is nearly 4 times that of the cows in olden days. Thus, it's not so bad to be a cow in some of the large farms these days—except for the ending.

MEGADROUGHT IN THE WEST

According to bioclimatologist Park Williams, the Western USA has been in a drought during the past 15 years, worse than any other 15-year period since about 1150, or 850 years ago (18). The megadroughts have been called "the great white sharks of climate: powerful, dangerous, and hard to detect before it's too late. They have happened in the past and they are still out there, lurking in what is possible for the future, even without climate change."

A megadrought is a threat to civilization and is defined more by its duration than its severity. It is an extreme dry spell that can last for a decade or longer. It has parched the West periodically, including present-day California, long before Europeans settled the region in the 1800s. Most of the USA's droughts of the past century, even the infamous 1930s Dust Bowl that forced migration of Oklahomans and others from the Plains, were exceeded in severity and duration multiple times by droughts during the preceding 2000 years. The difference now is the Western US is home to >70 million people who were not here for previous megadroughts. The implications are far more daunting. Droughts are cyclical and these long periods of drought have been commonplace in the past, according to a climatologist at the National Drought Migration Center in Lincoln, Nebraska. "We are simply much more vulnerable today than at any time in the past. People just can't pick up and leave to the degree they did in the past."

How do scientists know how wet or dry it was centuries ago? Though no weather records exist before the late 1800s, scientists can examine "proxy data" such as tree rings and lake sediment to find out how much or little rain fell hundreds or even thousands of years ago. These rings are wider during wet years and narrower during dry years.

Prolonged droughts, some of which lasted more than a century, brought thriving civilizations to starvation, migration, and finally collapse, wrote Lynn Ingram, a geologist at the University of California Berkeley in her recent book, *The West Without Water*. Decade-long droughts happen once or twice a century in the Western USA. But much worse droughts, ones that last for a century or more, occur every 500 years or so. Has California reached megadrought status? Not yet: "This one wouldn't stand out as a megadrought." But this is the state's worst consecutive 3 years for precipitation in 119 years of records.

As of August 28, 2014, 100% of the state of California was considered in a drought, according to the US Drought Monitor. More than 58% is in "exceptional" drought, the worst level. Record warmth has fueled the drought, as the state has seen its hottest year since records began in 1895. Because of the dryness, California Governor Jerry Brown declared a statewide emergency in 2014. Since then, reservoir storage levels have continued to drop, and as of late August 2014, they were down to about 59% of the historical average. Regulations restricting outdoor water use were put in place in July 2014 for the entire state. People are not allowed to hose down driveways and sidewalks, nor are they allowed to water lawns and landscapes. There are also reports of wells running dry in California. About 1000 more wildfires than usual have charred the state. The drought is likely to inflict over $2 billion in losses on the agricultural industry. If California suffered something like a multidecade drought, the best-case scenario would be some combination of conservation, technological improvements (such as desalinization plants), multistate economic-based water transfers from agriculture to urban areas, and other things like that to get humans through the drought. In the worst-case scenario, there might be all-out migration and/or ghost towns. We must learn how to use water more efficiently.

What role does climate change play in this or future droughts? Scientists apparently say that they don't have the tools to tease out how much of this specific drought might be attributed to climate change. As of now, probably very little of the California drought can be attributed to climate change with any certainty. Overall, past droughts have probably been due to subtle changes in water temperatures in the tropical Pacific Ocean. Colder water temperatures tend to produce drier conditions in the West. According to some computer models, California could actually see more, not less, winter rain and snow because of climate change. Overall, rising temperatures would tend to favor more droughts, however. During the 20th century, California's population increased from 1.5 to almost 40 million, and that increase may well have occurred during an outlier, an unusually wet century. Overall, the 20th century experienced less drought than most of the preceding 4 to 20 centuries, according to a study in *Science*.

Megadroughts are likely to hit the Southwest USA in this century. Megadroughts, according to an American Geophysical Union conference spokesman in 2014, could possibly be even worse than anything experienced by any humans who have lived in the Western part of the US in the last 1000 years! And we need rain badly here in Texas. If there is not enough water, medicines are hard to swallow.

PERFORMANCE OF HIGH SCHOOL STUDENTS

The highest SAT score available is 800. In *math*, the 2014 high school students across the nation registered 512 and those in Texas, 495; in *reading*, the US average was 496 and in Texas, 475; in *writing*, the US average was 487 and in Texas, 460

(19). Texas education officials have attributed the declining SAT scores in the state to an increase in the number of minority students taking the exams. Minorities generally perform worse than white students on standardized achievement tests, like the SAT and ACT, the nation's two leading college-entrance exams.

California students outperformed Texans by big margins in 2014: by 15 points in math and 22 in reading. Demographics of the student populations in the two states are similar: California is 53% Hispanic and 26% white, while Texas is 51% Hispanic and 30% white. Additionally, >60% of seniors in both states took the SAT.

The drop in SAT math scores in Texas might rekindle debate over the state's recent decision to no longer require all high school students to take algebra II. The College Board reported that just over one-third of the 179,036 Texas students who took the SAT met its college and career readiness benchmark, which requires a score of 1550 out of a possible total of 2400. That was well under the national average of 43% who hit the benchmark. Most minority students fell short of the benchmark: only 19% of Hispanic and 14% of black students in Texas met the college readiness standard. Both percentages trailed the national averages for those groups. We can do better in this great state!

ENDANGERED JOBS

According to a piece in *The Dallas Morning News,* the following are jobs expected to decline in the next few years: mail carrier, farmer, meter reader, newspaper reporter, travel agent, lumberjack, flight attendant, drill-press operator, printing worker, and tax examiner and collector (20). Technology killed the switchboard operator, the lamplighter, and the ice cutter, and it's now a threat for workers in a variety of other fields. When economics change, it kills opportunities, but it also brings other opportunities.

ADVERBS AND LAWYERS

A piece by Jacob Gershman indicated that no part of speech has had to put up with so much adversity as the adverb (21). It is supposed to be used sparingly, if at all, to modify verbs, adjectives, or other adverbs. Although it is generally believed that the adverb is not the writer's friend, there is one place where the adverb not only flourishes but wields power—the American legal system. Adverbs in recent years have taken on an increasingly important and often contentious role in courthouses. Their influence has spread with the help of lawmakers churning out new laws packed with them. Words such as "knowingly," "intentionally," and "recklessly," which deal with criminal intent, appear frequently in legal writings. Other adverbs like "substantially" or "indiscriminately" have been pivotal in some federal appeals court rulings. The word "quickly" has gotten some attention. Tax law allows the government to immediately freeze the assets of a suspected tax cheat who "appears to be designing quickly" to hide his or her wealth. A legal anthropology professor at the University of Kentucky College of Law recently stated, "Contrary to the ordinary view that adverbs are superfluous, law generally and criminal law especially, emerges through its adverbs."

The number of adverb-dense disputes over how to properly construe a criminal statute has surged since the 1980s. A US Supreme Court case in 2009 turned on the modifying reach of the word "knowingly," tucked into a federal statute defining the crime of aggravated identity theft. In 2013, House Republicans clashed with Justice Department attorneys over a Justice Department lawyer's use of fuzzy adverbs, like "traditionally," "typically," and "ordinarily" in his statements about the Obama administration's response to an investigation of the Fast and Furious gun-trafficking operation. Even among the most adverbially disinclined, virtually everyone recalls backtracking on promises not to use the adverb. Hemingway used few adverbs. Avoiding adverbs forces one to confront the significance of one's word choice, opined Justice Anthony Kennedy of our Supreme Court. Maybe those of us in medicine can learn something from the lawyers about our use of adverbs.

WILLIAM CLIFFORD ROBERTS, MD
November 4, 2014

1. Sachdeva A, Cannon CP, Deedwania PC, Labresh KA, Smith SC Jr, Dai D, Hernandez A, Fonarow GC. Lipid levels in patients hospitalized with coronary artery disease: an analysis of 136,905 hospitalizations in Get With The Guidelines. *Am Heart J* 2009;157(1):111–117.e2.
2. FDA undermines campaign against deadly painkillers. *USA Today*, September 30, 2014.
3. Hamburg MA. FDA combats opioid abuse. *USA Today*, September 30, 2014.
4. Landers J. Obesity link to cancer grows. *Dallas Morning News*, October 2, 2014.
5. Landers J. Texas obesity rate up a notch. *Dallas Morning News*, September 5, 2014.
6. Reddy S. Germs thrive at work, too. *Wall Street Journal*, September 30, 2014.
7. Potter E. 5 myths about germs on aircraft. *USA Today*, October 14, 2014.
8. Barker L. 10 simple steps can gain you time and quality. *Dallas Morning News*, September 30, 2014.
9. Emanuel EJ. Why I hope to die at 75: An argument that society and families—and you—will be better off if nature takes its course swiftly and promptly. *The Atlantic*, October 2014.
10. Gelles K. Crash test ratings help reduce highway deaths: Traffic fatalities. *USA Today*, September 23, 2014.
11. Almond S. *Against Football: One Fan's Reluctant Manifesto*. Brooklyn, NY: Melville House Publishing, 2014.
12. Associated Press. National Football League: 3 in 10 ex-players face Alzheimer's, dementia. *Dallas Morning News*, September 13, 2014.
13. Donlan TG. Oh please, not another czar: The Ebola crisis in West Africa creates a government crisis in the US. *Barron's*, November 3, 2014.
14. O'Donnell J, Unger L. CVS stops tobacco sales. *USA Today*, September 3, 2014.
15. Embree S. McKinney woman's nondrinking age was 21. *Dallas Morning News*, September 1, 2014.
16. Rockoff JD. Drug firms redirect pitch to hospitals. *Wall Street Journal*, September 25, 2014.
17. Bauers S. Cow of the future. *Dallas Morning News*, October 5, 2014.
18. Rice D. California's 100-year drought: Fierce fires, agricultural losses—severe water shortage a 'threat to civilization.' *USA Today*, September 3, 2014.
19. Stutz T. SAT math scores hit a 22-year low. *Dallas Morning News*, October 7, 2014.
20. Hirsch MM, Espinosa A. Turbulence ahead for 10 jobs? *Dallas Morning News*, September 1, 2014.
21. Gershman J. Lawyers, judges modify the view that adverbs are mostly bad. *Wall Street Journal*, October 8, 2014.

Chapter 18

April 2015

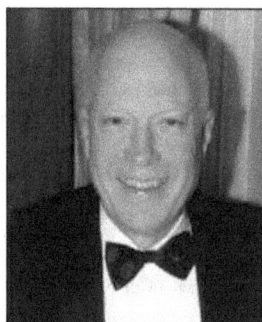

William C. Roberts, MD.

SERUM LOW-DENSITY-LIPOPROTEIN CHOLESTEROL <50 MG/DL

Boekholdt and associates (1) from multiple medical centers did a meta-analysis from 8 randomized controlled statin trials in which conventional lipids and apolipo-proteins were determined in all study participants at baseline and at 1-year follow-up. Among the 38,153 patients allocated to statin therapy, 6286 major cardiovascular events occurred in 5387 studied participants during follow-up. The authors found that >40% of the participants in these trials did not reach a low-density lipoprotein (LDL) cholesterol level <70 mg/dL despite being prescribed rosuvastatin 20 mg or atorvastatin 20 mg. There was a clear relation between LDL cholesterol level attained and cardiovascular risks, with the major cardiovascular event rate at 1 year increasing incrementally from 4.4% in those with LDL levels <50 mg/dL, 10.9% for those with LDL of 50 to <70 mg/dL, 16% for those with LDL of 70 to <100 mg/dL, and up to 34% in those with LDL >190 mg/dL. This relation, of course, supports the premise that "lower is better" when it comes to LDL goals.

US DEPARTMENT OF AGRICULTURE'S DIETARY GUIDELINES

Every 5 years our government has been issuing guidelines about healthy eating choices (2, 3). A panel that advises the Department of Agriculture submitted its latest draft recommendations in December 2014, and they include what foods are better not only for our health, but also for our environment. That means that when the latest version of the government's dietary guidelines come out (near the end of 2015), they may push even harder than in the past for people to choose more fruits, vegetables, nuts, whole grains, and other plant-based foods at the expense of meat. The study, as shown in *Table 1,* indicates that compared with other popular animal proteins, beef produces the most heat-trapping gases per calorie, produces the most water-polluting nitrogen, needs the most water for irrigation, and requires the most land. Once the recommendations of the advisory panel are finalized, they will be submitted to the

Departments of Agriculture and Health and Human Services, which will craft the final dietary guidelines. The guidelines are the basis for the US Department of Agriculture's "My Plate" icon that replaced the food pyramid in 2010 and is designed to help Americans with healthy eating. Guidelines also will be integrated into school lunch meal patterns and other federal eating programs.

Of course, the meat industry has fought for years to ensure that the dietary guidelines do not call for eating less meat. The present guidelines now recommend eating lean meats instead of reducing meat altogether. The new guideline recommendations featured in the December 2014 draft recommend fewer "red and processed meats."

The government's first food guide came in 1916 and established guidance based on food groups. Since then, the guide has come in many forms. The latest one is the circle broken into roughly 4 parts, named fruit, vegetables, grains, and protein, with a small circle for dairy on the side. A growing body of research has found that meat animals, and cattle in particular, with their belching of greenhouse gases, trampling of the landscape, and need for massive amounts of water, are a major factor in global warming.

Administration officials are already enmeshed in bitter fights with Republicans over coal-fired power plants, methane emissions from oil and gas production, and regulation of automobiles. Whether they have the stomach for adding a food fight to the list remains uncertain. The possibility that climate change

Table 1. Land and water needed to produce 1000 calories and resulting pollutants*

From	Land needed (square feet)	Water needed (gallons)	Greenhouse gases generated (pounds)	Nitrogen generated (ounces)
Beef	1,580	435	21	6
Pork	57	49	4	2
Poultry	44	38	4	1
Eggs	32	28	3	1
Dairy	94	45	4	1

*Source: *Dallas Morning News* (2, 3).

politics could affect nutrition guidelines serves as a reminder of how many parts of daily life the struggle to limit global warming can reach.

A revamp of the food pyramid to take climate into account would be a bold step. Despite a major push by the United Nations for countries to rework dietary policies with an eye on climate impact, no country has done so. The Netherlands is expected to be the first when it releases a new chart illustrating food guidelines this year.

This antimeat bandwagon has recently been rebuffed by Nicolette Hahn Niman, the author of *Defending Beef: The Case for Sustainable Meat Production* (4). Ms. Niman writes: "People who advocate eating less beef often argue that producing it hurts the environment. Cattle . . . have an outsized ecological footprint: they guzzle water, trample plants and soils, and consume precious grains that should be nourishing hungry humans. Lately, critics have blamed bovine burps, flatulence, and even breath for climate change." Ms. Niman, a long-time vegetarian and environmental lawyer, once bought into these claims. Her husband, Bill, founded Niman Ranch but left it in 2007, and they now have a grass-fed beef company. As a consequence, she has come to the opposite view. She claims that raising beef cattle, especially on grass, is an environmental gain for the planet.

Her arguments are as follows: she indicates that the Environmental Protection Agency argues that all of US agriculture accounts for just 8% of our greenhouse emissions, with by far the largest share owing to soil management—that is, crop farming. A Union of Concerned Scientists report concluded that about 2% of US greenhouse gases can be linked to cattle and that good management would diminish it further. The primary concern is methane, a potent greenhouse gas, but if cattle were fed certain nutritional supplements, the methane from cattle could be cut by half. She further argues that cattle are key to the world's most promising strategy to counter global warming: restoring carbon to the soil. One-tenth of all human-caused carbon emissions since 1850 has come from the soil, according to certain ecologists. This, she argues, is due to tillage, which releases carbon and strips the earth of protective vegetation, and to farming practices that fail to return nutrients and organic matter to the Earth. Plant-covered land that is never plowed is ideal for recapturing carbon through photosynthesis and for holding it in stable forms.

She further argues that most of the world's beef cattle are raised on grass. Their pruning mouths stimulate vegetative growth as their trampling hoofs and digestive tracts foster seed germination and nutrient recycling. These beneficial disturbances, like those once caused by wild grazing herds, prevent the encroachment of woody shrubs and are necessary for the functioning of grassland ecosystems. She states that research by the Soil Association in the United Kingdom showed that if cattle were raised primarily on grass and if good farming practices were followed, enough carbon could be sequestered to offset the methane emissions of all UK beef cattle and half its dairy herd. Similarly, in the US, the Union of Concerned Scientists estimated that as much as 2% of all greenhouse gases (slightly less than what's attributed to cattle) could be eliminated

by sequestering carbon in the soils of grazing operations. She indicates that grass is also one of the best ways to generate and safeguard soil and to protect water. Grass blades shield soil from erosive wind and water, while its roots form a net that holds soil and water in place.

Niman also argues that cattle are not voracious consumers of water. Some environmental critics of cattle assert that 2500 gallons of water are required for every pound of beef produced. But this figure (or the even higher ones often cited by advocates of veganism) are based on the most water-intensive situations.

Finally, she questions the thought that eating beef worsens world hunger. She indicates that this is ironic since a billion of the world's poorest people depend on livestock. Most of the world's cattle live on land that cannot be used for crop cultivation, and in the US, 85% of the land grazed by cattle cannot be farmed, according to the US Beef Board. She mentions that the bovine's most striking attribute is that it can live on a simple diet of grass, which it forages for itself. And for protecting land, water, soil, and climate, there is nothing better than dense grass.

A major concern of mine would be the fattening cattle farms where cows are placed when they weigh about 700 pounds and are fattened up to 1100 pounds. The ground is trampled, there is no grass around, and the feces slide off into the various water drainage sites.

FAST FOOD AND TEST SCORES

Some researchers at Ohio State University used data from a nationally representative sample of about 11,700 children to measure how fast food might be affecting classroom performance (5). This study measured how much fast food the children ate at age 10 and then compared the consumption levels with test results in reading, math, and science 3 years later. They found that even small increases in the frequency in which the students ate fast food were associated with poor academic test results. Habitual fast-food eaters—those who ate fast food daily—had test scores about 20% lower than those who didn't eat any fast food. The connection held true even after the researchers took into account more than a dozen other factors about the children's habits and backgrounds, including fitness, broader eating habits, socioeconomic status, and characteristics of their neighborhoods and schools. More than half the fifth graders ate fast food 1 to 3 times a week and nearly three-quarters of them ate fast food at least once a week. Nearly one-third of American children between the ages of 2 and 11—and nearly half of those aged 12 to 19—eat or drink something from a fast food restaurant every day according to a study published in 2008. Fast food still accounts for about 13% of total calories eaten by children and teenagers aged 2 to 18 in the USA.

GLOBESITY

Nearly a third of the world's population is overweight or obese, a percentage that is set to hit 50% by 2030 according to a recent report on "Globesity and Health and Wellness" by Sarbjit Nahal, head of thematic investing at Bank of America Merrill Lynch (6). He estimates the global impact of obesity is

$2 trillion, or 2.8% of global gross domestic product—on par with smoking, armed violence, war, and terrorism. US generals are calling the problem the biggest security threat facing the US today, since overweight recruits cannot pass the fitness requirements. Car makers have been forced to revamp the size of crash-test dummies because the safety implications are so fundamentally different. Although the US, China, and India are the countries with the greatest share of the world's obese, Greece and Italy have higher percentages of overweight and obese people than the US. It is not just a problem in the developed world. In the developing world, the lower rungs of the socioeconomic ladder have less time for physical activity and eat more processed food. Increasingly in emerging markets, people who are well off are eating fresh and healthy foods and going to the gym.

THE ANNUAL PHYSICAL EXAMINATION

In 2012, the Cochrane Collaboration, an international group of medical researchers who systematically review the world's biomedical research, analyzed 14 randomized controlled trials with over 182,000 people followed for a median of 9 years that sought to evaluate the benefits of routine, general health checkups, i.e., visits to the physician for general health and not prompted by any particular symptom or complaint (7). The conclusion was that checkups were unlikely to be beneficial. Regardless of which screenings and tests were administered, studies of annual health exams dating from 1963 to 1999 showed that the annual physical did not reduce mortality overall or for specific causes of death from cancer or heart disease. And the checkups consumed billions of dollars, although no one is sure exactly how many billions because of the challenge of measuring the additional screenings and follow-up tests. This lack of evidence is the main reason the US Preventive Services Task Force—an independent group of experts making evidence-based recommendations about the use of preventive services—does not have a recommendation on routine annual health checkups. The Canadian guidelines have recommended against these exams since 1979.

According to Ezekiel J. Emanuel, one explanation for the ineffectiveness of the annual exam in reducing the death rate is that it does little to avert death or disability from acute problems. Unintentional injuries and suicides are, respectively, the fourth and tenth leading cause of death among Americans. And, the annual physical does little for chronic conditions without significantly useful interventions, such as Alzheimer's, the fifth leading cause of death among older people.

TANNING BEDS

Twenty minutes in a tanning bed costs $7.00 (8). A publication in 2014 estimated that tanning beds account for as many as 400,000 cases of skin cancer in the USA each year, including 6000 cases of melanoma. The incidence in women <40 has risen by one-third since the early 1990s. In 2014, the US Food and Drug Administration (FDA) invoked its most serious risk warning, lifting tanning beds from a category that included Band-Aids to that of potentially harmful medical devices. The Obama administration's 2010 health care law imposed a 10%

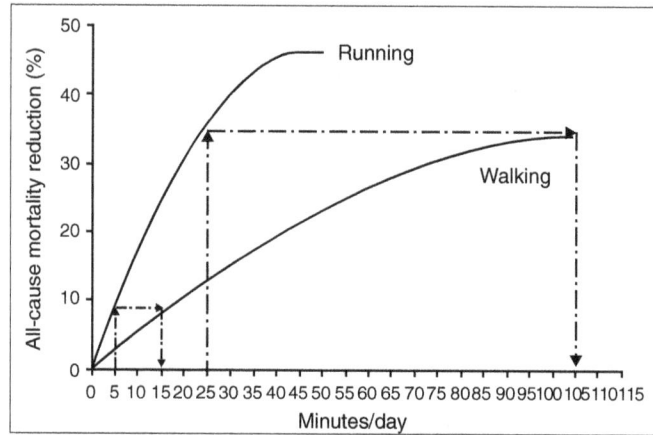

Figure 1. Comparison of benefits between walking and running. A 5-min run generates the same benefits as a 15-min walk, and a 25-min run is equivalent to a 105-min walk. Reprinted from Lee DC et al, 2014 (9), with permission from Elsevier.

tax on tanning salons. More than 40 states now have some restrictions on the use of tanning salons by minors. The use of indoor tanning among teenage girls dropped from 25% to 20% from 2009 to 2013. Stay away.

RUNNING AND MORTALITY

Lee and associates (9, 10), from a 15-year follow-up of 55,137 adults at the Cooper Clinic in Dallas, found that running as little as 5 to 10 minutes per day was associated with reduced mortality from all causes (30%) and from cardiovascular disease (45%) and could add 3 years of life expectancy (*Figure 1*). This minimal amount, half of that recommended in the guideline, is similar to the 15-minute per day of brisk walking reported in the *Lancet* in 2011 by Wen et al, one-half of the currently recommended 150 minutes per week, or 30 minutes per day. Both showed a 3-year extension of life expectancy, and both are good news of course to the sedentary, because finding 5 to 15 minutes per day to exercise is much easier than finding 30 minutes. Prior to these two studies, no conclusive timeline had been identified with sufficient statistical power to show definite health benefit.

DALLAS MURDER RATE

In 2014, the murder rate in Dallas was its lowest since 1930, the year that Bonnie and Clyde met (11). A total of 116 murders occurred in Dallas in 2014. That is also a drop from the 143 murders in 2013, and it's less than half the murders recorded in 2004. The number of murders in Chicago in 2014 was 407, and in Philadelphia, 248, both slight drops from the 2 previous years. For every 100,000 Dallasites, the city recorded just over 9 murders in 2014, slightly above the 2013 national average for cities of >1 million people. In contrast, in murder havens Flint and Detroit, Michigan, 48 and 45 people, respectively, of every 100,000 were murdered. The murder number does not include justifiable homicides, such as shootings by police or homeowners who shoot burglars. The City of Dallas peaked at 500 murders in 1991. The number of aggravated assaults in 2014 increased in Dallas compared to the previous year.

OUR HOTTEST YEAR

The Earth's hottest year on record was 2014 (12). Both the National Oceanic and Atmospheric Administration (NOAA) and NASA calculated that in 2014 the world had its hottest year in 135 years of recordkeeping. Earlier, the Japanese Weather Agency and an independent group from the University of California at Berkeley also measured 2014 as the hottest on record. Thus, the globe is warmer now than it has been in the last 100 years and, as one scientist mentioned, probably 5000 years. Furthermore, 9 of the 10 hottest years in NOAA global records have occurred since 2000, a reflection of the relentless planetary warming that scientists say is a consequence of human emissions and that has posed profound long-term risks to civilization and to the natural world.

NOAA indicated that 2014 averaged 58.24°F, 1.24° above the 20th century average. NASA, which calculates temperatures slightly differently, put 2014's average temperature at 58.42°F, 1.22° above the average of the years 1951 to 1980. Earth broke NOAA records for heat in 2010 and in 2005. The last time the Earth set an annual NOAA record for cold was in 1911. February 1985 was the last time global temperatures fell below the 20th century average for a given month, meaning that no one <30 years of age has ever lived through a below-average month.

The heat of 2014 was driven by record warmth in the world's oceans, and it did not just break old marks, it shattered them. Record warmth spread across far-eastern Russia, the western part of the US, interior South America, much of Europe, Northern Africa, and parts of Australia. One of the few colder spots was in the central and eastern US. Climate scientists indicated the most significant part of 2014's record is that it happened during a year when there was no El Niño weather isolation. During an El Niño when a specific area of the Central Pacific Ocean warms unusually and influences weather worldwide, global temperatures tend to spike. Previous records, especially in 1998, happened during El Niño years. The planet is warming and it is as simple as that.

SEA RISING

According to an article in the January 2015 issue of *Nature,* the current rise in sea level is 2.5 times faster than it was from 1900 to 1990 (13). The faster pace apparently is due to the melting of ice sheets in Greenland and Antarctica and shrinking glaciers, triggered by human-made global warming. Previous research had shown that between 1900 and 1990 the seas rose about two-thirds of an inch each decade. The new study recalculates that rate to less than half an inch a decade. Since 1990, however, seas have been rising about 1.2 inches a decade. While hundreds of tide gauges around the world have been measuring sea levels since 1900, they have mostly been in Europe and North America. Thus, estimates of 20th century sea level rise gave an incomplete picture of the global effect. The new method uses statistical analysis and computer models to better simulate the areas in the gap. The implications are that more and more sea level rise will occur in the future, perhaps at a faster rate than previously thought.

THE CASE FOR FOSSIL FUELS

Alex Epstein in a book entitled *The Moral Case for Fossil Fuels* argues that plentiful, reliable, affordable energy is necessary for human flourishing and, indeed, for human life, and at this point, that energy can best be provided by fossil fuels: coal, petroleum, and natural gas (14). The author drives home the idea that the crusade against fossil fuels stems less from a desire to ensure clean air and water for human use than from an idealization of "untouched" nature—the view that human nonimpact on the planet is to be striven for above all else. Epstein argues that if one is concerned about sea level rises or destructive hurricanes, one should cheer on industrialization all the more loudly. Prosperous economies are best able to manage the challenges Earth's climate throws our way. "It is only thanks to cheap, plentiful, reliable energy that we live in an environment where the water we drink and the food we eat will not make us sick and where we can cope with the often hostile climate of Mother Nature."

From air-conditioning to desalinization, it is industrial society—enabled by affordable and abundant energy—that allows humans to transform their environment and thrive in otherwise unpleasant climates. Epstein further emphasizes that climate crusaders who thwart developing world access to coal-fueled power plants perpetuate the misery. Cheap, 24/7 electricity is critical to economic development. While coal has become enemy #1 in large swaths of the West, access to cheap electricity from coal-fueled power plants vastly improves the length and quality of life of the world's poor. The vast numbers of people on this planet who do not have access to sufficient energy to cook 2 meals a day spend a significant portion of their waking hours gathering sticks and dung to burn for heat and cooking. They would benefit tremendously if they were connected to a large coal-fired power plant. Indeed, the quality of the very air they breathe would improve; every year millions of people die prematurely due to the inhalation of contaminants from indoor cooking fires.

STEVEN BRILL ON HEALTH CARE COSTS

Steven Brill is the author of *Time's* "Trailblazing Special Report on Medical Bills." His book, *America's Bitter Pill,* is a sweeping inside account of how Obamacare happened and what it does and does not do to curb the abuses (15). Brill's piece in *Time* was published in January 2015 and was adapted from his book.

Brill indicates the following: America's total health care bill for 2014 was $3 trillion. That's more than the next 10 biggest spenders combined: Japan, Germany, France, China, the UK, Italy, Canada, Brazil, Spain, and Australia. All that extra money produces no better results, and in many cases, worse results. There are 31.5 magnetic resonance imaging (MRI) machines per 1 million people in the US, and 5.9 per 1 million in the UK. We spend $86 billion treating back pain, which is as much as is spent on all the countries' state, city, county, and town police forces. Possibly half of that is unnecessary. We spend $17 billion a year on artificial knees and hips, which is 55% more than Hollywood takes in at the box office each year. We have created a system in which 1.5 million people work in the health insurance industry, while barely half as many physicians provide the actual care. And all those high-tech advances—pacemakers, MRIs, 3-D mammograms, etc.—have produced an ironically upside-down health care marketplace. Health care is the only industry in which technological advances have increased costs instead of lowering them.

Health care is America's largest industry by far, employing a sixth of the country's workforce. It is average Americans' largest single expense, whether paid out of their pockets or through taxes and insurance premiums. The health care industry spends four times as much on lobbying as the #2 Beltway spender, the military industrial complex.

Brill's solution includes cutting out the middleman, the insurance companies, which now account for 15% to 20% of private health care costs. As hospitals consolidate, something that is happening all over the country, they need to become their own insurance companies so they can cut out the middleman and align the incentives. The insurance company, then, would have not only every incentive to control the doctors' and hospitals' costs, but also the means to do so.

PERCENT OF INCOME SPENT ON HEALTH INSURANCE

The US average in 2013 was 9.6%, nearly double that in 2003. The percentage of income spent on insurance premiums and deductibles in 2013 was highest in Florida at 12.4% and second highest in Texas at 12.3% (16). The cost of the average employer-sponsored family health insurance plan was $16,049, or 27% of the annual income of working Texans in 2013! Many Texas companies have shifted more of the cost of these plans to their workers. Deductibles, the amount a worker has to spend on health care before insurance kicks in, went up sharply in Texas between 2003 and 2013. Single workers paid deductibles averaging $624 in 2003, and the average in 2013 was $1543. While employers once paid 80% of premiums, now companies typically pay a little over two-thirds of the premium cost for a family plan in 2013, leaving the workers with the other 31%. Health insurance premiums in Texas increased by 6.1% a year between 2003 and 2009, but slowed to 2.4% annually between 2010 and 2013. Premium hikes for workers during those 3 years, however, and deductibles went up by 7.4% annually. With median income at $49,500 in 2013, the average Texas family with a workplace insurance plan spent $6,088 on premiums and deductibles. In 2003, the cost was $2,960, or 7.4% of income. The result is that out-of-pocket costs are consuming a greater share of employee incomes.

MEDICARE PATIENT MALADIES

The most common chronic ailments in patients ≥65 years who are enrolled in Medicare are listed in *Table 2* (17). About two-thirds of Medicare beneficiaries have two or more chronic conditions, and they tend to visit different doctors for different diseases. Often, a single overseeing physician is not involved. Beginning in January 2015, Medicare will pay primary care physicians a monthly fee to better coordinate care for the most vulnerable seniors, those with multiple chronic illnesses, even

Table 2. Prevalence of the most common chronic ailments in Medicare patients

Ailment	Prevalence
Hypertension	57%
Hypercholesterolia	48%
Coronary disease	30%
Arthritis	29%
Diabetes mellitus	25%
Kidney failure	13%
Heart failure	13%
Depression	11%
Chronic obstructive pulmonary disease	10%
Cancer	9%
Alzheimer's disease/dementia	9%
Osteoporosis	7%

*Source: Centers for Medicare and Medicaid Services, 2012 data, as it appeared in *Dallas Morning News* (17).

if they don't have a face-to-face encounter. The goal is to help patients stay healthier between doctor visits and avoid hospitalization and nursing homes, which of course are quite expensive. Medicare's new fee is about $40 a month per qualified patient. Previously, the program paid only for services provided in the physician's office. To earn the new fee, physicians must come up with a care plan for qualified patients and spend time each month on such activities as coordinating their care with other health providers and monitoring their medications. Also, patients must have a way to reach someone in the care team who can access their health records 24 hours a day for proper evaluation of an after-hours complaint. The new fee could enable physicians to hire extra nurses or care managers to do more of the preventive work. Patients must agree to care coordination; the fee is subject to Medicare's standard deductible and co-insurance.

Being a care coordinator is like being a quarterback. Dr. Matthew Press described in a piece in the *New England Journal of Medicine* (18) the 80 days between diagnosing a man's liver cancer and his surgery. The internists sent 32 e-mails and had 8 phone calls with the patient's 11 other physicians. (This article was supplied to me by Dr. Joseph Rothstein.) The chronic care management fee is one of multiple projects Medicare has underway in hopes of strengthening primary care and, in turn, saving money.

AFGHAN OPIUM POPPY CULTIVATION

The United Nations estimates that the land area used to cultivate poppies in Afghanistan increased 7% in 2014 to 554,000 acres (19). The profits from opium and heroin are huge, and the UN Office of Drugs and Crime reported that in 2014, Afghan poppy farmers took in about $850 million, more than twice as much as 5 years earlier. Processing labs have sprung up there in several border provinces, and street sales of refined powder have become a major business in Kabul and several provincial capitals. Domestic law enforcement efforts have been limited and ineffective, with only about 2000 police nationwide assigned to any narcotic work. Corruption is so entrenched that a major drug trafficker, whose rare 20-year sentence was held as a success for the ambitious US Drug Enforcement support program, bribed his way out of an Afghan prison recently and vanished. The number of addicts in Afghanistan has soared, and there is little help for those who want to quit. There are 170 drug treatment facilities in Afghanistan, most built with foreign funds, but their total capacity is only 39,000 patients, and the few residential programs release addicts to the street after 40 days with little follow-up.

CANINE OVERPOPULATION

Melinda Beck in a piece in *The Wall Street Journal* indicates that there are an estimated 375 million stray dogs worldwide (20). She discusses methods of sterilization and suggests that the fastest and least expensive method of neutering male dogs is a quick injection of calcium chloride into the testicles, which makes them sterile. The dogs get a light sedative but no general anesthesia or incisions. They can be up and running again in minutes. The cost: about $1 per dog. Calcium chloride could be a boon to animal shelters in many impoverished areas, many of which lack the funds and facilities to sterilize dogs surgically. More than 3 million dogs and cats are euthanized in US shelters every year. But few veterinarians and shelter operators even know about calcium chloride. It has been stalled in a regulatory catch-22 that illustrates how products that do not have much profit potential can languish unused. Inexpensive, nonsurgical sterilization would be a godsend to countries like India, where packs of dogs run wild. And the stray dogs terrorize some neighborhoods, fighting over food and reproducing exponentially.

Research on calcium chloride goes back to the 1970s when it was tested as a sterilizing agent in calves, colts, and other animals. A number of studies now have described a variety of doses and solutions of calcium chloride and concluded that a 20% solution of calcium chloride in ethyl alcohol was optimal, rendering dogs "azoospermic" and reducing testosterone levels by 70%, with no adverse effects.

Calcium chloride is not approved by the FDA and probably never will be. It is such a common chemical that it cannot be patented. As a result, drug companies are not interested in investing the $10 million or more needed to run the required clinical trials. Without FDA approval, most veterinarians and animal welfare groups are leery of endorsing it.

Nevertheless, finding safe, nonsurgical ways to control animal reproduction has been a goal of animal researchers for decades, but progress has been slow. One nonprofit foundation that works to advance neglected medical research tried to start the FDA approval process for the use of calcium chloride in male cats in 2014 but the bid for a "barrier to innovation" waiver of the $87,000 application fee was denied on the grounds that the research was not "innovative" enough. I suspect that calcium chloride will slowly be adapted as an inexpensive, quick, relatively painless procedure that could make a big dent in canine overpopulation.

PLANNING FOR THE INEVITABLE

Jane Bryant Quinn, author of *Making the Most of Your Money Now*, described what to tell your adult offspring about your money (21). She strongly advised telling your offspring where to find your will, health care directive, financial records, and any life insurance policies. If the will leaves them uneven shares, explain that decision, either orally or by a thoughtful explanatory letter. Tell all of the offspring who has the power of attorney or is the executor of your will. She advises not telling the offspring exactly what you are worth, in case your assets get depleted later in life. The offspring shouldn't be planning on an inheritance they might not get. Conversely, up-front disclosure about your intentions can help prevent siblings' dishonesty in handling family assets, if that is a risk. Families manage better when one leaves no big surprises behind.

To prevent your family's scrambling to find documents during an emergency, she advises the following. 1) Inventory your assets and their location. Include the name of your physician, accountant, insurance agent, and financial advisor. 2) Make a list of passwords for your computer, mobile devices, and accounts. 3) Compile a list of the medications you take. 4) Prepare an advance directive, which often consists of two parts: a power of attorney that names someone to make medical decisions for you if you are incapacitated and a living will that details the life-sustaining measures you want if you are unlikely to recover. 5) Execute a durable power of attorney so someone can make financial decisions on your behalf if you are unable. 6) Don't put a will or advance directive solely in a safe deposit box, where family members might not have access to it. Give copies to trusted relatives.

COSTS OF MEDICAL CARE PER CAPITA IN VARIOUS DEVELOPED COUNTRIES IN 2013

When the costs of medical care per capita were compared in 12 developed countries, the USA led the list, with $2.91 trillion for health care in 2013, or $9,255 per American (22) *(Table 3)*. The increase in the US from 2012 to 2013, namely 3.6%, was the lowest since the government started counting medical expenses in 1960. In part, the US spends more because our prices are so much higher—for hospitals, drugs, medical devices, and medical salaries. Over 44 million US consumers have uncollected medical debt on their credit reports. The US also spends more than the other countries because our citizens as a whole are in worse shape than the citizens of most other countries, with obesity, high cholesterol levels, heavy salt and sugar in our diets, and smoking (although down to 17% presently). After Mexico, the US is the fattest country in the world. About 25% of our population doesn't exercise whatsoever. Indolence, of course, leads to diabetes mellitus, some cancers, elevated blood cholesterol levels, and other chronic conditions that drain the nation's wealth. The care for patients with chronic disease in the US accounts for $3 of every $4 spent on our health care.

PRACTICAL WISDOM FROM JOHN W. GARDNER

John Gardner (1912–2002), a great civic leader and Secretary of Health, Education, and Welfare under President Lyndon

Table 3. Per capital cost of health care in various developed countries in 2013*

Country	Cost (US dollars)
USA	$9,255
Norway	$6,758
Switzerland	$6,080
Netherlands	$5,178
Germany	$4,884
Canada	$4,602
Finland	$3,686
Iceland	$3,642
United Kingdom	$3,289
Italy	$3,183
South Korea	$2,411
Hungary	$1,803

*Source: *Dallas Morning News* (22).

Johnson, delivered the commencement address in June 1991 at Stanford University's 100th commencement ceremony. The speech is full of practical wisdom (23).

> As you settle into your adult lives, you cannot write off the danger of complacency, boredom, growing rigidity, imprisonment by your own comfortable habits and opinions. A famous French writer once said, "There are people whose clocks stop at a certain point in their lives." I could without any trouble name a half dozen national figures resident in Washington, DC, whom you would recognize, and I could tell you roughly the year their clock stopped.

> If you are conscious of the danger of going to seed, you can resort to countervailing measures. At any age. You can keep your zest until the day you die. If I may offer you a simple maxim, "Be interested." Everyone wants to be interesting, but the vitalizing thing is to be interested. Keep your curiosity, your sense of wonder. Discover new things. Care. Risk. Reach out.

> Learn all your life. Learn from your failures, from your successes. . . . We learn from our jobs, from our friends and families. We learn by accepting the commitments of life, by playing the roles that life hands us (not necessarily the roles we would have chosen). We learn by taking risks, by suffering, by enjoying, by loving, by bearing life's indignities with dignity.

> The lessons of maturity aren't simple things such as acquiring information and skills. You learn not to engage in self-destructive behavior, not to burn up energy in anxiety. You learn to manage your tensions, if you have any, which you do. You find that self-pity and resentment are among the most toxic of drugs. You conclude that the world loves talent but pays off on character. You discover that no matter how hard you try to please, some people in this world are not going to love you, a lesson that is at first troubling, and then really quite relaxing. . . .

> You bear with the things you can't change. You come to terms with yourself. As Jim Whitaker, who climbed Mount Everest, said: "You never conquer the mountain. You only conquer yourself." You master the arts of mutual dependence, meeting the needs of loved ones and letting yourself need them. You can even be unaffected—a quality that often takes years to acquire. You can achieve the simplicity that lies beyond sophistication. . . .

> One of the enemies of sound, lifelong motivation is a rather childish conception we have of the kind of concrete, describable goal toward which all of our efforts drive us. We want to believe that there is a point at which we can feel that we have arrived. We want a scoring system that tells us when we've piled up enough points to count ourselves successful. So you scramble and sweat and climb to reach what you thought was the goal. And when you get there, you stand up and look around and chances are you feel a little empty. . . .

> You wonder whether you climbed the wrong mountain. But . . . life isn't a mountain that has a summit. Nor is it . . . a riddle that has an answer. Nor a game that has a final score. Life is an endless unfolding and . . . an endless process of self-discovery, an endless and unpredictable dialogue between our own potentialities and the life situations in which we find ourselves. By potentialities I mean not just intellectual gifts but the full range of one's capacities for learning, sensing, wondering, understanding, loving and aspiring. . . . It is my hope that you will keep on growing, and that you will be the cause of growth in others.

WILLIAM CLIFFORD ROBERTS, MD
February 2, 2015

1. Boekholdt SM, Hovingh GK, Mora S, Arsenault BJ, Amarenco P, Pedersen TR, LaRosa JC, Waters DD, DeMicco DA, Simes RJ, Keech AC, Colquhoun D, Hitman GA, Betteridge DJ, Clearfield MB, Downs JR, Colhoun HM, Gotto AM Jr, Ridker PM, Grundy SM, Kastelein JJ. Very low levels of atherogenic lipoproteins and the risk for cardiovascular events: a meta-analysis of statin trials. *J Am Coll Cardiol* 2014;64(5):485–494.
2. Jalonick MC. Diet rules: eat less meat for Earth's sake. *Dallas Morning News*, January 3, 2015.
3. Halper E. Warming food fight: proposal to add meat's carbon effect to pyramid rankles industry. *Dallas Morning News*, January 25, 2015.
4. Niman NH. *Defending Beef: The Case for Sustainable Meat Production.* River Junction, VT: Chelsea Green Publishing, 2014 (288 pp.).
5. Ferdman RA. Fast food tied to lower test scores in kids. *Dallas Morning News,* December 27, 2014.
6. Blumenthal RG. Globesity on the rise. *Barron's,* December 29, 2014.
7. Emanuel EJ. Say ah, or just say no? *Dallas Morning News,* January 23, 2015.
8. Tavernise S. Experts double down on dangers of tanning beds. *Dallas Morning News,* January 11, 2015.
9. Lee DC, Pate RR, Lavie CJ, Sui X, Church TS, Blair SN. Leisure-time running reduces all-cause and cardiovascular mortality risk. *J Am Coll Cardiol* 2014;64(5):472–481.
10. Wen CP, Wai JP, Tsai MK, Chen CH. Minimal amount of exercise to prolong life: to walk, to run, or just mix it up? *J Am Coll Cardiol* 2014;64(5):482–484.

11. Hallman T. Murder rate is lowest since '30. *Dallas Morning News*, January 8, 2015.
12. Scientists: last year hottest ever. *Dallas Morning News*, January 17, 2015.
13. Borenstein S. Study: sea level rise accelerating faster than calculated. *Dallas Morning News*, January 15, 2015.
14. Epstein A. *The Moral Case for Fossil Fuels*. New York: Portfolio, 2014 (256 pp.).
15. Brill S. *America's Bitter Pill: Money, Politics, Back-Room Deals, and the Fight to Fix Our Broken Healthcare System*. New York: Brill Journalism Enterprises–Random House, 2015 (528 pp.).
16. Landers J. High cost of health. *Dallas Morning News*, January 9, 2015.
17. Neergaard L. Easing the physicians' juggling act. *Dallas Morning News*, January 8, 2015.
18. Press MJ. Instant replay—a quarterback's view of care coordination. *N Engl J Med* 2014;371(6):489–491.
19. Constable P. Heroin epidemic spreading again with alarming speed. *Dallas Morning News*, January 11, 2015.
20. Beck M. Too many dogs: a simple solution. *Wall Street Journal*, November 29–30, 2014.
21. Quinn JB. Kids and your money: It's important to have 'the talk.' *AARP Bulletin/Real Possibilities*, January-February 2015.
22. Landers J. U.S. health system is bleeding green. *Dallas Morning News*, February 1, 2015.
23. Gardner J. Commencement address at Stanford's 100th commencement ceremony, June 16, 1991. Available at http://jgc.stanford.edu/docs/JWGCentennialCommencementSpeech.pdf; retrieved January 9, 2015.

Chapter 19

July 2015

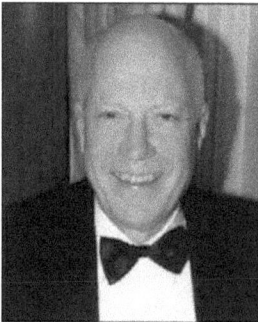

William C. Roberts, MD.

"THE PILL" AND ITS FOUR MAJOR DEVELOPERS

In 2012, Jonathan Eig published *The Birth of The Pill: How Four Crusaders Reinvented Sex and Launched a Revolution* (1). In 36 chapters the fascinating story is told.

She was already 71 years of age, had loved sex, and had spent 40 years seeking a way to make it better. She wanted a scientific method of birth control that would allow women to have sex as often as they liked without becoming pregnant. She was Margaret Sanger (1879–1966) *(Figure 1)*, one of the legendary crusaders of the 20th century. She was meeting with Gregory Goodwin Pincus (1903–1967), a scientist with a genius IQ but a dubious reputation. He was 47 and had been rejected as a radical by Harvard, humiliated in the press, and left with no choice but to conduct his oftentimes controversial experiments in a converted garage. He was a biologist and perhaps the world's leading expert in mammalian reproduction in the 1930s.

Pincus knew about Margaret Sanger; almost everyone in the US did. It was Sanger who had popularized the term "birth control" and almost singlehandedly launched the movement for contraceptive rights in the US. Women would never gain equality, she reasoned, until they were freed from sexual servitude. Sanger had opened the nation's first birth control clinic in 1916 and helped launch dozens more around the world. But all she had to work with were condoms and cervical caps, usually ineffective, impractical, and difficult to obtain. Sanger explained to Pincus that she was looking for an inexpensive, easy-to-use, and completely foolproof method of contraception, preferably a pill. It should be something biological, she said, something a woman would swallow every morning, with or without the consent of the man with whom she was sleeping; something that would make sexual intercourse spontaneous, with no forethought or fumbling, no sacrifice of pleasure; something that would not affect a women's fertility if she wished to have children later in life; something that would work everywhere from the slums of New York to the jungles of Southeast Asia; something 100%

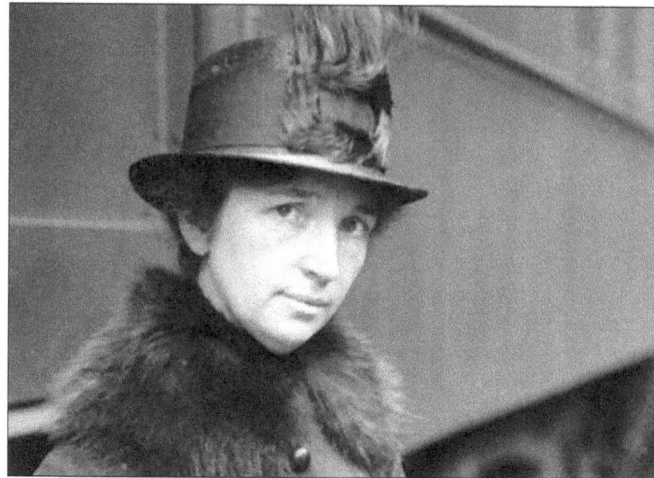

Figure 1. Margaret Sanger. Photo: Public domain.

effective. She asked Pincus, "Could it be done?" She had approached other scientists earlier and they said it could not be done. They had argued that it was dirty, disreputable work. And, even if somehow it could be done, they argued there would be no point. Thirty states and the federal government still had laws prohibiting birth control. Why go to the trouble of making a pill no drug company would dare to manufacture and no doctor would dare prescribe? But Sanger held out hope that Gregory Pincus was different, that he might be bold enough or desperate enough to try.

Also, times were changing. In 1948, only 2 years earlier, a college professor in Indiana named Alfred Charles Kinsey published a study called "Sexual Behavior in the Human Male" to be followed 5 years later by "Sexual Behavior in the Human Female," studies which disclosed that people were much freer with sex than previously admitted. Sex for the pleasure of women was an idea that was unthinkable in 1950. Worse, it was dangerous. What would happen to the institutions of marriage and family? What would happen to love? If women had the power to control their own bodies, if they had the ability to choose when and whether they got pregnant, what would they want next? Science, argued Sanger, would give women the chance to become equal partners with men.

Once Sanger asked Pincus to start working on a pill, he drove directly to his office at the Worcester Foundation for

Experimental Biology, an institution he had founded with one of his colleagues, Hudson Hoagland, to speak with one of his researchers, M. C. Chang. While the foundation started out in a renovated barn in Worcester, by 1950, it had moved to an ivy-covered brick home in a residential section of nearby Shrewsbury. Pincus had known of Chang and enticed him to join the foundation for a salary of $2000 a year ($26,000 by today's standards). Chang, who knew Pincus by reputation, thought he would be working in one of America's prestigious institutions and that his fellowship would include free lodging. He did get free lodging, but his room was at the YMCA. He and Pincus would travel to and from work by bus. Later, Chang would move to the foundation, sleeping on a small bed in a corner of a converted laboratory using Bunsen burners to heat his meager meals. As a strict Confucian, Chang apparently did not mind. Pincus told Chang that he had spoken to Margaret Sanger about her desire for a pill to prevent pregnancy. It had to be a pill, not an injection, jelly, liquid, or foam, and not a mechanical device used in the vagina. When Pincus talked in this way with a sense of purpose, his colleagues paid attention. Pincus knew from the beginning that it would be one thing to build a birth control pill and another to persuade the world to accept it.

Pincus and Chang already knew that injections of the hormone progesterone prevented ovulation in rabbits. Nevertheless, for many reasons, scientists had not tried to explore the implications for humans. There were too many risks. Also at the time, progesterone was very expensive. Pincus and Chang knew how progesterone functioned. When an egg is fertilized, progesterone prepares the uterus for implantation and shuts down the ovaries so no more eggs are released. In effect, Pincus recognized, nature already had an effective contraceptive. Now the task was to see if they could produce it, modify it, and put it to use. Fortunately, new technology was making progesterone less expensive to obtain. If Sanger would pay for it, Pincus thought he had a good idea of how to proceed.

He and Chang began by repeating their experiments done in Pennsylvania 13 years earlier, adjusting the dosages and means of delivery to get a feel for progesterone and how it worked. They started with rabbits. Pincus sent a request for funding to the Planned Parenthood Federation of America, the women's health and advocacy group that Sanger had helped form. He asked for $3100: a $1000 stipend for Chang, $1200 for the purchase of rabbits, $600 for animal food, and $300 for miscellaneous supplies. Sanger wrote to Pincus that they had $2000 but Pincus and Chang got to work.

The first results were what they had expected: the animals receiving progesterone did not appear to ovulate! They next moved to rats, and once again the experiment worked: there were no pregnant rats and once again larger doses had a longer-lasting effect. Within a relatively brief period, the Worcester Foundation had about 20 scientists and operated on an annual budget of $300,000, about $63,000 of which was contributed by local residents.

Fortunately, it was a time of enormous growth in the pharmaceutical industry. By the late 1940s and early 1950s, drug makers like G.D. Searle & Company were competing fiercely to discover and market new ones. In the 1940s, Searle, a small pharmaceutical company based in Skokie, Illinois, and other drug companies were looking for ways to synthesize cortisone, which had recently been demonstrated to relieve arthritic pain. Pincus persuaded the drug company that he could synthesize cortisone by pumping serum through the adrenal gland of sows and spent $500,000 of Searle's money trying to prove it. But before Searle could make use of Pincus' new technology, researchers at the Upjohn Company found a simpler and less expensive way to do the job.

In the fall of 1951, hoping to repair the relation with Searle and secure their help on Margaret Sanger's progesterone project, Pincus went to Skokie to meet with Albert L. Raymond, the drug company's director of research. Pincus failed in his initial attempt to acquire money from Searle.

Sanger. Who was Margaret Sanger? She was from a family of 11 children. She was number 6, born in 1879, in Corning, New York. Her mother was frail and submissive and died of tuberculosis at age 50. Her father was a charming stonecutter. Maggie, as she was known, left home at an early age and enrolled at Claverack College, a boarding school in New York's Hudson Valley. She earned her way through and began speaking out on suffrage and women's emancipation. She enrolled in nursing school at White Plains Hospital in Westchester County, New York. Though she considered marriage "akin to suicide," at the age of 22 she met a handsome young painter and architect named William Sanger. They fell in love, married, and built a home in Hastings-on-Hudson, Westchester County, New York. Soon came three children, two boys and a girl.

Not happy with either suburbia or marriage, in 1912, Margaret and her family moved to New York City and she began spending time in Greenwich Village. There she discussed sexual freedom, voluntary motherhood, and the need for women to have more autonomy in the bedroom and in society. During this time, Sanger worked for William Wald's visiting nurse service, a group of nurses sent out by the Henry Street Settlement House to care for poverty-stricken women, and often helped the women through childbirth. Sanger was astonished by the poverty and misery: children sick, dirty, and underfed; tuberculosis rampant; and women seemingly unaware of how their bodies worked and the risk of repeated pregnancies and venereal disease. In the 1920s, the state health department distributed circulars warning women that pregnancies occurring too close together were dangerous, predisposing mothers to tuberculosis. But the same department barred women from receiving information about how to prevent pregnancy.

Doctors estimated that one-third of all pregnancies in the US at the time ended in abortion. Sanger became convinced that women should have the right to contraception. In 1913, she wrote a 12-part series of articles about sex and reproduction for *The Call*, a radical newspaper. Sanger rejected the idea of full-time motherhood. She became involved in the right to vote for women and the drive to prohibit the sale of alcohol, with the idea that if men stopped drinking, they would be less abusive and less likely to force their wives to have sex.

In 1914, soon after the publication of Sanger's newspaper, *The Woman Rebel,* the US Post Office Inspector issued a warrant for her arrest, charging her with four counts of violating US obscenity laws. Sanger, now 34 years old, chose not to appear in court. Instead, she jumped bail, left her family, and moved to Europe, where she fell in love with 55-year-old Henry Havelock Ellis, one of the world's preeminent sexual psychologists. Ellis had made it his mission to solve the mysteries of sex, collecting histories from men and women in an effort to prove that physical intimacy was natural and varied. Ellis introduced Sanger to more intellectuals, including the science fiction writer H. G. Wells, George Bernard Shaw, Bertrand Russell, and Lorenzo Portet.

Ellis mentored Sanger. Now for the first time she had a plan. At first she had seen contraception primarily as a way to help women control the size of families. Now she was beginning to believe that if sex were disconnected from childbirth, women might be liberated in ways they had never imagined: there would be changes in marriage, in the meaning of family, and in career and educational opportunities for women.

While Sanger was in Europe, her husband was arrested by Anthony Comstock, a special agent for the Postal Service, for distributing pamphlets about birth control. Comstock made it his mission to fight smut in America, almost singlehandedly creating a strict set of antiobscenity laws. Comstock was appointed special agent for the YMCA Committee for the Suppression of Vice. While leading raids and smashing up sex devices, pornographic pictures, and contraceptives, Comstock became famous for guarding America from pornography and disease. In 1873, he had persuaded Congress to pass a bill banning the use of the mail for transporting "any obscene, lewd, lascivious, or filthy book, pamphlet, picture, paper, letter, writing, print or other publication of an indecent character." After that, every state had its own antiobscenity laws, many of which made it illegal to sell or disseminate information on contraceptives. To enforce the federal law, Comstock was appointed a special obscenity agent of the US Post Office. Soon after, he was authorized to carry a gun. The Comstock Law defined immorality so broadly that it could have included nearly anything. Thus, it was not surprising that it was deemed to ban not only the sale of contraceptive devices but also the transmission of information regarding contraception. The law influenced policy and kept women from getting birth control for decades!

Soon after her arrival in England, Sanger wrote to her husband that she considered their 12-year marriage over. She asked for a divorce, but he did not feel the same way. In 1915, however, Sanger's husband was convicted on obscenity charges with a judge saying he had violated not only the laws of man,

but the law of God in his scheme to prevent motherhood. He served 30 days in prison. Only then did Margaret agree to return home. Soon afterwards, her 5-year-old daughter Peggy developed pneumonia and died. For the rest of her life she was tormented by dreams of babies. This tragedy, however, did not compel her to pay more attention to the care of her two surviving children. Instead, Sanger went back to work. She began by posing for publicity photos, wearing a wide Quaker collar with her young son by her side, looking like a respectable young mother. It was about this time that she began using the phrase "birth control" instead of contraception. The key word in the phrase was "control." If women truly got to control when and how often they gave birth, they would hold a kind of power never before imagined. Without control, women were destined to be wives and mothers and nothing more.

In 1916, Sanger opened her first birth control clinic in Brooklyn, where a team of nurses distributed condoms and pessaries (flexible rubber caps that were commonly sold in drug stores as a "womb support" but in reality functioned similarly to a diaphragm or cervical cap). The clinic, of course, operated in direct violation of New York state law, so no one was surprised when police raided the place 10 days after it opened, confiscating contraceptive devices and arresting Sanger. She served 30 days in the penitentiary charged with illegal distribution of birth control products.

Sanger gradually became more sophisticated in her radicalism. Instead of challenging society's conservative views on sex and challenging obscenity laws, she tried to recruit physicians, scientists, and corporate leaders to join her crusade, emphasizing the benefits to public health. She encouraged women to see their doctors to get fitted for diaphragms, hoping that doctors would be valuable allies in her fight. One of her allies at the time was a wealthy widower named James Noah Slee, who met Sanger and quickly fell in love with her. Slee was 20 years older than Sanger and had been president of the 3-in-1 Oil Company, makers of the product that almost every American at the time kept on hand to grease typewriters, bicycle chains, and sewing machines. Sanger had been separated from her first husband 7 years when she met Slee. In 1922, she finally divorced William Sanger and married the crusty aristocratic Slee. Slee gave Sanger all the money she wanted for her cause. She and her husband now owned their own company to design and market birth control devices.

By 1925, more than 1000 doctors from around the world sought admission to Sanger's annual birth control conference held in New York City. British economist John Maynard Keynes, as well as Norman Thomas, W. E. B. Du Bois, Upton Sinclair, and Bertrand Russell attended. The birth control movement was clearly gaining visibility in the US and spreading quickly around the world. Overall, the birth rate in the US fell 30% between 1895 and 1925, even though women had begun to marry at younger ages. By 1930, the Birth Control League, the organization Sanger founded, was overseeing 55 clinics in 23 cities.

In 1932, US Custom officials, citing obscenity laws, seized a box of experimental diaphragms sent to Sanger by a Japanese physician and father of 12 who believed his new design would make contraceptives more effective. Sanger and her allies challenged the seizure, arguing that the law was blocking scientific progress and hindering the advancement of medicine. In a landmark decision, a New York State Board of Appeals judge agreed. After that, as long as physicians were involved, it would be legal to use the mail to spread information about contraception or to ship contraceptive devices. The decision opened the door for the American Medical Association to recognize contraception as preventive medicine.

Pincus. In January 1952, Pincus filed a report to Planned Parenthood stating that 10 mg doses of progesterone administered orally had suppressed ovulation in 90% of the rabbits tested. The results were good enough to justify tests on women, and he was ready to begin. When her second husband died in 1942 at the age of 83, Sanger inherited $5 million. She gave some of the money to the birth control movement, some to friends, and spent much of it on lavish vacations. Planned Parenthood had grown rapidly in the 1940s, adding branches across the country. It was led mostly by businessmen and male physicians. Prescott S. Bush, a Connecticut businessman whose son and grandson would both become US presidents, served as treasurer for Planned Parenthood's first national fundraising campaign in 1947. The organization unfortunately was frightened by the idea of doing something that had never been tried before: giving medicine to healthy women simply to improve their lifestyles. A scandal or a lawsuit could sink the entire organization. Planned Parenthood was not ready to go out on a limb and certainly not for Pincus.

Gregory Goodwin Pincus *(Figure 2)* fancied himself a poet, philosopher, tiller of the soil, and lover of women. His passion for life and ideas was great. As a teenager he wrote in his diary, "Our one duty is self-development; man's job is to get the most out of his talents and to help others do the same." It was not sex, money, or fame that guided Pincus. It was his quest for greatness, a desire that never ebbed as long as he lived. The Pincus family arrived in New York City in 1891 from Odessa, a cosmopolitan Russian city. The anti-Jewish pogroms were sweeping Russia at the time and the Pincuses fled. They moved to a New York City slum and from there to Colchester, Connecticut, and then to a kibbutz.

In 1902, Lizzie Lipman and Joseph Pincus married, and six offspring followed. Gregory ("Goody") was the first, arriving in 1903. He worked his way through Cornell University washing dishes and waiting tables. One day during his senior year, Pincus returned home to find a visitor with his family. Her name was Elizabeth Notkin, 4 years older than he. The five Pincus boys had never seen anyone like Lizzie. She cursed, drank, and chain-smoked cigarettes. In 1923, she and Goody married before a judge while she visited him at Harvard where he was doing a PhD in biology. It wasn't long before she was pregnant with her first child. At age 27, Goody Pincus was appointed an instructor in the department of general physiology at Harvard. A year later he was promoted to assistant professor of biology. At Harvard he experimented mostly with rats, studying how they responded to heat and light. When he graduated, he had a postdoctoral fellowship, studying for 2 years at Harvard and 1 year in Europe.

In Europe for the first time, Pincus began researching the eggs of mammals, the subject that would become his life's work. He returned to Harvard as a professor in 1930. Pincus' interest was how animals passed along genetic traits, and that led him to the study of mammalian eggs, specifically how they were fertilized and how they developed in vitro. He tried hormone injections to see how they affected rabbits and at one point noted that estrogen injections prevented pregnancy. In 1934, Pincus announced to the National Academy of Sciences that he had fertilized rabbit eggs in a test tube, transplanted them into the body of a host mother, and brought the baby rabbits to term. This was radical research at the time. He also wrote in a grant application that his goal was to apply his in vitro technique to humans. His work began to attract an unusual amount of attention beyond the academic community. The *New York Times* cited his work for the first time in a 1934 article. The newspaper unfortunately went on to portray Pincus as a sinister scientist trying to grow babies in bottles. After fertilizing rabbit eggs and restoring them to their mother, Pincus took another step: letting the eggs become embryos while remaining in the glass. In 1936, Pincus achieved parthenogenetic development of a rabbit ovum; they had begun the reproductive process without any fertilization, simply by manipulating the environment surrounding the egg. Not long after that, Pincus transplanted the egg successfully into surrogate female rabbits. The press called this "immaculate conception." In the same year Harvard marked its 300th anniversary with a pamphlet listing the greatest scientific discoveries made

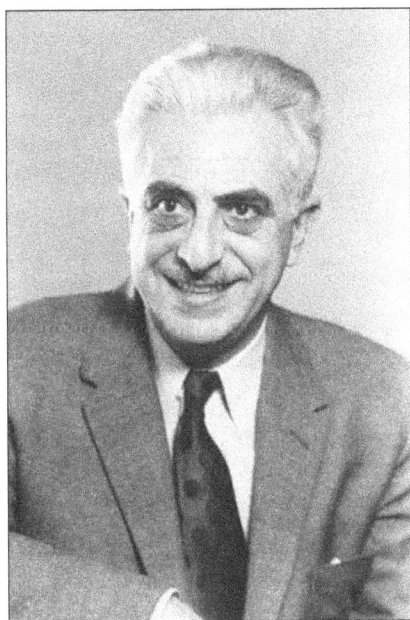

Figure 2. Dr. Gregory Pincus. Photo from Images from the History of Medicine, Library of Congress, ID 186672.

by its faculty in three centuries of study. Pincus' work made the list. The same year he published his groundbreaking book, *The Eggs of Mammals*.

With each new discovery, each audacious claim, and each speech before a scientific body, Pincus attracted more attention in the mainstream press. Newspapers all over the country carried reports of his research. In 1937, *Collier's Magazine* published a feature story on Pincus' work. A critic was quoted as saying, "If babies were made in test tubes, it would be the ruin of women." Pregnancy not only improved a woman's looks, the critic noted, but also improved her nervous system. Suddenly, Pincus was being portrayed as a revolutionary or, worse, a deviant. Soon after the *Collier's* article, Harvard gave Pincus the news: He would receive a grant to study for one more year at the University of Cambridge in England and then he would be finished. Thus, at age 34, Pincus had already published a groundbreaking book and a number of attention-grabbing scientific studies and was on the cusp of what appeared to be a brilliant career, teaching and conducting research at one of the wealthiest and most prestigious universities in the world. But, suddenly, he was gone.

Pincus probably was the victim of small-mindedness and anti-Semitism, but he was also undone by his own outsized ego. He couldn't find another college willing to hire him. His classmate, Hudson Hoagland, who had left Harvard and gone to work in Clarke University in Worcester, rescued him. The Pincuses arrived in Worcester in the fall of 1938, and Pincus went back to work on hormones. In 1944, he and several other scientists organized a major conference on hormones. They called it the Laurentian Hormone Conference. Pincus became the chairman of the conference, a position he maintained for the rest of his life.

In 1944, he and Hoagland made a move almost entirely unheard of in the American scientific community. They founded their own laboratory, calling it the Worcester Foundation for Experimental Biology. Hoagland and Pincus proved to be excellent salesmen, and the people of Worcester responded generously. Hoagland in particular had a gift for raising money. He had come from an affluent family and projected an image of sophistication. He was no slouch as a scientist, but it was clear from the start that Pincus was the real genius and Hoagland the organization man. At first the two scientists operated out of a room at the Worcester State Hospital, but they soon had enough money to hire a dozen workers and purchase a 12-acre estate in nearby Shrewsbury. By 1951, the foundation employed 57 men and women, making it by some accounts the largest privately owned independent scientific research institution in the country.

The family had little money and lived in several crowded apartments and finally found a place at the Worcester Lunatic Asylum, a frightening and dangerous place, but it saved money on rent and enabled Pincus to concentrate more completely on his work. He did not own a car or drive one until in his 40s. He would take a bus or hitch a ride with another scientist to get to work each day. Pincus was an accomplished Scrabble and chess player and devoured mystery novels. At the beach he would swim more than a mile out to sea. In the early 1950s, with the Worcester Foundation being more stable, the Pincus family bought a house. It looked more like an old hotel than a house, and Pincus paid $30,000 for it (about $260,000 today). The red brick structure had a dozen bedrooms, 10 fireplaces, and a furnished basement where Pincus sometimes offered free lodging to visiting scholars. They had parties lasting late into the night and leaving nearly everyone drunk. Inebriated or sober, Lizzie was razor sharp, every bit her husband's intellectual equal when conversations were not so scientific. She spoke French and Russian fluently.

Despite his exile from Harvard, Pincus was beginning to establish a reputation for leadership among his peers. He was not only a brilliant scientist but he had a gift for organizational work. The Laurentin Hormone Conference became the biggest and most important hormone conference in the world and, as a result, Pincus, with no university or corporate affiliation and no landmark discovery to call his own, became an influential player in the scientific community. He helped decide which scientists would be invited to the conference each year, who would be permitted to present papers, and whose papers would be cited in the yearly conference report.

McCormick. In the fall of 1950, shortly before Gregory Pincus first met Margaret Sanger, Sanger received a letter from a 75-year-old woman named Katharine Dexter McCormick (1875–1967) *(Figure 3)*. It read, "I want to know a) where you

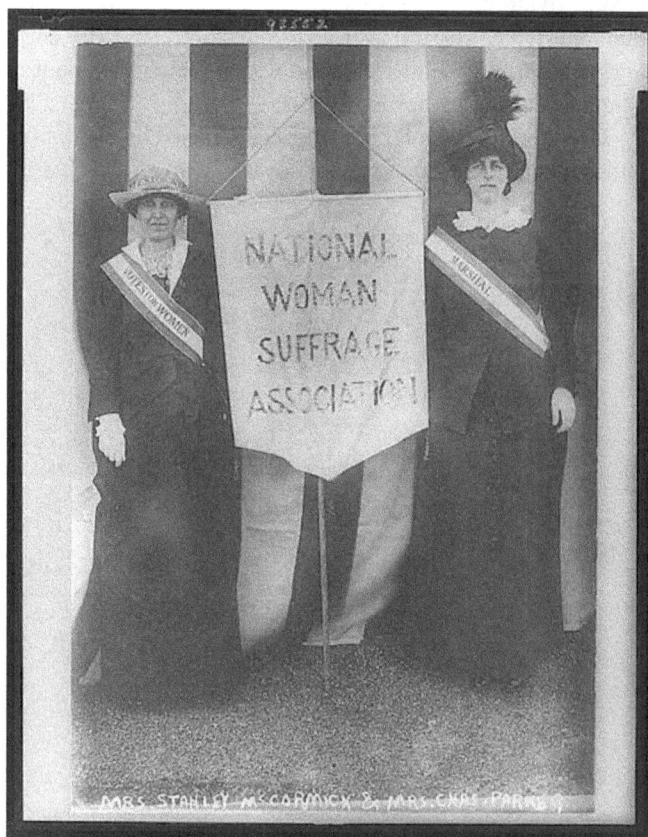

Figure 3. Suffragists Katharine McCormick and Mrs. Charles Parker, April 22, 1913. Photo: Library of Congress (LC-USZ62-93552).

think the greatest need of financial support is today for the National Birth Control Movement; and b) what the present prospects are for further birth control research, and by research, I mean contraceptive research." For Pincus and Sanger, the timing of the letter could not have been more fortuitous. McCormick was one of the world's wealthiest women, and after years of personal struggle and tragedy (her husband was schizophrenic) she was at last free to spend that wealth. McCormick was the recently widowed wife of Stanley Mc-Cormick, the youngest son of Cyrus McCormick, inventor and manufacturer of the mechanized reaper and one of the wealthiest men in the world. Katharine was 29 years old at the time of her wedding, fierce and lovely, a leader in the women's movement and one of the first women to graduate with a degree in science from the Massachusetts Institute of Technology. She had intended to go to medical school, but marriage changed that.

With her husband ill, she sensed that hormones, a word coined in 1905, may have been responsible for her husband's condition and she became a student of these chemical messengers. In 1909, she began volunteering with the Women's Suffrage Movement and by 1921 began collaborating with Sanger, who was busy planning the first American birth control conference in New York. When her husband died in 1947, Mrs. McCormick inherited more than $35 million, including almost 32,000 shares in the McCormick-owned company International Harvester. Sanger too was now a widow, her husband having died in 1943. McCormick knew exactly what she wanted to do with her money.

In January 1952, Sanger stopped to visit Katharine McCormick in her mansion in Santa Barbara, California. Just before the visit, Sanger had received a report from Pincus indicating the results of the experiments he and Chang had performed on rabbits and rats, explaining the effects of hormone injections versus administration by mouth. He confirmed that the oral doses were 90% effective and said he hoped to experiment with different progesterone compounds that might work better. Pincus concluded that the experiments "demonstrate unequivocally that it is possible to inhibit ovulation in the rabbit and successful breeding in the rabbit with progesterone. . . . It has been demonstrated furthermore that following the sterile period, normal reproduction may ensue." In June 1952, McCormick made plans to visit the Worcester Foundation to see firsthand what was happening there. She met with Hoagland and Chang and learned about the progesterone work underway, but she did not see Pincus who was out of town. After that visit, McCormick became Sanger's leading expert on the Pincus plan for contraceptive research.

Rock. Pincus recognized that what the pill project needed now was not necessarily a biologist but a product champion—someone who could build a team to do the scientific work, forge alliances with manufacturers needed to supply chemicals, and if all went well, spread the news of the coming invention so it might have a chance of acceptance. He knew what to do next: test progesterone in women. To do that he would have to

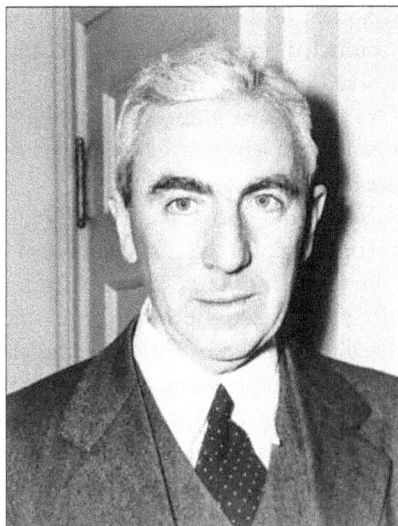

Figure 4. Dr. John Rock. Photo: Library of Congress (LC-USZ62-128825).

add a player to his team—a physician, preferably a gynecologist, someone who could reassure the patients involved in the experiments that they were safe and would convey to the drug companies supplying the progesterone that no one would be harmed by the experiments. He considered several but came down to a physician named John Rock (1890–1984) *(Figure 4)*, who like Pincus was a Harvard man. Rock was respected by his peers and adored by his patients. He was tall, slender, and silver-haired with a gentle smile and a calm, deliberate manner. Even the name connoted strength, solidity, and reliability, and he was a Catholic.

Born in 1890 in Marlborough, Massachusetts, Rock was a son of an Irish saloonkeeper, and although he was big, strong, and athletic, he preferred playing with his sisters, and his brothers sometimes called him "sissy." He gained admission to Harvard and attended not only college there but also medical school. In 1926, he became director of the sterility clinic at the Free Hospital for Women in Boston. While the Catholic Church opposed abortion, Rock believed a woman's health was more important than the health of her fetus and that pregnancies should be terminated when they imperiled patients' lives. "Religion," he used to tell his daughter, "is a very poor scientist." Over time Rock underwent a fundamental change as compassion for his patients overwhelmed his compulsion to tow the church's line. He sympathized with women who came to his office who said they were afraid of becoming pregnant again, whether it was because their bodies were worn out or because they couldn't imagine caring for more children. Rock began seeing that many couples wanted contraception because they wanted to delay, not avoid, becoming parents. In 1931, he was one of 15 Boston doctors (and the only Catholic) to sign a petition calling for the repeal of the state's ban on contraception.

In 1925, Rock married Anna Thorndyke, a Boston woman who shared his sense of adventure, having served as an ambulance driver in France during World War I. He was 35 and she 29 at marriage. They had five children together. He adored his wife and had no fear of showing his affection publicly. In his practice, he counseled pregnant women and delivered babies but he also worked with women who could not conceive and came to believe that sexual intercourse offered an important bond for husbands and wives as they struggled unsuccessfully to have children.

Although Sanger did not want Pincus to include Rock on his team investigating progesterone because of her mistrust of the Catholic Church, Pincus saw in Rock not only a talented scientist but also an important promoter of his new, as yet unrealized, birth control pill. Rock had already gained a small measure of fame as the Catholic doctor who dared defy his own church. In 1944, he made headlines when he achieved the first successful in vitro fertilization of human ova. In 1948, Rock had published a book called *Voluntary Parenthood* stating: "Nothing in a life of a man and woman is going to be as important to themselves or society as their parenthood."

Gregory Pincus and John Rock had met in the 1930s when Pincus was still at Harvard. In the 1940s when Rock began experimenting with in vitro fertilization of human ova, one of his first steps was to send his research assistant to Pincus for guidance. Rock was unusual among fertility specialists at the time because he also asked husbands to have their semen tested. He suspected (and his suspicions were confirmed in later years) that men were responsible for a large percentage of infertility problems. He was also unusual in that he operated a rhythm clinic down the hall from the fertility clinic. Rock's rhythm clinic was the first free clinic in Massachusetts to offer birth control advice. The women visiting his rhythm clinic were asked to chart their menstrual cycles and sex lives for 3 months. After that, Rock tried to instruct the women who had regular cycles when they could safely have sex with little risk of fertilization. He knew that many of the women were using diaphragms, douches, and condoms, but the law would not allow him to prescribe or even discuss those items unless the woman's health was in serious jeopardy! Rock had long believed that the church and the state of Massachusetts were wrong for rejecting birth control.

In 1952, Pincus and Rock attended the same scientific conference and chatted between sessions about their work. When Rock described his work with the pregnant women, Pincus suggested to him that he try progesterone without estrogen. Rock experimented with different combinations of hormones in different methods of delivery, trying to find the medicine that worked best and caused the fewest side effects. He did not ask his patients to sign consent forms but he did explain to the women that the medicine they were about to take would not directly help their infertility. This was how experiments were done at the time. He started the women on 50 mg of progesterone and 5 mg of estrogen and escalated gradually to 300 mg of progesterone and to 30 mg of estrogen. When the first round of treatments ended, no one had died and no one had become seriously ill. Thirteen of the 80 women in Rock's care became pregnant. Rock told col-

leagues about this promising result which came to be known as "The Rock Rebound." The women taking the hormones were often convinced they were pregnant because the hormones produced many of the same symptoms as pregnancy. The women were desperate to have children since most had been trying for years.

When he learned of Rock's work, Pincus was pleased but not surprised that the progesterone was having a contraceptive effect. The important thing to Pincus was the fact that Rock's patients were not dying. Here was proof, it seemed to him, that it was safe to give progesterone to women. Rock told Pincus that he was encouraged by his work with progesterone, but that he had a big problem: patients receiving the hormone believed that they were pregnant, no matter how much he assured them they were not. And they were crushed when the truth finally became clear to them.

Pincus proposed an elegant solution and one that would have enormous consequences for his own work and for the future of women around the world. To keep the women from ovulating while permitting monthly menstruation, the simplest solution was to have the women stop taking the progesterone pills for 5 days each month. It made sense to both men.

Early clinical trials. One company supplying hormones for his progesterone experiments was G.D. Searle. Although the drug maker had had no success with Pincus a year earlier, company officials had never given up on the brilliant but unpredictable scientist. Searle officials continued to believe that Pincus might come up with something useful, and it was a lot less expensive for the drug company to write grants for the Worcester Foundation than it would have been to hire its own researchers. For these reasons, despite Pincus' failures, Searle agreed to pay the foundation $62,400 for a 12-month period beginning in June 1953. In addition, Pincus would receive shares of Searle's stock starting with 19 shares valued at $921.50. Officials at Searle had not committed to a new contraceptive, and they asked Pincus not to publicize their involvement in his project. They told Pincus that they would not have anything to do with a birth control pill that interfered with the menstrual cycle.

Because Massachusetts law banned all forms of contraception, Pincus devised a method to test a birth control formula by calling it a "fertility treatment." If he had still been on the faculty of Harvard or even if he had still been operating in affiliation with Clarke University, he never would have gotten away with it. Pincus saw himself as more than a research scientist now. He was an activist, a crusader, and a businessman. He was also a builder of coalitions.

In the 1950s, there was still no law requiring physicians to inform patients that they were being included in an experiment. Rock told his patients that the progesterone they were receiving would shut down their ovaries and make it impossible to get pregnant, that the treatment would simulate pregnancy and might cause nausea, and that they would have a better chance of becoming pregnant when the experiment was complete.

Beginning in 1953, Pincus and Rock enlisted 27 of Rock's patients at the Free Hospital for a 3-month trial. Because Pincus wanted to be certain that the hormone was effective in halting ovulation, women who failed to ovulate regularly were not included. The women enlisted were still infertile, but Rock did not know what was causing their infertility. Instead of the progesterone-estrogen mix that Rock had used in the past, the women in this experiment received only progesterone and they received the tablets daily for 3 weeks of each month, stopping for a week to allow them to menstruate. The tests were demanding and the testing was referred to as "the Pincus progesterone project" or PPP because so many urine specimens were tested. Pincus tested the urine specimens in Shrewsbury. Pincus also included a gynecologist in Worcester, Dr. Henry Kirkendall, and asked him to recruit 30 women for a study similar to Rock's. The women would need to take their own temperature every day and record their findings. They also were expected to take daily vagina smears and collect their own urine for hormone analyses. The progesterone dosage would be high, between 250 and 300 mg a day. The women were not paid for their participation, nor were they informed that the results might lead to the invention of a new form of birth control. Most of them were doing it simply because a trusted doctor had asked them to.

In the first year of the trials, Pincus, Rock, and Kirkendall enrolled 60 women. Unfortunately, half of the women enrolled dropped out either because the test procedure was too demanding or because the side effects were too disturbing. Unfortunately, in that experiment 15% of the women showed signs of ovulation while taking progesterone, significantly worse results than Pincus had seen with rabbits and rats.

In the meantime, Russell Marker, George Rosenkranz, and Frank Colton had developed synthetic progesterone (progestin), which was 4 to 8 times more potent than the natural progesterone, and the new compound was able to survive absorption in the digestive tract, which meant it could be taken orally. This was the compound that Pincus was searching for.

In May 1953, as Pincus and Rock were launching their first round of tests on humans, Sanger and McCormick met with Pincus and see if he was someone McCormick might wish to support. The women were not put off by the cheaply furnished offices, the poor ventilation in the animal rooms, or the jerry-rigged appearance of the laboratories. If anything, they seemed captivated by the place's strappy charm and were especially enthusiastic about Pincus' plan for testing John Rock's patients. As the tour concluded, McCormick asked Pincus how much money he needed. Pincus had already negotiated a grant of $17,500 from Planned Parenthood to cover the first year of clinical trials. McCormick had agreed to pay half that amount. McCormick now asked how much it would take to fund the entire research project. How much to get the pill? Pincus answered $125,000. The next day McCormick phoned Pincus to say she would write a check for $10,000 with more to come. By this time, Searle was funding the Worcester Foundation at a rate of about $5600 a month, making it the foundation's biggest private backer by far and accounting for about 8% of the foundation's total income. Also Searle at this time was paying about one-third of Pincus' $15,000 annual salary, when the median family income in the US was $5,000.

By the fall of 1953, the Worcester Foundation had 46 grants providing a total of $622,000 in income. All but 11% was spent on research. Fortunately, Pincus received $50,000 from McCormick to build an animal testing center which was needed desperately. Meanwhile, he continued to try different progesterone compounds to see which one worked best and continued to look for ways to test on women.

More than ever, McCormick was taking charge. Sanger was in poor health, low on energy and increasingly cantankerous. While Sanger at times was distracted or incapacitated by illness, it was McCormick who urged the work forward. She was beholden to no one and was free to speak her mind. McCormick alone among the team of developers had the courage and independence to declare that all women, married or not, should have access to the pill.

About half of the women in Rock's and Kirkendall's study dropped out. Testing a birth control pill was more difficult than testing other drugs. It was one thing to try a new medication in sick people who wanted to get better, but these were healthy young women volunteering for experiments. Pincus told McCormick that he would need to test hundreds if not thousands more women and have more staff—doctors, nurses, and clerks—as well as more examining rooms. After a year of work and a dropout rate of about 50% in their first round of testing, Pincus and Rock had completed research on only about 30 women.

In March 1954, Pincus and his wife went on a trip to Puerto Rico where he lectured at medical schools and before groups of doctors. He was impressed by the quality of work done on the island and encouraged to learn that dozens of birth control clinics were in operation. He concluded that experiments could be done in Puerto Rico on a relatively large scale. Best of all, birth control had been legal in Puerto Rico since 1937! In Puerto Rico, overpopulation and poverty had long been serious issues. The island was poor and crowded and family sizes were large. By age 55, the average mother in Puerto Rico had given birth to 6.8 children. Just over 8% of married Puerto Rican women under the age of 50 had volunteered for sterilization. Although abortion was illegal in Puerto Rico, it became so commonplace in the 1950s that Puerto Rico developed an international reputation as a place where the procedure could be obtained, no questions asked. Finally, McCormick and Rock agreed with Pincus that Puerto Rico was the place to go to study the women they needed.

As Pincus began planning Puerto Rican trials for the birth control pill in 1954, another scientist, Jonas Salk, was launching the first trials of his polio vaccine. Salk would spend tens of millions of dollars on his vaccine trial, while Pincus would operate on a first-year budget of less than $20,000. Salk would go on to test his drug on 600,000 children during field trials while Pincus was hopeful that he could round up 300 subjects. Neither Salk nor Pincus were concerned with profiteering from their inventions. In 1954, as Pincus negotiated with Planned Parenthood for support and funding and arranged with Searle and Syntex for supplies of the necessary progesterone compounds, he, like Salk, focused on the scientific work, not on the money. While the public clamor for birth control hardly equaled the clamor for a polio vaccine, the growing concern was about population growth.

When Pincus first visited the island in February 1954, he met Dr. Edris Rice-Wray, medical director of Puerto Rico's Family Planning Association. She was not from Puerto Rica but from Detroit. She had earned a bachelor's degree at Vassar College and her medical degree at Northwestern University. In 1949, she had moved to San Juan with her two children after divorcing her husband in Chicago. Dr. Rice-Wray became the point person for Pincus' study in Puerto Rico.

In the meantime, Pincus had found another site to acquire women for his study, namely, Worcester State Hospital, an asylum more than a century old. It was not difficult for Pincus to obtain permission to experiment on patients at the asylum. No permission slips needed to be signed. The directing physician, Dr. Bardwell Flower, a Harvard graduate, was pleased to have a few more physicians on hand in his enormous hospital. It helped too that McCormick offered money to paint and refurbish some of the asylum's wards in exchange for cooperation in the progesterone study. They administered progesterone and estrogen in varying doses to women diagnosed with paranoia, schizophrenia, melancholia, manic depression, chronic alcoholism, Alzheimer's disease, Pick's disease, and others. Pincus managed to enroll 16 women—all of them classified as psychotics—for the first round of progesterone testing. He also gave the hormone to 16 men to see how it would affect their sterility. (Sanger and McCormick, however, had made it clear that they did not trust men to take responsibility for contraception, and they wanted women to possess control of their own bodies and their own fertility.) The pill in the men had varying results, and that side of the study was soon discontinued.

In February 1955, Pincus visited McCormick in Boston to bring her up to date. In late 1954, Pincus began experimenting on animals with a new group of progestins that were many times more powerful than natural progesterone. Two of the compounds seemed especially promising. One, called norethindrone, had been developed by Syntex, and the other, named norethynodrel, had been developed by Searle. Pincus and Chang preferred the Searle product because the female animals with it did not develop slightly masculine characteristics. Pincus informed Searle that he wanted to use the compound norethynodrel and intended to try it as an oral contraceptive for women. Searle agreed to send the experimental drug under the condition that the bottles were unlabeled and Searle was not mentioned as the supplier.

Pincus brought McCormick up to date on the advantages of doing clinical trials in Puerto Rico. This time he would begin a new experiment with nurses and medical students on that island. He would drop the endometrial biopsies, which were extremely uncomfortable and scared off participants. In addition, the students would be required by the faculty to participate as part of their studies. If the young women were worried about the stigma of being birth control subjects, Pincus had a solution: he would label the project a "study of the physiology of progesterone in women." And once the nurses and students enrolled, word would spread that the substances were safe and effective. From there it would get easier. Pincus told McCormick the new drugs would cost about 50¢ a gram, which would mean expenses of about $5000 for the treatment of 100 women during the first year of testing. In addition, he would need money for physicians, nurses, secretaries, travel, and printed materials. For the first year the total operating expenses would probably be about $10,000. McCormick assured him that money would not be a problem.

In late 1955, John Rock reported to Searle preliminary results of his tests with the new progestin compound norethynodrel. Rock's test showed that progestins stopped the pituitary gland from producing the hormones that signaled the ovaries to release eggs. But the pill had other effects that were not yet clearly understood. It appeared to change the consistency of the cervical mucus, making it more hostile to sperm. Rock indicated that he was relatively confident that the Searle progestin was safe and that it would not affect the woman's ability to get pregnant. He was optimistic enough to encourage Searle to promote the drug more widely, but he was nowhere near as optimistic as Pincus. Additional results by Rock showed that both norethynodrel and norethindrone appeared effective. Best of all, they worked at doses of only 10 mg per day, which was one-thirtieth of the progesterone dose Pincus and Rock had been giving earlier.

In October 1955, Pincus and Sanger went to Japan to attend a meeting where he initially had planned to announce that an oral contraceptive for humans was nearly ready when, in fact, he had not yet decided which form of the contraceptive worked best and at which dose. Sanger was greeted as a hero in Tokyo. The number of reported abortions in Japan had increased from 246,000 in 1949 to just over 800,000 in 1952, and the number of sterilization operations jumped from 6000 in 1949 to more than 44,000 in 1956. Sanger opposed abortion as a method of birth control and believed that Japan needed an oral contraceptive more desperately than most nations. She also believed that the country was well positioned to take advantage of innovations in contraception. Literacy rates, for example, were high. Midwives were active even in remote villages. If it worked in Japan, Sanger strongly hoped it would work all over Asia and the world.

In February 1956, Pincus flew to Puerto Rico to see if he could salvage the trials. The university students and nurses had all quit. He needed a new approach. He met with Dr. Rice-Wray who was both the medical director of the Family

Planning Association and director of the training center for nurses at the Department of Health's Public Health Unit, in a poverty-stricken district of San Juan. These dual roles made her an ideal guide to Puerto Rico for Pincus and Rock. She knew her way around the communities where the field trials would be taking place, and she was a rebel who had given up a comfortable medical practice in Chicago because she believed that women should have access to contraception. Rice-Wray began by visiting the superintendent of the housing development, a man who saw first hand the effects of overpopulation and the burdens it placed on young mothers. He turned over a detailed list of all the community's residents and promised that his staff would help Rice-Wray recruit subjects. She enlisted a strong, smart, ebullient nurse whom everyone in the area knew. Puerto Rican government officials approved the study.

By the end of March 1956, Rice-Wray and her nurse associate had selected a group of 100 women as well as a control group of another 125. Though almost all were Catholic, Rice-Wray encountered only one woman who said her religion prohibited her from enrolling in the study. The subjects receiving the birth control pill were told that they were taking an experimental new contraceptive. The women in the control group were told they were part of a survey on family size. They used Searle's compound, norethynodrel. The subjects were supposed to take one pill a day for 20 days before stopping. Dr. Rice-Wray began distributing birth control pills in April 1956. She gave each woman a full bottle, enough to last 20 days. She told her patients to wait 5 days after completing one bottle before starting another. Even though she tried to keep the instructions simple, mistakes occurred. One patient went home and took all the pills at once. Others shared them with friends. Doctors, nurses, and social workers tried handing out calendars. They tried giving women beads on a string to help them count. Nothing worked.

A newspaper got wind of the study and reported it. Afterwards, 30 women dropped out of the trial, some because their husbands objected, others because they were worried about what their priest would say, and still others because they were experiencing unpleasant side effects. After 6 months, an additional 48 patients had quit, leaving only about 20 of the original 100. After a slow start, the study was never again at a loss for volunteers. By the end of 1956, 221 women had participated. Seventeen of those women had gotten pregnant—a fact that might have been troubling to some scientists but not to Pincus. The pregnancies had nothing to do with the pill, he told Katherine McCormick. Women were getting pregnant because they weren't following instructions. They either forgot to take the pill every day or chose not to take it because the side effects were becoming too much to bear. Among the first 221 women in the study, 38 (17%) reported negative reactions to the drug and at least 25 women withdrew from the study specifically because of the side effects. In December 1956, Dr. Rice-Wray and Pincus traveled to Skokie, Illinois, to present their findings to the officials at G.D. Searle, which had already

patented norethynodrel and had recently trademarked a new name for the drug, calling it Enovid.

By 1957, Pincus and Rock both felt confident that the pill worked and that it worked safely. Their biggest challenge was to get more women to try it and at the same time see if they could do something about the side effects. Pincus believed that most of the side effects were psychosomatic. To test that theory, he designed a simple experiment. One group of women was given Enovid with the usual warnings about possible reactions. Another group was told they were getting Enovid but was given a placebo instead along with the same warnings on side effects given to the first group. The third group received the real Enovid and no warnings about the side effects. The side effects were 23% in the first group, 17% in the second group, and 6% in the third group. Pincus' experiment violated two basic rules of modern medical research: his patients were not informed of the purpose of the study, nor were they warned of the risks. The results nevertheless convinced him that he was right. Many of the side effects were imaginary.

Pincus sought more patients. He contacted Clarence Gamble of Proctor & Gamble fame who had been sponsoring research in Puerto Rico for years, and Gamble offered to fund a second trial. He connected the Pincus team with the medical director at Ryder Memorial Hospital in a city 35 miles from San Juan. The women came to the hospital for two reasons: to have babies and, immediately afterward, to get sterilized. If it were not for the latter procedure, they would have delivered at home by midwives. The area chosen by Gamble was a slum region with no toilets or sewers and housing so crowded there was scarcely room for a squeezed pedestrian. Gamble hired a woman to take a census of La Vega, going door to door asking mothers how many children they had, whether they were sterilized, and what type of birth control they were using, if any. Enovid was offered to the women who had been denied sterilization at the hospital. There was no trouble finding willing patients, but once again side effects complicated the work. Women complained of breakthrough bleeding, nausea, and headaches. Nevertheless, women desperate to avoid pregnancy continued to enroll in the studies.

With trials now underway in two Puerto Rican communities, Pincus and his team began to work on a third location in Port au Prince, Haiti. Increasing numbers of patients gave Pincus and Searle hope that they might have enough information to prove Enovid's safety.

At one point, Pincus and Chang discovered that Searle's compound had accidentally been contaminated with a tiny amount of synthetic estrogen, also known as mestranol. Pincus had always tried to avoid the estrogen, and when he learned of this accidental contamination he ordered the drug company to get rid of estrogen—not only because he felt it might be unsafe but also because he thought the estrogen might have been responsible for some of the side effects. To his surprise, however, not only did the nausea persist, but women began experiencing even more breakthrough bleeding. As a consequence, it dawned on Pincus that the accidental contamination might have been a good thing. With more experimentation, he found that breakthrough bleeding increased when the estrogen dose fell, and nausea and breast pain increased when it rose. He also discovered that when the estrogen levels were too low, the pill was less effective in preventing pregnancy. Now, instead of purifying the pill, he suggested that Searle intentionally make it 10 mg tablets with 1.5% mestranol. The side effects did not disappear completely but the bleeding almost stopped.

Still in the first months of 1957, the dropout rates remained high and the number of women enrolled in this study was low—too low, Pincus believed, to win approval from the Food and Drug Administration (FDA). In an effort to remove emphasis on the number of patients enrolled in the trial, Pincus stopped talking about women altogether. Instead he talked about the number of menstrual cycles observed: in the 1279 cycles when the regime of treatment was meticulously followed, there was not a single pregnancy. Simply put, 1279 menstrual cycles sounded a lot more impressive than 130 women.

Searle faced difficult questions: What were the rules for testing the pill in healthy people? How far did a company have to go to prove such a product? Was 1 year of testing enough to measure long-term effects? Pincus urged Jack Searle not to get bogged down. In the end, there was no way to answer such questions because no one had ever done anything like this. There were risks with any drug, but the rewards for this drug in particular were like no other. This was a drug that had a chance to make money, change lives, change the culture, and combat massive world problems, such as hunger, poverty, and overcrowding. Childbirth also was dangerous, especially for women who were sick or weak or starving. There was no way to measure how many lives might be saved by a reliable contraceptive. In the end, Jack Searle concluded that the potential rewards outweighed the risks.

FDA submission. Searle did hedge its bet in one important way: Instead of seeking approval from the FDA for a birth control pill, the company applied for the approval of Enovid as a treatment for menstrual disorders. Searle's application to the FDA in 1957 made no mention of contraception. Amenorrhea, dysmenorrhea, and menorrhagia were the menstrual problems Enovid was said to combat. The company also claimed that the new drug would be used to treat infertility, because even though the number of cases was small, tests showed that women resting the ovaries for several months were more likely to become pregnant when they stopped taking the drug. The FDA inspectors could not reject the drug as a contraceptive because Searle was not asking for approval as a contraceptive. The only question was whether it worked safely and effectively in treating menstrual disorders.

On June 10, 1957, after taking 2 months to review the application filed by G.D. Searle and company, the FDA approved the sale of Enovid for infertility and menstrual irregularities. About the same time, the drug was approved for the same uses in England under the brand name Enavid. It turned out that Searle did not have to market the pill as birth control because men and women were learning for themselves what it could do. It did not hurt that the FDA had required the drug company to include a warning on each bottle that said that "Enovid prevented ovulation"; in other words, the real purpose of the drug was listed as if it were a side effect. That statement was like a free ad.

In 1958, 17 states still had laws banning the sale, distribution, or advertisement of contraception. Gradually, one state at a time, the laws were being overturned. Those in place were largely unenforced. It was clearer than ever that most Americans favored some type of birth control.

In 1959, drugs came with labels and nothing more. There were no informational inserts to tell patients how the drug should be used or to warn them of possible side effects. If patients needed instructions beyond those printed on the bottle, they asked their physicians. For good reason, Searle was more worried than usual about how this drug would be received if they had received permission to sell it as birth control. For one thing, women would be taking it by choice rather than by necessity. They would be trying it for replacement of other forms of birth control, not to ease pain or cure an illness. Searle wanted to set the right tone, striking a balance between the pill's medical uses and its social benefits. Searle invited John Rock who believed strongly in Enovid to help them with their pitch. He suggested the company use phrases such as "child spacing," "postponement of pregnancy," and "suppression of ovulation" in its writings rather than contraception or birth control. Searle would settle eventually on "family planning" as its euphemism of choice. In a brochure prepared for physicians, Rock spent 1.5 pages describing the menstrual cycle for general practitioners who were perhaps not as familiar with it as gynecologists. Enovid, he wrote, "completely mimics" the natural action of progesterone in suppressing ovulation. In a separate brochure for patients, he wrote: "Enovid is an artificially made hormone that is chemically quite similar to the two hormones, estrogen and progesterone, naturally produced in the human ovary."

On July 23, 1959, G.D. Searle asked the FDA to approve Enovid for birth control. (Though it was not yet officially recognized as birth control, more than 500,000 women were taking the pill.) Though the number of women enrolled in clinical trials for the pill remained small, Searle submitted the biggest new drug application in American history at that time, with 20 volumes of data. In 1959, the FDA had only four full-time and four part-time physicians assigned to investigate the 369 new drug applications submitted that year. Those seven investigators were under extreme pressure to keep up with applications, but they had little time to conduct their own research or maintain their professional education. The Enovid application wound up on the desk of one of the part-timers, Pasquale DeFelice, a 34-year-old obstetrician-gynecologist, who was still completing his residency at Georgetown Medical Center in Washington, DC. He was Catholic, and he was on his way to becoming the father of 10 children.

DeFelice seriously questioned the validity of the use of a progesterone and the small number (n ≈ 130) of patients studied and asked Searle for more data. Searle went back to work to collect more data. In the meantime, DeFelice sent a questionnaire to 61 US physicians who had considerable experience with the drug. The response barely favored release of Enovid as a birth control agent. Despite considerable FDA hesitancy, DeFelice phoned Searle on April 7, 1959, indicating the agency's approval. The official announcement was May 9, 1960. The world has not quite been the same since.

Soon after the pill was accepted, Pincus began working on a pill with lower hormone levels, and by 1964 Searle began selling Enovid-E, with a hormone dose of only 2.5 mg, reducing the cost for consumers to only $2.25 a month and reducing or eliminating the side effects for many.

Looking back more than a half century, it seems unbelievable that a group of brave, rebellious misfits—Sanger, Pincus, McCormick, and Rock—made such a radical breakthrough and did it with no government funds and comparatively little corporate money. Pincus made relatively little money on his invention—only his wages from Searle and the company stock he purchased. He never patented the drug, but he had no regrets. He was a pure scientist.

If there was one problem with Pincus' invention, it was that even educated women sometimes had difficulty using it. Healthy young women were not accustomed to taking medicine every day. Sometimes they forgot or they lost track of how many tablets they had taken since the start of the menstrual cycle. Nervous men found themselves reminding their wives and girlfriends, which led to friction. The men wondered if the women might secretly be trying to get pregnant, and the women suspected that the men cared more about the women's sexual availability than their health. After one such marital spout, David T. Wagner of Geneva, Illinois, decided not to leave the matter entirely in his wife's hands. Wagner took a piece of paper and put it on the dresser in their bedroom. On the paper he wrote the days of the week; he then placed one pill atop each day. When Doris swallowed a pill, the day of the week would be revealed and husband and wife both would have confirmation that she had taken it. Wagner said that this did wonders for their relationship. Wagner, a product engineer for

Illinois' Toolworks, began sketching a pill box that would also function as a calendar. In 1962, he applied for a patent on a circular pill dispenser. Searle declined interest in his invention, but Ortho's contraceptive pill hit the market in February 1963, and it arrived not in a bottle but in a beautiful "Dialpack." Eventually, all the pill producers used the distinctive package that Wagner had devised.

In 1967, *Time* magazine put the pill on its cover, reporting that "in a mere 6 years it has changed and liberated the sex and family life of a large and still growing segment of the US population: eventually, it promises to do the same for much of the world."

In 2010, British scientists released the results of a 40-year study, "Mortality among contraceptive pill users," that showed that women taking the birth control pill were less likely than other women to die of heart disease, cancer, and other ailments [2]. The study, which tracked 46,000 women, helped ease concerns about elevated risks of cancer or stroke. The women who took the pill were 12% less likely to die of any cause during the study.

In 2011, Laura Pincus Bernard, Goody's daughter, walked through the empty halls of the ivy-covered building where her father once worked, where Chang once slept, and where animals once mated or attempted to mate before giving their lives to science. The place was deserted except for a lone woman tapping a computer keyboard at her desk. That something so big and world-changing had come from so humble a place seemed a little short of a miracle.

William C Roberts

WILLIAM CLIFFORD ROBERTS, MD
May 20, 2015

1. Eig J. *The Birth of the Pill: How Four Crusaders Reinvented Sex and Launched a Revolution.* New York: W. W. Norton & Company, 2014 (388 pp.).
2. Hannaford PC, Iversen L, Macfarlane TV, Elliott AM, Angus V, Lee AJ. Mortality among contraceptive pill users: cohort evidence from Royal College of General Practitioners' Oral Contraception Study. *BMJ* 2010;340:c927.

Chapter 20

October 2015

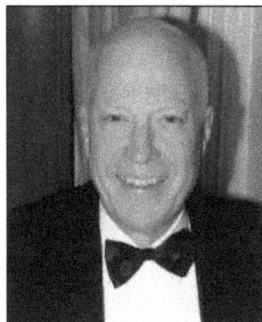

William C. Roberts, MD.

ALZHEIMER'S

About 5.2 million Americans had Alzheimer's in 2014 (1). By 2050, an estimated 13.5 million are predicted to have the disease. Alzheimer's care cost $226 billion in the last fiscal year, and some $150 billion fell to Medicare and Medicaid; the remainder mostly was handled by patients and families. Alzheimer's disease is escalating as baby boomers—a generation of 76 million Americans born between 1946 and 1964—turn 65 at a rate of roughly 10,000 a day. The risk of Alzheimer's of course increases with age, and as baby boomers get older the number of people developing the disease will rise to levels far beyond anything we've seen before. The disease is more prominent in women than in men. At age 65, seemingly healthy women have about a 1 in 6 chance of developing Alzheimer's during the rest of their lives, compared with a 1 in 11 chance for men.

Lauren Neergaard of the Associated Press suggested five tips to help guard against Alzheimer's (2). 1) *Get plenty of sleep:* poor sleep can spur the brain-clogging protein amyloid that is a hallmark of Alzheimer's. 2) *Exercise the gray matter:* working crossword puzzles, taking music lessons, or learning a new language keeps the brain engaged. Learning and complex thinking strengthen connections between nerve cells, building up "cognitive reserve" so that as Alzheimer's brews the brain can withstand more damage before symptoms become apparent. 3) *Get plenty of physical activity:* the least active have the worst cognition when they are middle-aged. Sedentary behaviors increase the chances of Alzheimer's. 4) *Maintain mental health:* depression and loneliness accelerate cognitive decline. Experiencing stress is one thing, but how we cope with it is more important. 5) *Eat healthy:* diets high in fruits and vegetables and lower in fat and sugar are good for the arteries that keep blood flowing to the brain. Diabetes mellitus and excessive weight raise the risk of dementia.

THE GOLDEN RULE FOR STATIN THERAPY: STAY ON THE DRUG

The European Atherosclerosis Society Consensus Panel statement on assessment, etiology, and management of statin-associated muscle symptoms was published in February 2015, and several of the panel members were interviewed thereafter (3). Dr. Erik Stroes of Amsterdam stated, "Let's start with the Golden Rule: never stop using your statin." His thesis was that if statins reduce the risk of major vascular events 20% with every 39 mg/mL reduction in low-density lipoprotein (LDL) cholesterol, that risk returns if the lipid-lowering drugs are stopped. He mentioned a recent article showing that patients who had had a myocardial infarct who stopped their statins had a 4- to 7-fold increase in risk of cardiac death over the following 4 years. Stroes stressed that "stopping a statin is not just an important decision, but pivotally important." He mentioned at least 7 studies where discontinuing a statin had unwanted consequences. His view: Before abandoning a statin because of muscle symptoms, physicians need to be absolutely certain the muscle-related events are attributable to the drug. When a statin is discontinued in a patient, that discontinuation is liable to do the patient harm.

The panel statement indicated that the rate of myopathy is 0.5 events per 1000 patients over a 5-year period. This event frequency is based on data from randomized controlled clinical trials. The risk of rhabdomyolysis is 0.1 events per 1000 patients over a 5-year period.

When experts began preparing the consensus statement, a number of the contributors blamed the media for sensational headlines trumpeting risks with statins. Several believe the media was responsible for blowing the potential side effects out of proportion and led to patients' stopping the drug needlessly. Some contributors to the report found fault not only with the media but also with research universities or institutions that trumpeted data from observational studies where data are not as consistent or as reliable as those from randomized controlled clinical trials. The consensus panel recommended that if a patient is identified with statin-associated muscle symptoms, the first task is to rechallenge the patient with another statin after stopping the first drug for 2 to 4 weeks. One Cleveland Clinic study showed that more than 70% of patients who stopped their statin because of side effects could be successfully restarted with a different statin. A Boston-based study showed that 92% of patients who stopped their statin were successfully rechallenged with statin therapy and still taking the drug 12 months later. If the rechallenged patient is still not able to tolerate a statin, the panel recommended that physicians try again, aiming for a lower dose with a particularly potent statin or advising the patient to take a statin every other day or twice weekly. If still unsuccessful, the remaining step may involve trying again with the highest maximally tolerated dose of statin and then adding ezetimibe.

PCSK9 INHIBITOR APPROVED

In June 2015, a Food and Drug Administration (FDA) advisory panel recommended that the agency approve the cholesterol-lowering drug Praluent (alirocumab) (4–6). The drug is produced by Sanofi SA and Regeneron Pharmaceuticals and is the first of these PCSK9 inhibitors approved. This new class of medicines blocks a protein called PCSK9, which interferes with the liver's ability to clear LDL cholesterol from the bloodstream. Praluent is an injectable medicine only and is administered every 2 weeks. It will probably be recommended only for patients with heterozygous or homozygous familial hypercholesterolemia, the former occurring in 1 of 500 people and the latter in 1 in 1,000,000 people. The drug is expected to cost about $1000 monthly or $500 for each injection. The two companies state they already have a study underway to see if cardiac outcomes improve with the drug, and the results are expected in 2017. In clinical studies evaluated by the FDA and the advisory committee, Praluent showed "no marked disparities in deaths, serious adverse events, or adverse events leading to discontinuation of the drug." The studies showed patients with the drug had their LDL cholesterol lowered by 40% to 60%.

NEW BLOCKBUSTER DRUGS

In 2014, the FDA gave the green light to 41 new drug compounds for a wide range of diseases, including viruses, cancer, and skin infections (7). It was also the year of the most successful drug launch in history, *Sovaldi*, the new hepatitis C drug from Gilead Sciences ($10.3 billion in sales). The class of 2015 brings promising new treatments for high cholesterol levels, cystic fibrosis, and heart failure. Although it is never easy to predict which drugs will win approval by the FDA, Barrons considered the following drugs to have a high probability of regulatory approval in 2015 and the potential to deliver annual sales of $1 billion or more.

Novartis has a new blockbuster with *LCZ696*. In the US alone, just over 5 million people have chronic heart failure. Data have shown that, compared with current treatments, use of LCZ696 has led to a 20% lower risk of death caused by a "cardiac event" and fewer hospitalizations.

Regulators approved a drug in January 2015 from Novartis that offers a new way to treat psoriasis. Known as *Cosentyx*, the drug blocks a protein that plays a role in inflammation. In four clinical trials, more than 80% of patients taking it saw at least 75% of their symptoms disappear.

Vertex Pharmaceuticals became the first drug maker in more than a decade to launch a new treatment for cystic fibrosis when the drug *Kalydeco* won regulatory approval. This drug is effective in only a small fraction of patients, but when paired with an experimental drug, also from Vertex, the new combination was more effective.

CYSTIC FIBROSIS DRUGS

Boston-based Vertex Pharmaceuticals' newest cystic fibrosis drug, *Orkambi*, is a combination of Kalydeco (ivacaftor) with another compound called lumacaftor (8). It treats the most common form of cystic fibrosis but at an annual wholesale cost of $259,000 per patient. It is administered twice daily in an oral tablet. Vertex already sells Kalydeco, which treats a different genetic type of cystic fibrosis and has an annual price of $311,000 per patient in the US. The FDA advisory committee of 13 independent physicians, scientists, consumers, and patient representatives recommended approval in May 2015 by a vote of 12 to 1. The new drug appears to be only modestly effective. That's a lot of money for modest effectiveness.

COST OF CANCER

Jim Landers had an extensive piece on the cost of cancer care recently in *The Dallas Morning News* (9, 10). Prescription drug costs for new cancer treatments are soaring at unsustainable rates. By 2020, the cost of specialty drugs for cancer and other diseases could reach $400 billion a year, about $100 billion more than the entire prescription drug industry today. Cancer now is the second leading cause of death in the US behind cardiovascular disease and is heading rapidly toward the number one spot. Worldwide, annual cancer cases are expected to rise over the next 2 decades from 14 million diagnoses to about 22 million. In 2015, nearly 2 million Americans will be diagnosed with cancer. Drug companies, of course, need to recoup research investments, which can run more than $1 billion for development of a new drug. Medicare, the federal health insurance program, is prohibited from negotiating with the pharmaceutical industry over prices! Although many hospitals receive discounts on cancer drugs under Medicare rules, they are not required to share those discounts with patients. Also, it is illegal to import the same drug at a less expensive price from pharmacies abroad!

JONAS SALK AND HIS POLIO VACCINE

When I was a youngster, my mother kept my brother and me out of public swimming pools in the 1940s because of fear of polio. In post-World War II, polio struck seemingly out of the blue each summer as temperatures rose. The virus hit kids particularly, causing paralysis and breathing only by iron lungs. Apart from the atomic bomb, America's greatest fear after World War II was polio. As a result, scientists were in a frantic race to find a way to prevent or cure the disease. In 1938, a US president, Franklin D. Roosevelt, the world's most recognized victim of the disease, founded the National Foundation for Infantile Paralysis (later known as the March of Dimes Foundation), an organization that would fund the development of a vaccine. As described in the recent book by Charlotte DeCroes Jacobs entitled *Jonas Salk: A Life*, Salk (1914–1995) in 1947 accepted an appointment to the University of Pittsburgh School of Medicine (11). In 1948, he undertook a project funded by the National Foundation for Infantile Paralysis to determine the number of different types of polio virus. He extended the project towards developing a vaccine against polio and devoted himself to this work for the next 7 years. The field trials set up to test the Salk vaccine were considered the most elaborate program of its kind in history, involving 20,000 physicians and public health offices, 64,000 school personnel, and 220,000 volunteers. Over 1,800,000 school children took part in the trial. When news of the vaccine's success was made public on April 12, 1955, Salk was hailed as a miracle worker and the day almost became a national holiday. Around the world, an immediate rush to vaccinate began. Almost overnight Salk became the most adored man in the nation. Fan letters and awards poured in for the rest of his life.

The Jacobs book concerns primarily Salk's career after developing the safe and effective vaccine for polio. Salk's vaccine was a killed version of the polio virus, and it coaxed a person's antibodies to protect against the live virus. Although the country accepted Salk's work with great adoration, other researchers were not as approving. Salk's great rival, Albert Sabin (1906–1993), had developed a different virus, one that relied on a live version of the polio virus. For the rest of their careers, Salk and Sabin battled over which vaccine was safer and more reliable. In the end, both approaches proved crucial to slowing polio worldwide. To date, the disease is endemic only in Afghanistan, Nigeria, and Pakistan, and public health experts continue to push full eradication.

The polio fight for Salk was just the beginning. Having established his vaccine at the age of 40, he struggled to have the rest of his life mean as much. There was some family turmoil. In 1968, he divorced his first wife (with three children) and married French artist Francoise Gilot, the mother of two of Pablo Picasso's children. Toward the end of his career, he worked on an AIDS vaccine. Although he did not succeed, his fame brought attention to the fact that AIDS was an important disease that should not be shunted to the sidelines as some kind of distasteful gay epidemic.

EXTENDING LONGEVITY

A recent piece by Ariana Eunjung Cha described what is happening in Silicon Valley about the possibility of living many decades longer than presently (12). In 2004, Peter Thiel, who had recently made a fortune selling PayPal, which he cofounded, to eBay, gathered in San Francisco with a group of tech titans who founded Google, Facebook, eBay, Napster, and Netscape with the desire of convincing them to use their billions to rewrite the nation's science agenda and transform biomedical research. Their objective was using the tools of technology—chips, software programs, algorithms, and big data, which they had used in creating the information revolution—to understand and upgrade what they considered to be the most complicated piece of machinery in existence, namely the human body. The entrepreneurs want to rebuild, regenerate, and reprogram patients' organs, limbs, cells, and DNA to enable people to live longer and better. The work they are funding includes hunting for the secrets of living organisms with insanely long lives, engineering microscopic nanobots that can fix the body from the inside out, figuring out how to reprogram

the DNA we are born with, and exploring ways to digitize our brains based on the theory that our minds could live long after our bodies expire. Oracle founder Larry Ellison, who wishes to live forever, has donated more than $430 million to aging research. Sean Parker, the Napster cofounder, has donated millions to finding a cure for allergies and cancer therapies. Google's Sergey Brin has proposed a new kind of science that starts with masses of DNA and a community of people with certain genes. He apparently has the Parkinson's disease gene and has donated $150 million to the effort. Pam Omidyar, a biologist and former research assistant in an immunology lab, cofounded the Omidyar Network with her husband, eBay's Pierre Omidyar, who became a billionaire at 31. They have donated millions to research on resiliency—the trait that helps people bounce back from illness or other adversity. And Page, who is now 41 and chief executive of Google, has made the biggest bet on longevity yet, founding Calico, short for California Life Company, a secretive antiaging research center, with an investment of up to $750 million from Google. Microsoft cofounder Bill Gates and his wife, Melinda, the wealthiest couple in the world with an estimated worth of $79 billion, believe that charitable giving is the key element to close the gap between the poor and the rich.

Of course, there are many who are ambivalent about using new medical treatments to live radically longer lives. A survey indicated that nearly two-thirds worry that radical life extension would strain natural resources, that only wealthy people would get access to new treatments, and that medical scientists would offer the treatments before they fully understood how it affected people's health.

MEDICINE FROM THE PULPIT

A piece in the *AARP Bulletin* recently described a strategy of the Reverend Sean Dogan, pastor of the Long Branch Baptist Church in Greenville, SC (13). The article indicated that Reverend Dogan had given over 400 eulogies for his parishioners, most of whom had died from heart disease, diabetes mellitus, obesity, or stroke, and after each funeral he would sit with friends and families of the deceased to a meal of fried chicken, mac and cheese, and collard greens boiled in fatback. Then one day 4 years ago, Dogan had a revelation. It was the food that was killing his people. Thus, one Sunday morning he stepped up to the altar with a weight scale in hand for all to witness as he weighed himself. Like many in his congregation, he was overweight. "The time for change," he declared, "has come." With that passionate appeal, Dogan joined scores of African American ministers around the country who, from their powerful perches, have been making the health of their congregation a priority. Nationally, nearly 48% of African Americans are obese compared with 33% of European Americans. Perhaps nowhere are these problems more evident than in the rural South. Not only Reverend Dogan's church, but a number of similar churches are now trying to turn the tide. They are enlisting community foot soldiers to give them a hand. Good for Reverend Dogan!

ADDING BODY MASS INDEX TO VITAL SIGNS

The vital signs, of course, include blood pressure, heart rate, respiratory rate, and body temperature. I don't believe many physicians count the respiratory rate. Recently, after throwing the ball to my granddaughter's pitbull in the backyard, I noticed that her respiratory rate was well over 100 breaths per minute. Dogs, of course, in contrast to humans cool their bodies by panting. Like other carnivores, they have no capacity to sweat. If a human being was breathing over 100 times a minute, I think that recording would be worthwhile, but for people breathing normally, the number of breaths per minute is infrequently counted. I recently attended a conference where a patient was discussed nearly 30 minutes and at the end it was brought out that the patient weighed 350 pounds and was only 64 inches tall. If that information had been provided initially, the whole discussion would have changed. Body mass index (BMI) will determine many of our fates and is more important than the respiratory rate.

FASHION, BODY MASS INDEX, AND MORE

Most of the world is getting heavier. About two-thirds of adults in the USA are overweight, and half of them are obese (BMI ≥30 kg/m²). The fashion models have the rare problem of too little weight. In 2007, Spain enacted regulations that barred models below a BMI of 18.5 from being featured in fashion shows (14). In the same year, Italy started insisting on health certificates for models as well as banning models under 16 years old from its runways. In 2013, Israel enacted similar BMI rules for models. In 2015, French lawmakers voted in favor of a measure that would ban excessively thin fashion models from the runways and potentially fine their employers in a move that prompted resistance in the modeling industry. Those who hire underweight models could be fined as much as $82,460 and face up to 6 months in prison. The point of the bill was to combat anorexia. The image of so-called "ideal beauty" augments the risk of eating disorders. The amendment is part of a broader bill that still requires approval by France's Senate before becoming law, but it is expected to pass and to be enforced by the end of 2015. The modeling industry in France, of course, opposes the proposal.

The National Assembly, Parliament's lower house in France, also voted in the same bill to alter the packaging of cigarettes such that the package would be less attractive and help discourage young people from starting to smoke (15). About 30% of the French smoke. Additionally, people who encourage minors to drink excessively could face a year behind bars and a 15,000 euro ($16,000) fine. The sale to minors of products inciting people to get drunk, such as t-shirts, would be forbidden. Also, the same bill would require changes to the business model of some fast-food chains. The bill would ban free soda refills in restaurants in a move aimed at fighting obesity. Also, amid concerns about skin cancer, the bill would bar tanning salons from selling sun-bed services to customers under age 18 or to engage in advertising targeting minors. The bill also would allow for a 6-year test period in which intravenous drug users would be given access to clean needles under medical supervision and in the presence of drug counselors. Medicine is moving not only into the pulpit but certainly into the legislative halls of numerous countries.

OBESITY AMONG POLICE OFFICERS

Robert Atcheson, a former captain in the Washington, DC, Metropolitan Police Department, wrote a piece entitled "Why Real Men Don't Eat Meat" (16). He indicated that "law enforcement is the fattest profession in the world" according to a study published in *The American Journal of Preventive Medicine*. Police officers are 25 times more likely to die from weight-related disorders such as heart disease than from fighting crime. Atcheson, who retired at age 50 after 25 years in the DC police force, switched from a meat-eating lifestyle to 100% vegan, thanks to encouragement from his daughter. After examining the benefits of the vegetarian-plant lifestyle and thinking about the preventable chronic diseases in his family, he made the switch. He indicated that approximately 75% of the nation's $2 trillion health care bill in 2012 was treating diet-related chronic diseases such as heart disease, diabetes mellitus, high blood pressure, and obesity. He wrote:

> It's ludicrous that those responsible for protecting the people of this country are themselves in dire need of protection—and from entirely preventable diseases, no less. Because I don't eat animal products my risk of cancer is a fraction of the average. I weigh the same today as I did at 21. I bet my life savings that unlike many of my family members—and fellow jarheads and cops—I will never get heart disease or diabetes. . . . Once I went vegan I gave my officers a message I'd like the whole country to hear: When you eat meat and other animal products, you are playing a losing game of chicken with your health. It takes courage and discipline to ditch that crap and clean up your plate. Do what I did, and what many of my best officers eventually did, too: trade in that morning donut for a smoothie. Swap that chicken sandwich for a black bean burger. Your health—and your family—will thank you.

He also indicated that obesity is the #1 cause of military ineligibility, and according to Mission:Readiness, a group of 300 retired military generals and admirals, it costs the Pentagon about $1 billion annually. Chronic diseases also disproportionately affect veterans: One in four have diabetes, and nearly 80% are overweight or obese.

OBESITY AND NATIONAL GROWTH

Morgan Stanley recently prepared a 70-page report warning that sugar consumption might sharply curtail economic expansion around the world (17). Many countries, the firm said, will experience slower growth than expected over the next 20 years as diabetes mellitus and obesity take a toll on workers' productivity. The US's 2.5% annual growth, projected by the Organization for Economic Cooperation and Development, falls to 1.8% when the full cost of sugar is factored in. Per capita sugar consumption worldwide has climbed nearly fivefold over the past century to 53 pounds a year as American diets take hold overseas. Some health experts call sugar the new tobacco, addictive and lethal. The problem is particularly pressing in the emerging markets, indicated Carmen Nuzzo, a Morgan Stanley European economist who coauthored the report. Rising middle classes show a clear penchant for sugary drinks and foods—the higher the income, the higher the rate of sugar consumption and the greater the rate of sedentary living. Now, more than 40% of the world's 3.87 million diabetics live in India and China. But, the greatest danger to economic growth rates, according to Morgan Stanley, is in Chile, the Czech Republic, Mexico, the USA, and Australia because of the very high rates of diabetes and obesity.

HIGH-SPEED POLICE CAR PURSUITS

Since 1979, more than 11,500 people have been killed in police chases, including 6301 fleeing drivers, 5066 nonviolators, and 139 police (18). Most bystanders were killed in their own cars by fleeing drivers. US police chase tens of thousands of people each year—usually for traffic violations or misdemeanors—and drivers often speed away recklessly. These police chases lead to many injuries and too many deaths. Pursuit of fleeing drivers is probably the most dangerous job law enforcement officers do. The Justice Department in 1990 urged police departments to adopt policies listing exactly when officers can and cannot pursue someone. Police chases have killed nearly as many people as justifiable police shootings.

Despite the Justice Department's warning, the number of chase-related deaths in 2013 was higher than the number in 1990—322 compared with 317. Many police departments let officers make on-the-spot judgments about whether to chase based upon their perception of a driver's danger to the public. Officers continue to violate pursuit policies concerning when to avoid or stop the chase. Some departments allow chases only of suspected violent felons; others let officers chase anyone if they decide the risk of letting someone go outweighs the risk of a pursuit.

Injuries are more difficult to determine than fatalities. Records from six states show that 17,600 people were hurt in chases from 2004 through 2013—an average of 1760 injuries a year in those states, which make up 24% of the US population. Those numbers suggest that chases nationwide may have injured 7400 people a year, more than 270,000 since 1979.

Some of the chases are for relatively small crimes. California records of 63,500 chases from 2002 through 2014 showed that more than 89% were for vehicle code violations, including speeding, vehicle theft, reckless driving, and nearly 5000 instances of a missing license plate or an expired registration. Just 5% were an attempt to nab someone suspected of a violent crime, usually assault or robbery; 168 sought a known murder suspect. Nearly 1000 were for safety violations that endangered a driver only, including 850 drivers not wearing a seatbelt and 23 motorcycle riders not wearing a helmet. In 90 instances, police chased someone for driving too slowly. Most dangerous are chases on slippery roads and pursuits of inexperienced, risk-prone teenage drivers and of motorcyclists, who have little crash protection. In Michigan since 2004, 74% of motorcyclists

fleeing police were killed, injured, or possibly injured when they crashed; in contrast, just 18% of chased car drivers were killed, injured, or possibly injured in a crash. Police departments routinely warn officers about hazardous road conditions and high-risk drivers. Some bar motorcycle policemen from pursuits because of the danger if an officer crashes.

Police departments that resist chases have faced resistance from officers. In 2012, the Florida Highway Patrol stopped letting officers chase anyone and allowed pursuits only of suspected felons, drunken drivers, and reckless drivers. The number of pursuits fell almost in half, from 697 in 2010–2011 to 374 in 2013–2014. Dallas' crime rates have plummeted since restricting police chases.

TELEDOC

It is the Dallas provider of phone-based medical care where doctors diagnose and prescribe medications over the phone for unknown and unseen patients. Teledoc is the largest telemedicine provider in the country. In the first 3 months of 2015, it provided more than 150,000 remote visits for patients across the country seeking routine medical care (19). Patients whose employers or insurers have deals with Teledoc can call one of the company's referral centers, day or night, 365 days a year. The referral center tracks down the patient's medical record and shares it with a physician on duty, and the physician calls the patient back, usually within 10 minutes. The physician and patient can use a video service, like Skype, exchange digital images, or just talk on the phone. Once the doctor interviews the patient and has made a diagnosis, he or she suggests remedies and may prescribe medicine. No controlled substances, like opiates, are allowed to be prescribed, and no lifestyle drugs, like Viagra, are either. The cost to the patient is no more than $40. Depending on insurance arrangements, it might be less.

The Texas Medical Board has fought Teledoc over this model since 2011. In April 2015, it voted that it was okay for patients to have remote visits with their regular physicians or on-call physicians who work in the same office, but the board's ruling against Teledoc, by a 13 to 1 vote, means that a patient unknown to a doctor must be examined in person before a physician can issue a diagnosis or a prescription. The Texas Medical Association supported the ruling.

"NO JAB, NO PAY" POLICY

The Australian government has ramped up pressure on parents who oppose vaccinations by threatening to withhold child care and other payments from families who do not immunize their children (20). The government announced in April 2015 that families could lose up to 15,000 Australian dollars (about $11,000) per child per year in tax and child care benefits from January 1, 2016, unless their children were vaccinated under a "no jab, no pay" policy. The government is removing a category of "conscientious objector" that allowed parents to remain eligible for full welfare benefits despite not immunizing their children. Although 97% of Australian families that claim tax benefits for their offspring are vaccinated, the number of children under 7 years old who are not vaccinated because their parents are objectors has increased by about 24,000 over the past decade to 39,000. Parents, however, will still be able to resist immunizing their children on medical and religious grounds without financial penalties.

GETTING TO YOUR DOCTOR

The federal government has 42 programs run by six different departments to help people get to their doctors' offices, according to the findings of a Government Accountability Office report released in April 2015 (21). The Department of Agriculture has a grant program to help assisted living facilities in rural areas buy vans; the Department of Housing and Urban Development provides bus tokens and taxi fares for people with AIDS; and the Department of Veterans Affairs provides mileage reimbursement or bus, train, boat, or even airplane tickets. The largest program, administered by Medicaid, spends more than $1.3 billion a year to get people to the doctor. Because medical transportation at other agencies is so fragmented, there's no accounting of how much the government spends in all.

BIRTH TOURISM

According to a piece in the *USA Today* by Calum MacLeod (22), business is booming in Beijing, China, for companies that coach pregnant women on how to deceive US immigration authorities so that they can enter the US for the sole purpose of giving birth to an American citizen. At least 500 companies offered "birth tourism" services in China in 2014. The number of Chinese citizens heading to the USA to give birth is not entirely clear, but it appears to be in the tens of thousands each year. The cost of the trip, including medical expenses, runs from $20,000 to $80,000. The business is legal in China, but the tactics for entering the US are not. The women apparently are coached to lie about the purpose of their visit by listing "tourism," which makes it easier to get a visa. They also are told to hide their pregnancies when going through US Immigration and avoid declarations that they are traveling for medical treatment. The US State Department says there is no law barring foreigners from traveling to the US for the purpose of giving birth. The tourism visa they usually travel on, known as a B-2 visa, allows foreigners to enter the US for "medical treatment." As long as the applicants are truthful about their intentions, prove they can afford their medical care, explain why they can't have the procedure done in their home country, and assert that they will abide by the time restrictions of their visa, such travel is generally allowed under US law.

Birth tourism is expected to grow. The main attraction: when children born in the USA turn 21, they can sponsor their parents to become legal US residents so the family can immigrate to the USA. The Chinese apparently admire America's clean air, safe food, and its respect for human rights; they seek a better education and environment for their children and hope to evade China's "one-child" policy. Expectant mothers typically arrive 2 months before birth and stay one more for postpartum recovery. They then return to China where government officials don't punish the parents for violating birth control rules because a second child is considered an American. At 18, however, the child must choose whether to be a US or a Chinese citizen. Birth tourism has become more popular than a US immigration program that lets wealthy applicants gain American residency by investing at least $500,000 in a US business.

JOGGING AND IMMORTALITY

Some investigators from Copenhagen, Denmark, recently compared the mortality of joggers running 1 to 2.4 hours per week with that of sedentary nonjoggers (23). The joggers were divided into light, moderate, and strenuous joggers. The lowest mortality was found in the light joggers followed by moderate joggers and, lastly, the strenuous joggers. The findings show a U-shaped association between all-cause mortality and the dose of jogging as calibrated by pace, quantity, and frequency. Light and moderate joggers had lower mortality rates than sedentary nonjoggers, whereas strenuous joggers had a mortality rate similar to that of sedentary nonjoggers. Thus, a little but not too much.

MILES RUN DURING PROFESSIONAL NATIONAL BASKETBALL GAMES

The NBA has SportVU Player Tracking technology in every NBA arena (24). The system includes cameras and STATS proprietary software, which tracks the movements of all the players and the ball on the court. During the 48-minute scheduled games, each of the 30 NBA teams as a group run just over 1000 miles. The distance covered per 48 minutes for the individual players is just over 3.0 miles per game. The average speed of each of the players averages 4.0 miles per hour. Most of the players in the starting lineup of NBA games average just over 30 minutes per game, and nearly all of them play in about 60 games per year. A number of the starters put in about 150 miles during the 72 regular season games.

MEDICARE'S 50TH BIRTHDAY

Medicare of course was part of Lyndon B. Johnson's great society expansion in the 1960s. In its first year, 1966, Medicare spent $3 billion. In 1967, the House Ways and Means Committee predicted that the program would cost $12 billion by 1990. It ended up costing $110 billion that year (25, 26). In 2014, the program cost $511 billion, and 7 years from now it will be $1 trillion. The latest projections from Medicare's trustees, released in July 2015, are that the program's main trust fund, for hospital care, will be exhausted by 2030. To keep Medicare's spending under control, payments to health care providers by the program have consistently been lower than those made by private insurers. The American Hospital Association reported that hospitals took in $0.88 for every $1.00 spent caring for Medicare beneficiaries in 2013. Now, nearly 3 in 10 seniors on Medicare struggle to find a primary care physician who will treat them.

Maybe a partial fix to the problem could start with increasing the age when Americans can enter Medicare. In 1965, eligibility for Medicare was set at age 65 because life expectancy then was 70 years. Today, life expectancy is 79 years of age and could reach 84 by 2050. The number of Medicare beneficiaries also has skyrocketed since the program's inception. It initially served 19 million people. Today, the program serves almost 50 million, and every day 10,000 baby boomers join the program's ranks. Raising the eligibility age for Medicare by just 2 years would save $19 billion by 2023. Some have figured that changing the eligibility age will not be enough to save Medicare. One proposal is to convert the open-ended entitlement to a system of means-tested vouchers. The government would give every senior a voucher based on health status, income, and age. Seniors in better health and those with the most money would receive smaller vouchers, and sicker or needier seniors would receive large ones.

But there is some good news for Medicare, according to an article by Krumholz and colleagues (27). From 1999 to 2013, mortality rates among Medicare patients fell 16% (from 5.3% to 4.5%); hospitalizations during the same period fell (from 35,274 to 26,930 per 100,000 person-years); and costs per patient fell (from $3290 to $2801 per patient). Among fee-for-service from 1999 to 2013, in contrast, hospitalization rates fell 24% (>3 million fewer hospitalizations); mortality rates fell 45% during hospitalization, 24% within a month of hospitalization, and 22% within a year of hospitalization; and costs for hospitalized patients fell by 15% during the 14-year period. Thus, not all Medicare news is bad news.

FEDERAL SPENDING AND FEDERAL TAXES

The US government spent $3.5 trillion in fiscal year 2014 (28). Of that, 86%, or about $3 trillion, was financed by tax revenue (income tax, payroll tax, corporate income tax, and other taxes). The rest came from borrowing. The federal spending breakdown is the following: Social Security, 24%; Medicare, Medicaid, CHIP, and marketplace subsidies, 24%; defense and international security, 18%; safety net programs, 11%; interest on debt, 7%; and other programs, 17%. The sources of federal tax revenue in 2014 were income tax, 46%; payroll tax, 34%; corporate income tax, 11%; and excise and estate taxes and others, 9%. Federal taxes are paid by 59% of American households; 41% of American households do not pay federal income tax. US charitable donations in 2013 totaled $335 billion, of which $241 billion was from individual donors. The largest charitable donations in 2013, namely $106 billion, went to religious groups, and $52 billion went to education institutions, most to 4-year colleges and universities. A survey of taxpayers receiving tax refunds this year indicated that 34% planned to use the money to pay down debt, another 33% to save the money or invest it, 26% for necessities, 3% for vacations or shopping, and 3% for other items. Thus, medicine accounts for nearly a quarter of our federal government's spending!

MORE ON THE AFFORDABLE CARE ACT

Scott W. Atlas, a physician and a senior fellow at Stanford University's Hoover Institution, writing in *The Wall Street Journal*, indicated that in 2013, 107 million people in the US were on Medicaid or Medicare, and that number will increase to 135 million by 2018, a growth rate tripling that of private insurance (29, 30). At the same time, private health care insur-

ance premiums are expected to skyrocket in 2016, many by more than 30%. Private insurance, of course, is superior for both access and quality of care. Insurance without access to medical care is a sham, he argued, and that is where the country is heading. According to a 2014 Merritt Hawkins survey, 55% of physicians in major metropolitan areas in the US refuse new Medicaid patients. The harsh reality awaiting low-income Americans is dwindling access to quality physicians, hospitals, and health care. Simultaneously, while the population ages into Medicare eligibility, a significant and growing proportion of physicians do not accept Medicare patients. According to the nonpartisan Medicare Payment Advisory Commission, 29% of Medicare beneficiaries who were looking for a primary care physician in 2008 already had a problem finding one. Articles in several medical journals, including *The American Journal of Cardiology*, clearly show that patients with private insurance have better outcomes than similar patients on government insurance. It is highly likely, Dr. Atlas argued, that restrictions in access to important drugs, specialists, and technology account for these differences.

Of the many negative effects of the Affordable Care Act, the increasing unaffordability of private insurance might be the most damaging. Thanks to its regulations on pricing and coverage, the law has already forced termination of private health insurance for more than 5 million Americans. That is projected to be as many as 10 million by 2021, a tenfold increase from 2011 projections at the onset of the law. Atlas concluded that reforming America's health care rests on reducing costs while improving access to the best physicians and hospitals. That comes from private insurance, not government insurance.

SUNSCREENS VERSUS VITAMIN D

We all know how important sunscreen is to decrease exposure to the sun's ultraviolet radiation, which causes skin aging, wrinkling, and skin cancer. We also know that vitamin D, made in the skin from sun exposure, is vital for good health. According to Joe and Teresa Graedon, in places like Phoenix and Tampa, just 6 minutes of sun exposure midday offers enough ultraviolet for fair skin to make 1000 IU of vitamin D (31). These authors suggest that 15 to 20 minutes of sun without sunscreen several times a week allows a good production of vitamin D. After that, lather up with sunscreen.

PATIENT MODESTY

Patient modesty might seem like an oxymoron when those seeking medical care are routinely told to remove their clothes, put on a flimsy gown, lie back, and let the professionals do their work (32). To many people, everything about those instructions induces anxiety and sometimes anger. They fear the vulnerability that comes with it. They can't relax when they're ceding control over what is happening to them, and it's irrelevant that physicians and nurses have seen thousands of bare bottoms and private parts. I was surprised to learn that there is a website on Medical Patient Modesty (www.patientmodesty.org), a fledgling nonprofit based in North Carolina that offers emotional support and practical resources.

COMPETENCE OF OLDER PHYSICIANS

One of every four US physicians is now >65 years of age (33). In June 2015, the American Medical Association (AMA) adopted a plan to help decide when it's time for senior physicians to bring down their shingle. The nation's largest organization of physicians agreed to spearhead an effort to create competency guidelines for assessing whether older physicians remain able to provide safe and effective care for patients. Physicians, of course, have no mandatory retirement age, unlike pilots, military personnel, and a few other professions. Physicians must meet state licensing requirements, and some hospitals require age-based screening. But there are no national mandates or guidelines on how to make sure older physicians can still do their job safely. The AMA agreed it's time to change that view. The plan it adopted noted that US physicians aged ≥65 has quadrupled since 1975 and now number 240,000. The AMA agreed to convene groups to collaborate in developing preliminary assessment guidelines. The report says that "testing should include an evaluation of physical and mental health and a review of physicians' treatment of patients."

ALCOHOL CONSUMPTION INCREASING

Average alcohol consumption in Europe, North America, and Northeast Asia is roughly 10 liters a year (34). That's the equivalent of 100 bottles of wine or 200 liters of beer (23.5 cases) for each person. Most of that consumption is accounted for by heavy drinkers. In the USA, 20% of drinkers account for three-fourths of alcohol consumed. Just over 4% of US deaths stem from alcohol use. In contrast, in Russia, it is 30%. Worldwide, alcohol use is responsible for 3.3 million deaths annually—more than HIV, tuberculosis, and violence combined. Between 1990 and 2010, alcohol rose from the eighth to the fifth leading cause of death. In 2006, the US Centers for Disease Control and Prevention (CDC) estimated that alcohol use costs the nation $223 billion, mostly for loss of productivity at work, but including $25 billion for direct medical expenses. In contrast, crime and justice costs were estimated at $38 billion. A 2013 study estimated the cost of alcohol abuse in Texas at $27 billion, or $703 for every resident. Federal officials in June 2015 reported a decline in teen binge drinking—having five drinks or more on one occasion within a month—between 2002 and 2013. The National Institutes of Health reported in June 2015 that as many as one-third of American adults have alcohol use disorder at some point in their lives. The Organization for Economic Cooperation and Development (OECD) in June 2015 found that alcohol taxes help discourage alcohol drinking. The US has the lowest taxes on alcohol among the OECD's 34 members, with an average of 14¢ per drink. Many studies on cigarette smoking have shown that higher taxes on a pack of cigarettes lead to lower smoking rates.

SNAKE BITES AND THEIR COSTS

In an average year in the USA, an estimated 7000 to 8000 people are bitten by poisonous snakes. The record rain in Texas in the springtime of 2015 pushed water out of the rivers and into people's homes and displaced snakes, which increased their biting opportunities. Joan Schulte, a pediatrician and public health service physician who works at the North Texas Poison Control Center at Parkland Health & Hospital System, writing in *The Dallas Morning News* in July 2015, detailed the experiences of several Texas victims of snake bites (35). One was a 65-year-old woman bitten by a rattlesnake. She was on Medicare. The federal government will pay up to $2493 per antivenom vial in the case of a snake bite. This particular woman received 18 vials at a cost of nearly $45,000. A 10-year-old girl put her arm on the railing of a bridge and immediately received a bite from a copperhead. Fortunately, she didn't need antivenom, which is the case in about 20% of those bitten by poisonous snakes in the US.

Why is the antivenom so expensive? The current version has been around 10 years and is considered more effective and safer than older antivenoms that were made with horse serum. A new antivenom, intended only for rattlesnake bites, was approved in spring 2015 by the FDA, and it may reduce prices when it becomes widely available in the next 2 years. The least expensive treatment is to avoid being bitten in the first place. If you are out in tall grass or hiking, wear real shoes, not flip-flops. Use a hiking stick and poke around before going into a weed bank. Don't get out of a boat in a muddy bank of water plants because cottonmouths and copperheads like that habitat. If you pick up firewood or rocks, first poke around with a long stick, and if you see a rattlesnake, don't try to pick it up to see if it really rattles.

PHARMAPHOBIA

Some physicians see pharmaceutical and device representatives frequently, and others do not see them at all. I favor physicians having good relations with pharmaceutical and device persons. I don't know any physician who has come up with a new drug in the past few decades. The new drugs come about through research almost entirely by the pharmaceutical industry. Dr. Thomas Stossel, who is the American Cancer Society Professor of Medicine at Harvard Medical School, a senior physician at Brigham and Women's Hospital in Boston, and a member of the National Academy of Sciences and the Institute of Medicine, has recently written a book entitled *Pharmaphobia: How the Conflict of Interest Myth Undermines American Medical Innovation* (36). He stated the following:

> The case underlying the conflict-of-interest movement is a mixture of moralistic bullying, opinion unsupported by empiric evidence, speculation, simplistic and distorted interpretations of complicated and nuanced information, superficially and incompletely framed anecdotes, inappropriately extrapolated or irrelevant psychological research results, and emotionally laden human-interest stories.

The reality of modern medicine, Dr. Stossel argued, is that private industry is the engine of innovation, with productivity and new advances dependent on relationships between commercial and academic and research interests. Companies, not universities or research with federal funding, run 85% of the medical-products pipeline. "We all inevitably have conflicts all the time. . . . The only conflict-free situation is the grave," he argued.

Dr. Stossel had much to say about the leading medical journals, which he called "mere magazine, not holy scripture." He pointed out the irony that most peer-reviewed studies could never survive the FDA's withering scrutiny, yet they are usually taken to be more rigorous and disinterested than the clinical trial data that drug makers generate for FDA approval. The medical journals maintain their prestige and brands by creating false scarcity and rejecting original and high-quality papers.

The *New England Journal of Medicine*, possibly the world's most influential medical periodical, in the spring of 2015 had a three-part series by a physician and correspondent, Liza Rosenbaum, encouraging a rethink of the conflict-of-interest doctrine, introduced with a piece by editor Jeffrey Drazen (37). Dr. Rosenbaum's measured, thoughtful essays called for a more rational approach to managing conflicts and "to shift the conversations away from one driven by indignation toward one that better accounts for the diversity of interactions, the attendant trade-offs, and our dependence on industry in advancing patient care."

MEDICAL EMERGENCY WHEN TRAVELING ABROAD

Though many travelers take important steps against infectious disease, including vaccinations, malaria pills, and diarrhea remedies, often overlooked are other physical dangers (38). From July 2013 to June 2014, a total of 802 US citizens died in foreign countries from "nonnatural" causes: vehicular accidents, 213; homicide, 184; suicide, 134; drowning, 108; drug related, 20; aviation, 18; terrorism, 13; maritime, 10; and all other, 102. A sudden catastrophic illness when traveling abroad might warrant prior membership in one of the transportation companies that provide flights back to the US. Global Rescue Grid membership, for example, based on trip length and the extent of services, starts at $119 for 7-day trips, and annual membership starts at $329 for an individual and not quite double that for a family. Other companies also offer travel evacuation and medical assistance services when abroad, including MedjetAssist and Medex. The CDC and the State Department offer free travel websites and apps to help travelers assess health and security risks when abroad. The CDC's TravWell includes destination-specific recommendations, checklists, and packing lists. It also has an app that lets users search for health risks by country and food type, called "Can I Eat This?" CDC's *Health Information for International Travel*—also known as the Yellow Book (because of the color of the cover)—is primarily aimed at health professionals who advise patients about travel risks, but it can also help consumers. The State Department offers "Smart Traveler," an app with frequently updated country information, travel alerts, warnings, maps, and US Embassy locations.

PATIENT-PARTICIPATING HEALTH CARE

Scott Burns in *The Dallas Morning News* recently had a piece on wearable devices that provide some inkling of our bodily functions (39). He mentioned the *Tricorder v1.0*, which costs about $150, much less expensive than the *iWatch*. He mentioned the *Fitbit Charge HR*, part of a new wave of health and fitness tools, that records heart rate from the wrist. Press a button on the band once and it tells the time, press again and it tells the total steps you've taken today, press it once more and the heart rate appears. Since the band detects motion, the FitBit app also tells how long one has slept and how often the sleep was restless or awake. It calculates resting heart rate, total calories burned for the day, and time spent in "fat burn" heart rate. One can enter the food eaten screen and watch the balance between calories ingested and calories burned. (He mentioned that dancing for 2 hours is the best calorie burner for him.) Another company, *AliveCor*, makes a tiny $75 device that will do a 30-second electrocardiogram any time you want it. At the end of 30 seconds, an algorithm reviews the reading and identifies atrial fibrillation if you have it. If it is atrial fibrillation, you can make notes on the condition that might have induced it. The device comes with an adhesive back so you can attach it to your smartphone, and then an email of your electrocardiogram, from the app, can be sent to your physician. He also mentioned the *Stroke Riskometer* app, which provides Framingham Heart Study risks of stroke. All of this, of course, will create a whole new mode of health research: medical data crowd sourcing. It will also build a world of participant patients rather than passive patients.

FRUGAL PHYSICIANS

Thomas J. Stanley and William D. Danko published in 1996 *The Millionaire Next Door: The Surprising Secrets of America's Wealthy* (40). Stanley, who obtained his PhD in economics from the University of Georgia and was a professor for many years at Georgia State University in Atlanta, was killed earlier this year in an automobile accident near his home in Marietta, Georgia (41). He and Danko interviewed hundreds of low-profile millionaires. They wrote: "Wealth is not the same as income. If you make a good income each year and spend it all, you are not getting wealthier. You are just living high. Wealth is what you accumulate, not what you spend."

According to the two authors, there are a lot of rich pretenders. They spend on prestige products and services but are two or maybe even one paycheck away from financial disaster. Typical millionaire couples don't buy clothes at upscale stores. They don't swap cars frequently. Many don't live in upscale neighborhoods. They live below their means. Warren Buffett apparently said that the best way to accumulate wealth is not to have a divorce and/or to have a frugal spouse. Physicians who are living on the edge—spending what they bring in—may be more prone to order that expensive test for their patient or perform that procedure or operation if in a bit of financial trouble. Herb Shriner stated: "Our doctor would never really operate unless it was necessary. He was just that way. If he didn't need the money, he wouldn't lay a hand on you."

BIG TOBACCO AND MARIJUANA

Tobacco companies for generations have talked privately about getting into the weed business (42). In the summer of 2014, researchers pouring through millions of pages of previously secret tobacco industry documents found that big tobacco has long had an interest in pot. Since at least the 1970s, the tobacco companies have been interested in marijuana and marijuana legalization as both a potential and a rival product. As public opinion shifted and government relaxed laws pertaining to marijuana criminalization, the tobacco companies modified their corporate planning strategies to prepare for future consumer demand. In many ways, the marijuana market of 2014 resembles the tobacco market before 1880, before cigarettes were mass-produced and marketed. According to Trevor Hughes, writing in *USA Today*, the legalization of marijuana opens the market to major corporations, which have the financial resources and product design technology to transform the marijuana market. Stay tuned!

MARRIAGE DECLINING

According to the Pew Research Center, 72% of Americans aged 18 years or older were married in 1960, and in 2015 the percentage was down to 50% (43). As someone indicated, "Marriage takes four 'C's': companionship, communication, cooperation, and commitment." All of this may be too much for some today.

INCOME OF DALLAS LAWYERS

Of the 29 law firms with operations in Texas, most provided financial data to *The Texas Lawbook* (44). Six of the law firms, which included 981 lawyers, had an average revenue per lawyer of over $1 million annually, including two with revenues >$1,240,000/lawyer annually. The other 23 firms had revenue per lawyer ranging from $489,000 annually to $999,000 annually. Most of the public, I suspect, believe that physicians make a lot of money, but I can assure you that very few practicing physicians in the USA make incomes approaching the average of these law firms. Only a handful of physicians make $1 million a year in Dallas. The list compiled by *The Dallas Morning News* did not include all law firms because some declined to provide any financial information. If one needs a lawyer, too often it is very difficult to increase one's total worth.

INCOME VARIABILITY BY REGIONS

Jo Craven McGinty described regional differences in cost that affect how far a dollar will stretch and shape how people in different parts of the country can achieve their goals (45). The basic aspirations of the middle class seem simple: *earn enough to purchase a home; sock away a sufficient amount for retirement; cover the cost of the children's education; have one or two family trips each year.* Although there are vast differences in how far a dollar will go in various parts of the country, top earners are classified by the federal government as individuals who make more than $200,000 a year or households bringing in >$250,000 annually, irrespective of where they live. The cost for goods and services in different metropolitan areas varies by as much as 40%, and the disparity in rents is even greater. Until recently, data on relative purchasing power have not been readily available. In 2014, for the first time, the US Bureau of Economic Analysis published differences in the cost of goods and services across states and metropolitan areas. The results illustrate stark

regional differences in purchasing power, and they help explain why some top earners don't feel rich and why some in the middle class feel especially strapped for cash.

The Bureau calculated the average prices paid by consumers for more than 200 different goods and services divided into categories including apparel; education; food; housing expenses, such as utilities and furniture; medical costs; recreation; transportation; and rents, which also included costs for homeowners. The percentage difference from the national average in prices for goods and services, including shelter, in 2012 varied from +18% in the District of Columbia to −14% in Mississippi. Hawaii was the next most expensive followed by New York, New Jersey, California, Maryland, Connecticut, Massachusetts, Alaska, New Hampshire, Virginia, Washington, Delaware, Colorado, Vermont, and Illinois. The remaining states were below average. Texas was 3.5% below average and 10th among the 35 states below average. The spread among all the states and the District of Columbia was nearly 32%, and the range in rents was even wider, varying by almost 97%. Hawaii's rents were 59% more than the national average; Mississippi had the least expensive rents, 38% below the national average. If the national average was $1000, someone in Mississippi would pay $621 and someone in Hawaii would pay $1590 for the same type of dwelling. Such disparities may also occur within the same state. These differences show why it is so difficult to pin down a definition for the middle class that feels right to all Americans. One size does not fit all.

RELIGIOUS SHIFTS

The present size and projected growth of religious groups, as a percentage of the world's population, will change considerably from 2010 to 2050 (46) *(Figure).* Presently, Christians make up about 31% of the world's population and Muslims, about 23%. From 2010 until 2050, the Muslim population around the world is expected to increase by about 73%; the Christian population, 35%; Hindu, 34%; Jewish, 16%; folk religions, 11%; unaffiliated, 9%; other religions, 6%; and Buddhism, −0.3%. The world population during these 40 years is expected to increase about 35%.

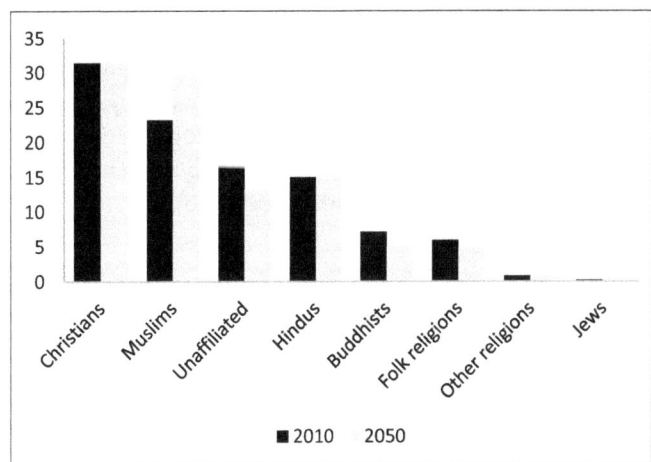

Figure. Size and projected growth of religious groups, as a percentage of the world's population, in 2010 and 2050. Data from Zoroya, *USA Today* (46).

GLOBAL GARBAGE

In an accounting of global garbage, researchers in the US and Australia, led by Jenna Jambeck, an environmental engineer at the University of Georgia, calculated the share that each of 192 countries could have contributed to plastic waste in the oceans (47). Dr. Jambeck and her colleagues calculated that people living within 30 miles of the coast in these countries generated a total of 275 million metric tons of plastic waste in 2010. A small but alarming fraction of it—between 4.8 million and 12.7 million tons of discarded bottles, bags, straws, packaging, and other items—ended up in the oceans. If the amount of plastic waste fouling the seas remains unchecked, they predicted that it may double by 2025, reaching levels "equal to 10 bags full of plastic per foot of coastline." The worst offender was China. Its coastal population generated 8.82 million metric tons of mismanaged plastic waste in 2010, about 28% of the world's total; of that, between 1.32 and 3.53 million metric tons ended up as marine debris. Indonesia, the world's fourth most populous nation, generated about 3.22 million tons of mismanaged plastic waste in 2010, about 10% of the world's total; of that, between 0.48 and 1.29 million metric tons ended up as marine waste. Thus, China and Indonesia alone account for more than one-third of the plastic bottles, bags, and other detritus washed out to sea. The US, ranked 20th, was responsible for just under 1% of the mismanaged plastic waste. Good for us!

DROUGHT IN THREE CONTINENTS

California is experiencing its worst drought in 40 years, and it has brought unprecedented water shortages, increased threats to wildlife and crops, higher electric bills, and huge economic losses. Brazil is experiencing its worst drought in 50 years, and it is impacting a fifth of Brazil's 200 million people, including those of the megacities of São Paolo and Rio de Janeiro. Additionally, water in Brazilian cities and reservoirs is extremely polluted. In Brazil, wastewater is not treated but just dumped into rivers. South Africa is experiencing its worst drought in 20 years. Food production for much of Central and Southern Africa is likely to be lower in 2015 than last year because of the drought. Water shortages have reached crisis levels in some of South Africa's eastern provinces. North Korea is said to be undergoing its worst drought in 100 years. Deaths of young children increased markedly in the first 6 months of the year in the drought-affected provinces. The country is experiencing electric shortages because of the drought and is reducing its hydroelectric generation capacity. Of all of the countries in the world, North Korea may be the one least capable of dealing with drought (48).

WILLIAM CLIFFORD ROBERTS, MD
August 11, 2015

1. Editorial. Baby boomer epidemic. *Dallas Morning News*, July 26, 2015.
2. Neergaard L. Mind your brain health. Associated Press, August 2, 2015.
3. Stroes ES, Thompson PD, Corsini A, Vladutiu GD, Raal FJ, Ray KK, Roden M, Stein E, Tokgözoğlu L, Nordestgaard BG, Bruckert E, De Backer G, Krauss RM, Laufs U, Santos RD, Hegele RA, Hovingh GK, Leiter LA, Mach F, März W, Newman CB, Wiklund O, Jacobson TA, Catapano AL, Chapman MJ, Ginsberg HN; European Atherosclerosis Society Consensus Panel. Statin-associated muscle symptoms: impact on statin therapy. *Eur Heart J* 2015;36(17):1012–1022.
4. Burton TM. Cholesterol drug gets cautious FDA nod. *Wall Street Journal*, June 10, 2015.
5. Winslow R. Cholesterol war gets pricey weapon. *Wall Street Journal*, July 25–26, 2015.
6. Silverman E. Price concerns follow news about cholesterol drug. *Wall Street Journal*, March 20, 2015.
7. Bennett J. Four new drugs in 2015. *Barron's*, March 9, 2015.
8. Burton TM, Armental M. New cystic-fibrosis pill to cost $259,000 a year. *Wall Street Journal*, July 3, 2015.
9. Landers J. Runaway cancer drug prices raise stakes for patients. *Dallas Morning News*, April 5, 2015.
10. Unknown. Cancer's high cost. *Dallas Morning News*, April 7, 2015.
11. DeCroes Jacobs C. *Jonas Salk: A Life*. New York: Oxford University Press, 2015.
12. Cha AE. Have cash, will seek longer lives. *Dallas Morning News*, April 12, 2015.
13. Jordan P. Preaching better health. *AARP Bulletin*, April 2015.
14. Chow J. France moves to ban ultrathin fashion models. *Wall Street Journal*, April 3, 2015.
15. Corbet S. Cigs, boozing, soda refills get a French kiss-off. *Dallas Morning News*, April 15, 2015.
16. Atcheson R. Why real men don't eat meat. *USA Today*, July 30, 2015.
17. Kim C. The price of sweetness. *Barron's*, March 30, 2015.
18. Frank T. High-speed police chases have killed thousands. *USA Today*, July 31–August 2, 2015.
19. Landers J. Does ruling on phone service benefit doctors or patients? *Dallas Morning News*, April 14, 2015.
20. McGirk R. Australia to cut benefits for families that skip shots. *Dallas Morning News*, April 15, 2015.
21. Korte G. US has 42 ways to get you to a doctor. *USA Today*, April 14, 2015.
22. MacLeod C. Chinese births on the rise in USA. *USA Today*, April 6, 2015.
23. Schnohr P, O'Keefe JH, Marott JL, Lange P, Jensen GB. Dose of jogging and long-term mortality: the Copenhagen City Heart Study. *J Am Coll Cardiol* 2015;65(5):411–419.
24. Sefko E. As playoffs near, keeping legs fresh is no easy task. *Dallas Morning News*, March 22, 2015.
25. Pipes SC. Medicare at 50: Hello, mid-life crisis. *Wall Street Journal*, July 30, 2015.
26. Troy T. Democrats roll out 'Mediscare' again. *Wall Street Journal*, July 31, 2015.
27. Szabo L. Drastic drop in Medicare deaths, costs. *USA Today*, July 29, 2015.
28. Murphy J, Carey AR, Loehrke J. April is always a taxing time. *USA Today*, April 14, 2015.
29. Atlas SW. Repairing the Obamacare wreckage. *Wall Street Journal*, June 29, 2015.
30. Unknown. The unaffordable care act. *Wall Street Journal*, July 11–12, 2015.
31. Graedon J, Graedon T. Vitamin D: how much sun do you need? *Dallas Morning News*, June 7, 2015.
32. Manning K. Undressed can be cause of stress for patients. *Dallas Morning News*, June 7, 2015.
33. Unknown. AMA to test older doctors' competence. *Dallas Morning News*, June 9, 2015.
34. Landers J. Drinking up, and so are the costs. *Dallas Morning News*, June 16, 2015.
35. Schulte J. Beware of snakes—and bills. *Dallas Morning News*, July 4, 2015.
36. Stossel T. A cure for 'conflict of interest' mania. *Wall Street Journal*, June 27–28, 2015.

37. Rosenbaum L. Conflicts of interest: part 1: Reconnecting the dots—reinterpreting industry-physician relations. *N Engl J Med* 2015;372(19): 1860–1864.

38. Landro L. How to prepare for trouble on a trip abroad. *Wall Street Journal*, June 1, 2015.

39. Burns S. Devices aim to get patients participating in care. *Dallas Morning News*, June 7, 2015.

40. Stanley TJ, Danko WD. *The Millionaire Next Door: The Surprising Secrets of America's Wealthy.* Marietta, GA: Longstreet Press, 1996 (272 pp.).

41. Hart A. 'Millionaire Next Door' author dies in crash. *Atlanta Journal-Constitution,* March 1, 2015. Available at http://www.ajc.com/news/news/millionaire-blockbuster-author-dies-in-crash/nkLxS/.

42. Hughes T. Pot industry wary of big tobacco. *USA Today*, April 14, 2015.

43. Unknown. Is opting out of marriage a smart or foolish move? *USA Today*, June 5, 2015.

44. Curriden M. Elite law firms take Texas by storm. *Dallas Morning News*, May 24, 2015.

45. McGinty JC. Why 'wealth' isn't defined simply. *Wall Street Journal*, February 21–22, 2015.

46. Zoroya G. Islamic faith is fastest-growing. *USA Today*, April 3, 2015.

47. Hotz RL. Asia leads world in dumping plastic in seas. *Wall Street Journal*, February 13, 2015.

48. Rice D. Drought: a global issue. *USA Today*, July 28, 2015.

www.ingramcontent.com/pod-product-compliance
Lightning Source LLC
Chambersburg PA
CBHW080149310326
41914CB00090B/1009